Essential Physical Medicine and Rehabilitation

Essential Physical Medicine and Rehabilitation

Edited by

Grant Cooper, MD

Department of Physical Medicine and Rehabilitation
New York-Presbyterian Hospital, The University Hospital
of Columbia and Cornell, New York, NY

Foreword by

Nancy E. Strauss, MD

Director of Residency Training in Physical Medicine
and Rehabilitation, New York-Presbyterian Hospital,
The University Hospital of Columbia and Cornell,
New York, NY

HUMANA PRESS ✺ TOTOWA, NEW JERSEY

999 Riverview Drive, Suite 208
Totowa, New Jersey 07512

humanapress.com

This publication is printed on acid-free paper. ∞

ANSI Z39.48-1984 (American Standards Institute) Permanence of Paper for Printed Library Materials.

Production Editor: Melissa Caravella

Cover design by Patricia F. Cleary

For additional copies, pricing for bulk purchases, and/or information about other Humana titles, contact Humana at the above address or at any of the following numbers: Tel.: 973-256-1699; Fax: 973-256-8341; E-mail: orders@humanapr.com; or visit our website at www.humanapress.com.

Printed in the United States of America. 10 9 8 7 6 5 4 3 2 1
1-59745-100-2 (e-book)
Library of Congress Cataloging in Publication Data

Essential physical medicine and rehabilitation / [edited] by Grant Cooper;
foreword by Nancy E. Strauss.
p. ; cm.
Includes bibliographical references and index.
ISBN 1-58829-618-0 (alk. paper)
1. Medicine, Physical. 2. Medical rehabilitation.
[DNLM: 1. Physical Medicine--methods. 2. Diagnostic Techniques and Procedures.
3. Rehabilitation--methods. WB 460 E78 2006]
I. Cooper, Grant, M.D.
RM700.E83 2006
615.8'2--dc22

2005028370

Dedication

To all medical students and residents of good heart—it's a long journey but, I trust, a good and noble one. I hope this book helps you navigate the path, and makes it a little less arduous.

—G.C.

Foreword

Essential Physical Medicine and Rehabilitation is the product of a creative and highly innovative resident, Dr. Grant Cooper. Dr. Cooper realized that our specialty was in need of a basic introductory book geared toward a medical student and junior resident population that would provide the information needed at the start of a physical medicine and rehabilitation (PM&R) rotation. As the title implies, it offers essential concepts and enables residents/students to build the backbone of their PM&R knowledge base and thus maximize their early clinical experience. This book provides a "jump start" so students/residents can begin from a strong and knowledgeable vantage point. The fact that PM&R remains a specialty that may not be easily definable by many medical students ensures even greater value of this book.

What is a physiatrist? What is PM&R? How can one specialty treat both the most physically fit and the most debilitated patients? How can one specialist treat both the youngest infants and the oldest patients? How can one specialty demand knowledge of nearly every organ system? Why would a physician need to know so much about so many aspects of a patient's lifestyle and environment? The answers to these questions lie in the core principles of our field.

Our expertise is in maximizing functional independence in patients with disability. The common denominator of our patient population is "loss of function." A physiatrist uses a wide array of interventions to rehabilitate their patients including, but not limited to, exercise, physical modalities (cold, heat, electrical stimulation), external devices (braces, artificial limbs), gait aids, assistive devices for activities of daily living, communication aids, seating and mobility systems, counseling, and specialized techniques (injection, manipulation, traction, and massage).

PM&R is a goal-oriented specialty that involves many health professionals. The physiatrist leads the team, which may include any or all of the following members: physical therapist, occupational therapist, speech therapist, recreational therapist, prosthetist, orthotist, rehabilitation nurse, vocational counselor, social worker, and rehabilitation engineer. Additionally, we may work closely with school staff, employers, architectural staff, insurance companies, or other individuals who may affect the patient's functional gains and achievement of independence.

As you read through *Essential Physical Medicine and Rehabilitation* and are introduced to core areas of our field, think like a physiatrist: ask yourself, "What is the functional limitation and how can I aid the patient in overcoming that limitation?" A common thread binds these diverse chapters, just as a common thread binds the diverse areas of our specialty. The common thread is functional disability. The common goal is to maximize functional independence.

In Chapters 1 and 2, we learn that the spectrum of brain injury includes minimal subtle findings to severe cognitive dysfunction. Identifying the deficits is critical in formulating a rehabilitation plan because even minimal changes in memory and concentration may have devastating effects on daily life functions. In Chapter 3, we see that spinal cord injury can affect nearly every organ system and serves as a model condition to demonstrate the principles of our specialty. Orthotics and prosthetics are described in Chapter 4 and demonstrate how the use of an external support or artificial limb can improve safety, stability, cosmesis, mobility, independence, and overall function. Chapters 5 and 6 discuss rehabilitation of the cardiac and pulmonary systems and reinforce the principle that without efficient cardiopulmonary function, endurance, conditioning, and exercise capacity are greatly limited. Chapter 7 introduces pediatric rehabilitation and suggests that when the developing body is affected with an insult, the body may learn early compensations and adaptations. Neuromuscular rehabilitation is described in Chapter 8 and refers to interventions used for disability that results from either acquired or inherited disorders of the anterior horn cell, peripheral nerve, neuromuscular junction, or muscle, which may lead to impairments of strength, sensation, and/or muscle tone. Cancer rehabilitation is discussed in Chapter 9. Malignancy can affect any part of the body, by direct invasion, associated pathology, or the effect of treatment. Chapters 10 and 11 describe orthopedic rehabilitation and spine and musculoskeletal medicine, respectively. These chapters demonstrate that we require intact structure (bones, joints, tendons, ligaments, and muscles) for correct posture, movement, and locomotion. Additionally, painful soft tissue disorders can be functionally limiting. Electrodiagnostic medicine, discussed in Chapter 12, is a diagnostic tool that school staff, employers, architectural staff, insurance companies, or other individuals who may affect the patient's functional gains and achievement of independence.

As you read through *Essential Physical Medicine and Rehabilitation* and are introduced to core areas of our field, think like a physiatrist: ask yourself, "What is the functional limitation and how can I aid the patient in overcoming that limitation?" A common thread binds these diverse chapters, just as a common thread binds the diverse areas of our specialty. The common thread is functional disability. The common goal is to maximize functional independence.

In Chapters 1 and 2, we learn that the spectrum of brain injury includes minimal subtle findings to severe cognitive dysfunction. Identifying the deficits is critical in formulating a rehabilitation plan because even minimal changes in memory and concentration may have devastating effects on daily life functions. In Chapter 3, we see that spinal cord injury can affect nearly every organ system and serves as a model condition to demonstrate the principles of our specialty. Orthotics and prosthetics are described in Chapter 4 and demonstrate how the use of an external support or artificial limb can improve safety, stability, cosmesis, mobility, independence, and overall function. Chapters 5 and 6 discuss rehabilitation of the cardiac and pulmonary systems and reinforce the principle that without efficient cardiopulmonary function, endurance, conditioning, and exercise capacity are greatly limited. Chapter 7 introduces pediatric rehabilitation and suggests that when the developing body is affected with an insult, the body may learn early compensations and adaptations. Neuromuscular rehabilitation is described in Chapter 8 and refers to interventions used for disability that results from either acquired or inherited disorders of the anterior horn cell, peripheral nerve, neuromuscular junction, or muscle, which may lead to impairments of strength, sensation, and/or muscle tone. Cancer rehabilitation is discussed in Chapter 9. Malignancy can affect any part of the body, by direct invasion, associated pathology, or the effect of treatment. Chapters 10 and 11 describe orthopedic rehabilitation and spine and musculoskeletal medicine, respectively. These chapters demonstrate that we require intact structure (bones, joints, tendons, ligaments, and muscles) for correct posture, movement, and locomotion. Additionally, painful soft tissue disorders can be functionally limiting. Electrodiagnostic medicine, discussed in Chapter 12, is a diagnostic tool that

Foreword

Essential Physical Medicine and Rehabilitation is the product of a creative and highly innovative resident, Dr. Grant Cooper. Dr. Cooper realized that our specialty was in need of a basic introductory book geared toward a medical student and junior resident population that would provide the information needed at the start of a physical medicine and rehabilitation (PM&R) rotation. As the title implies, it offers essential concepts and enables residents/students to build the backbone of their PM&R knowledge base and thus maximize their early clinical experience. This book provides a "jump start" so students/residents can begin from a strong and knowledgeable vantage point. The fact that PM&R remains a specialty that may not be easily definable by many medical students ensures even greater value of this book.

What is a physiatrist? What is PM&R? How can one specialty treat both the most physically fit and the most debilitated patients? How can one specialist treat both the youngest infants and the oldest patients? How can one specialty demand knowledge of nearly every organ system? Why would a physician need to know so much about so many aspects of a patient's lifestyle and environment? The answers to these questions lie in the core principles of our field.

Our expertise is in maximizing functional independence in patients with disability. The common denominator of our patient population is "loss of function." A physiatrist uses a wide array of interventions to rehabilitate their patients including, but not limited to, exercise, physical modalities (cold, heat, electrical stimulation), external devices (braces, artificial limbs), gait aids, assistive devices for activities of daily living, communication aids, seating and mobility systems, counseling, and specialized techniques (injection, manipulation, traction, and massage).

PM&R is a goal-oriented specialty that involves many health professionals. The physiatrist leads the team, which may include any or all of the following members: physical therapist, occupational therapist, speech therapist, recreational therapist, prosthetist, orthotist, rehabilitation nurse, vocational counselor, social worker, and rehabilitation engineer. Additionally, we may work closely with physicians use to help localize a lesion of the neuromuscular system, determine severity of the lesion, as well as time course and prognosis.

PM&R is a diverse medical specialty based on teamwork, optimism, creativity, and confidence in our patients. Overcoming disability and maximizing function are among the most rewarding values that medicine has to offer. The field of PM&R is at the forefront of this goal.

Nancy E. Strauss, MD
Director of Residency Training in Physical Medicine and Rehabilitation, New York-Presbyterian Hospital, The University Hospital of Columbia and Cornell, New York, NY

physicians use to help localize a lesion of the neuromuscular system, determine severity of the lesion, as well as time course and prognosis.

PM&R is a diverse medical specialty based on teamwork, optimism, creativity, and confidence in our patients. Overcoming disability and maximizing function are among the most rewarding values that medicine has to offer. The field of PM&R is at the forefront of this goal.

Nancy E. Strauss, MD
Director of Residency Training in Physical Medicine and Rehabilitation, New York-Presbyterian Hospital, The University Hospital of Columbia and Cornell, New York, NY

Preface

When I was a medical student interested in physical medicine and rehabilitation (PM&R), I found several excellent detailed texts for PM&R and I also encountered a few good, quick reference materials. What I felt was lacking was a comprehensive but high-yield, focused review of the most important points that I could read before and during my rotation. As a junior resident in PM&R, I again encountered the same frustration. What I was looking for was a book that would slice through the minutiae and offer me the critical information that I would need to know during a PM&R clinical rotation. Such high-yield review texts exist in other fields and I was never quite sure why they did not exist for ours. I suppose it is in part because we are a relatively young and small specialty. Additionally, the breadth and scope of our field, from treating the most debilitated patients to professional athletes, might seem daunting at first glance. And yet, as Dr. Strauss has eloquently laid out in her foreword to this book, there is a unifying theme of function that pervades the diverse aspects of our field.

In *Essential Physical Medicine and Rehabilitation*, I have aimed to create the book that I had sought as a medical student and junior resident. Each chapter is written by recognized experts and educators in their respective fields. Each chapter is written as though telling a medical student or junior resident, in concise terms, everything he or she should know before—and during—a first rotation in the given subspecialty. I believe this book accomplishes that goal. I hope you will agree.

Grant Cooper, MD

Acknowledgments

Essential Physical Medicine and Rehabilitation is a wonderful example of a true collaborative effort. It is a pleasure and a privilege for me to take a moment and acknowledge some of the people who helped make it possible. Humana Press and its Editor of Life and Biomedical Sciences, Don Odom, have been a pleasure to work with. Don's drive and commitment to excellence is inspiring. I would like to also extend a special thank you to Dr. Nancy E. Strauss and Dr. Michael O'Dell for their help and encouragement. Finally, this book would not have been possible without the hard work of its many distinguished authors who believed in the need for it.

—*G.C.*

Contents

Contributors

MATHEW N. BARTELS, MD, MPH • John Alexander Downey Associate Professor of Clinical Rehabilitation Medicine, Department of Rehabilitation Medicine, Columbia University College of Physicians and Surgeons, Medical Director of Human Performance Laboratory and Cardiopulmonary Rehabilitation, Columbia Campus, New York-Presbyterian Hospital, New York, NY

MONIFA BROOKS, MD • Spinal Cord Injury Medicine, Kessler Institute for Rehabilitation, West Orange, NJ

GRANT COOPER, MD • Resident, Department of Physical Medicine and Rehabilitation, New York-Presbyterian Hospital, The University Hospital of Columbia and Cornell, New York, NY

CHRISTIAN M. CUSTODIO, MD • Assistant Attending, Rehabilitation Service, Memorial Sloan-Kettering Cancer Center; Assistant Professor, Department of Rehabilitation Medicine, Weill Medical College of Cornell University, New York, NY

JOSEPH FEINBERG, MD • Associate Attending, Physiatry Department, Hospital for Special Surgery, New York, NY

STEVEN KIRSHBLUM, MD • Professor, UMDNJ/New Jersey Medical School, Newark, NJ; Medical Director and Director of Spinal Cord Injury Services, Kessler Institute for Rehabilitation, West Orange, NJ

C. DAVID LIN, MD • Assistant Professor, Department of Rehabilitation Medicine, Weill Medical College of Cornell University, New York, NY

GREGORY E. LUTZ, MD • Physiatrist-in-Chief, Hospital for Special Surgery and Associate Professor, Clinical Rehabilitation Medicine, Weill Medical College of Cornell University, New York, NY

BRENDA S. MALLORY, MD • Associate Clinical Professor, Department of Rehabilitation Medicine, Columbia University College of Physicians and Surgeons, New York, NY

STANLEY J. MYERS, MD • A. David Gurewitsch Professor, Clinical Rehabilitation Medicine, Vice Chair, Department of Rehabilitation Medicine, Columbia University College of Physicians and Surgeons; Adjunct Professor, Clinical Rehabilitation Medicine, Weill Medical College of Cornell University, New York-Presbyterian Hospital, New York, NY

MICHAEL W. O'DELL, MD • Professor of Clinical Rehabilitation Medicine, Weill Medical College of Cornell University, Associate Chief and Attending Physiatrist, New York-Presbyterian Hospital, Weill Cornell Medical Center, New York, NY

SHIKHA SETHI, MD • Resident, Department of Physical Medicine and Rehabilitation, New York-Presbyterian Hospital, The University Hospital of Columbia and Cornell, New York, NY

RAMNIK SINGH, MD • Chief Resident, Department of Physical Medicine and Rehabilitation, New York-Presbyterian Hospital, The University Hospital of Columbia and Cornell, New York, NY

JENNIFER SOLOMON, MD • Assistant Attending, Physiatry Department, Hospital for Special Surgery; Clinical Instructor, Department of Rehabilitation Medicine, Weill Medical College of Cornell University, New York, NY

NANCY E. STRAUSS, MD • Associate Clinical Professor of Rehabilitation Medicine, Columbia University College of Physicians and Surgeons, Associate Professor of Clinical Rehabilitation Medicine, Weill Medical College of Cornell University, Director of Residency Training in Physical Medicine and Rehabilitation, New York-Presbyterian Hospital, The University Hospital of Columbia and Cornell, New York, NY

MICHAEL D. STUBBLEFIELD, MD • Assistant Attending, Rehabilitation Service, Memorial Sloan-Kettering Cancer Center; Assistant Professor, Department of Rehabilitation Medicine, Weill Medical College of Cornell University, New York, NY

YUSUF TATLI, MD • Fellow, Physiatry Department, Hospital for Special Surgery, New York, NY

HEIKKI UUSTAL, MD • Medical Director, Prosthetic and Orthotic Team, JFK-Johnson Rehabilitation Institute, Edison, NJ; Clinical Assistant Professor, Department of Physical Medicine and Rehabilitation, UMDNJ-Robert Wood Johnson Medical School, Piscataway, NJ

JILDA N. VARGUS-ADAMS, MD, MS • Assistant Professor, Division of Pediatric Rehabiliation, Clinical Pediatrics and Clinical Physical Medicine and Rehabilitation, Cincinnati Children's Hospital Medical Center, University of Cincinnati College of Medicine, Cincinnati, OH

1 Traumatic Brain Injury

Ramnik Singh and Michael W. O'Dell

Background

Patients with traumatic brain injury (TBI) pose an enormous clinical, emotional, and intellectual challenge to rehabilitation professionals. For public policymakers, the cost of care for approximately 6 million survivors of TBI is measured in the billions of dollars. In addition to the motor, sensory, and language deficits commonly seen in nontraumatic etiologies, the patient with TBI often experiences cognitive and/or behavioral manifestations that alter his or her ability to benefit from the rehabilitation process, and requires innovative treatment strategies on the part of the rehabilitation team. Beyond the core disciplines (physiatry, physical/occupational therapy, and speech/language pathology), neuropsychology services are added to provide cognitive and behavioral assessment, treatment, and guidance to the remainder of the treatment team.

TBI is not a single disease process, but a continuum of injury with clinical manifestations, differing not so much in quality as in degree. At one extreme, 70–80% of all TBI cases are classified as mild, the vast majority of which recover without event and often without seeking medical attention. However, 10% of that mild injury group will experience chronic, debilitating symptoms, such as headache, dizziness, and cognitive and mood deficits, despite a relatively normal physical examination. Ten percent of TBI cases are classified as severe, 5% of which may remain in a vegetative or minimally conscious state for days, months, or years with profound physical and cognitive impairment.

From: *Essential Physical Medicine and Rehabilitation*
Edited by: G. Cooper © Humana Press Inc., Totowa, NJ

Between these two extremes lie the remaining 15–20% of patients with moderate to moderately severe TBI. This group is cared for by rehabilitation professionals in a variety of settings ranging from the neurological intensive care unit, to acute, subacute, and outpatient rehabilitation, to community-based transitional living settings. Some patients will exhibit severe deficits during the initial course of injury and recover to remarkably functional, if not normal, levels. Other patients with seemingly similar injuries will lag behind in physical and cognitive recovery, ultimately requiring indefinite supervision and assistance. Unlike patients with spinal cord injury, where functional levels can be relatively confidently predicted once a neurological level has been established, prognostication of ultimate function in TBI remains a painfully inexact science. Despite this uncertainty, a large proportion of patients make dramatic and meaningful recovery in the weeks and months following injury.

Epidemiology

Approximately 50% of TBI cases occur as a result of moving vehicles (motor vehicle accidents [MVAs], motorcycle and bicycle accidents, or pedestrians struck by a vehicle) and 20% from violence (assault or gunshot wound). The remaining injuries occur as a result of falls, child abuse, and sports injuries. The distinction between "brain injury" and "head injury" is not clear and clouds the interpretation of the epidemiological literature. Although TBI hospitalization rates have dropped over the past several years, it remains unclear whether this reflects an absolute drop in the numbers of TBI or a trend toward greater outpatient management among those with mild injuries. Rates of TBI caused by vehicular etiologies may be decreasing.

Although generally thought to be a condition of young males, TBI impacts a wide variety of ages and socioeconomic circumstances. Figure 1 provides a summary of the impact of gender and age on the incidence of TBI. The largest peak occurs in males between the ages of 15 and 24 years, where MVA and violence are the most common etiologies, and females are outnumbered 2 or 3:1. TBI is also more severe in males, with a 300–400% greater fatality rate compared with females. Among children under 5 years of age and adults older than 75 years, gender distribution is even, but the etiologies differ. Falls, child abuse, and athletic injuries are common among the young, and falls are common among the elderly.

Pathophysiology

The pathophysiology of TBI is best viewed as either primary or secondary and either focal or diffuse. Recent evidence suggests that mechanical

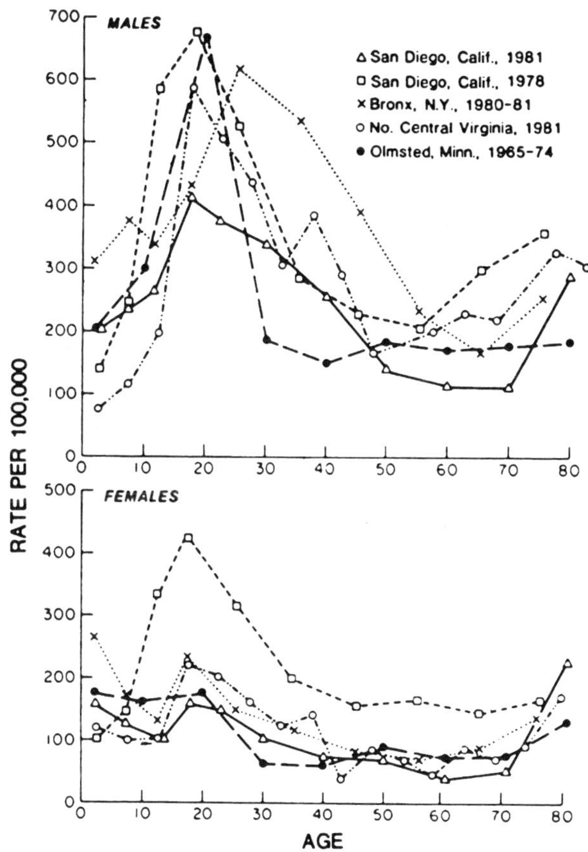

Fig. 1. Epidemiology of traumatic brain injury. Age-specific injury incidence rates per 100,000 individuals for males and females in selected US studies. Note the difference between male and female rate.

stretch of axons triggers calcium ion influx into axons, followed by alteration of other ions and neurotransmitters, such as glutamate and aspartate. These biochemical cascades can lead to further cellular damage and, although unsuccessful to date, pharmacological intervention to alter these biochemical and molecular cascades might one day prove effective in reducing secondary injury and improving clinical outcome. The best "treatment" for primary TBI, however, is prevention, including the use of airbags, improved safety technology, use of helmets, and enforcement of drunk-driving laws.

Diffuse axonal injury is a primary, diffuse brain injury, nearly pathognomonic for TBI. It is seen with high-velocity, large-amplitude acceleration–deceleration injuries, as seen in MVAs. Diffuse axonal injury is thought is to be responsible for immediate-onset, prolonged loss of consciousness, and is associated with a delayed recovery rate. Cerebral contusion is the primary, focal injury, and essentially represents "bruising" at the superficial cerebral cortex. Contusions tend to occur at the poles of the frontal and temporal lobes because of skull morphology, and account for the some of the common clinical symptoms following TBI, such as behavioral disinhibition and memory deficits, respectively.

Secondary injury occurs after the instant of impact, and is the basis for many acute neurosurgical interventions. Aggressive treatment of increased intracranial pressure has improved survival in patients with TBI. Cerebral edema in TBI, however, does not respond to steroid treatment. Intracranial hemorrhage results in local tissue damage and decreased cerebral blood flow. Epidural hematomas are located between the dura and skull and are associated with the tearing of the meningeal arteries, as seen with skull fractures. If evacuated quickly, prognosis tends to be good. Subdural hemorrhage occurs between the dura and brain parenchyma, and tends to expand slowly from low-pressure veins. Because there is no dura to protect the brain parenchyma, lasting neurological impairment may be more common. Subdural hygromas are subdural collections of cerebral spinal fluid associated with dural tears and bleeding. They occur days to weeks after injury and do not require treatment in many cases. Focal, secondary neurological deficits can also result from cerebral vasospasm/infarction after subarachnoid hemorrhage, infarction from local compression of cerebral vessels from brain swelling or hematomas, or brain abscess. Hypoxia is a type of diffuse secondary injury, and an independent predictor of poor prognosis following TBI. Cerebral hypoxia results from loss of blood flow to the brain, owing to either intracranial (trauma to the carotid arteries, increased intracranial pressure) or extracranial (hypotension and hypoxia from concomitant cardiac, pulmonary, orthopedic, or other visceral injury) factors. Other diffuse secondary injuries include hydrocephalus and meningitis, with the onset of the former often weeks after injury.

Commonly Used Assessments in TBI Rehabilitation

The severity of TBI is assessed using one or more of three measures: Glasgow Coma Scale (GCS; *see* Table 1), time of loss of consciousness (LOC), and length of posttraumatic amnesia (PTA). GCS score is determined in the field, where scores may be inaccurate because of any number

Table 1
Glasgow Coma Scale

Best eye response

1. No eye opening.
2. Eye opening to pain.
3. Eye opening to verbal command.
4. Eyes open spontaneously.

Best verbal response

1. No verbal response.
2. Incomprehensible sounds.
3. Inappropriate words.
4. Confused.
5. Oriented.

Best motor response

1. No motor response.
2. Extension to pain.
3. Flexion to pain.
4. Withdrawal from pain.
5. Localizing pain.
6. Obeys commands.

of factors, through the first few days post-TBI. Eye opening, verbal output, and motor function are evaluated on a scale of 3 to 15, with lower numbers indicating poorer function. Generally accepted ranges for TBI severity are mild (13–15), moderate (9–12), and severe (3–8).

Length of unconsciousness is generally considered to be the time from injury to the patient achieving a GCS score of 8 or greater. PTA can be measured prospectively using the Galveston Orientation Amnesia Test (GOAT) or roughly estimated by asking when consistent memory returned following the injury. Although not entirely clear, PTA over 2 weeks can probably be considered a severe injury. The Glasgow Outcome Scale is a very broad, five-level outcome measure used mostly in neurosurgical studies. The Rancho Los Amigos Scale of Cognitive Functioning (*see* Table 2) is a descriptive scale based on behavioral and cognitive observation of, and interaction with, the patient. The scale provides a brief clinical description of eight levels from unresponsive to near-normal. "Rancho" levels can be followed through the recovery process and serves as a useful short-hand for the rehabilitation team. However, patients do not always pass through all levels in order. The Functional Independence Measure is commonly used in the inpatient rehabilitation setting, but is considered a much better measure

Table 2
Rancho Los Amigos Level of Cognitive Functioning Scale

Level		*Description*
I	No response	• Deep sleep. Unresponsive to stimuli.
II	Generalized response	• Inconsistent and nonpurposeful.
III	Localized response	• Specific but inconsistent, e.g., turning head toward a sound or focusing on a presented object. • Follows simple commands in an inconsistent and delayed manner.
IV	Confused-agitated	• Severely confused, disoriented, and unaware of present events. • Inappropriate and bizarre behavior.
V	Confused-inappropriate	• Alert and responds to simple commands. • Nonpurposeful and random responses to complex commands. • Agitated response to external stimuli. • Can manage self-care activities with assistance. Memory is impaired and verbalization is often inappropriate.
VI	Confused-appropriate	• Goal-directed behavior, with cueing. • Can relearn old skills, such as ADLs, but memory problems interfere with new learning. • Has a beginning awareness of self and others.
VII	Automatic-appropriate	• Robot-like with appropriate behavior and minimal confusion. • Superficial awareness of, but lack of insight to, his or her condition. • Requires supervision because judgment, problem solving, and planning skills are impaired.
VIII	Purposeful-appropriate	• Alert and oriented, able to recall and integrate past and recent events. • Can learn new activities and continue in home and living skills. • Deficits in stress tolerance, judgment, abstract reasoning, social, emotional, and intellectual capacities may persist.

ADLs, activities of daily living.

Table 3
Modified Ashworth Scale

0	No increase in muscle tone.
1	Slight increase in muscle tone, manifested by a catch-and-release or minimal resistance at the end of the range when the affected part is moved in flexion or extension.
1+	Slight increase in muscle tone, manifested by a catch followed by minimal resistance throughout the remainder (less than half) of the ROM.
2	More marked increase in muscle tone through most of the ROM, but affected part easily moved.
3	Considerable increase in muscle tone, passive movement difficult.
4	Affected parts rigid in flexion and extension.

ROM, range of motion.

of physical, rather than cognitive, functioning. The Disability Rating Scale was designed specifically for TBI, and is purported to be useful throughout the continuum of recovery from coma to community re-entry. The Agitated Behavior Scale assigns a score of 1 to 4 in 14 different aspects of observed behavior. The Berg Balance scale is used in TBI rehabilitation, but was originally developed for elders. The Modified Ashworth Scale quantifies spastic hypertonia, and is often used to determine if interventions are successful (*see* Table 3).

History and Review of Acute Care Medical Records

Several aspects of the medical history are particularly important when assessing the patient with TBI who has been admitted to inpatient rehabilitation. Details on the mechanism and complications of injury should be documented, if available. Acute medical records should indicate if cervical spine radiographs were completed and read. If not, films clearly showing all cervical vertebrae should be obtained in rehabilitation. An understanding of concomitant fractures will help guide the physical examination in search of unrecognized injury, such as peripheral nerve damage. The physician should attempt to determine the initial GCS score and LOC, if possible. A premorbid history of alcohol and drug use is very common, as substance use is involved in 50% of injuries, and will become important in planning postdischarge services. Many times, this substance use history is an indication of premorbid self-medication for depression or anxiety.

Certain acute complications may predict problems in rehabilitation. For example, patients with subarachnoid hemorrhage or meningitis may be at higher risk for hydrocephalus. Evidence of cerebral contusion or intracranial hematomas may place the patient at higher risk for seizures and a basilar skull fracture for diabetes insipidus. Documentation of severe hypoxia or hypotension may impact prognosis in some cases.

Physical Examination

Vital Signs

An elevated temperature may signify an obvious or occult infection or may be associated with autonomic dysfunction or central fevers. Tachycardia may indicate infection, pulmonary embolism, pain, or severe deconditioning. Orthostasis may be caused by prolonged bed rest or medications.

General Appearance

Inspect any devices (tracheostomy, chest tubes, gastrostomy or jejunostomy tubes, second urinary catheter) or drains (Jackson-Pratt drain) that are present. Make a record of all peripheral (intravenous) and central access lines (percutaneous intravascular central catheter, internal jugular, or femoral) as well. Note whether the patient is hostile, tense, agitated, or uncooperative. Dystonia, myoclonus, or other movement disorders may be obvious on general inspection. In cases where the patient is confused, agitated, or unable to cooperate, a complete physical and neurological examination may not be possible.

Skin

Skin should be examined for ecchymoses, abrasions, and lacerations, which may indicate mechanism of injury or a previously unrecognized injury (fracture, etc.). Confirm that skin around any tubes or lines is dry, intact, and without breakdown or infiltration. Inspect areas of skin that may be macerated or compromised because of contractures (palm, antecubital fossa, axilla, and perineum). Skin overlying bony prominences should also be examined for erythema or breakdown. This includes the occiput, elbows, sacrum, ischial tuberosities, and heels.

Head, Ears, Nose, and Throat

The head and neck examination includes gentle palpation to search for step-off fractures, shunts, or other neurosurgical devices. The area over a bone flap may be diffusely swollen but should not be pulsating or pulling on suture lines. The eyes should be evaluated for erythema, inflammation, or conjuctival hemorrhage. Examine the ears for external trauma or otorrhea. Inspect the oral cavity for bruxism (grinding of the teeth), lacerations, candidal infection, or broken dentures. Facial bones should be inspected for evidence of trauma or fracture.

Neck

Neck examination should involve auscultation for carotid bruits and palpation of the trachea and surrounding structures, especially in cases of extensive head trauma. Document the size, make, fenestration, cuff status, and capping of a tracheostomy. If a cervical collar is in place, neck range-of-motion (ROM) examination should not be performed until consultation with the acute trauma or neurosurgical team.

Cardiopulmonary

The chest wall is palpated to elicit any undiagnosed rib, clavicular, or sternal fractures. The chest should be auscultated to rule out diaphragmatic elevation or pulmonary consolidation. Patients with a tracheostomy should be asked to cough, making note of the forcefulness of the effort. Cardiac evaluation should be performed, with attention given to arrhythmias. Peripheral vascular exam includes inspection of extremities for chronic skin changes, absent pulses indicative of arterial occlusion or compartment syndrome, and swelling or erythema indicative of venous thrombosis.

Abdomen

Abdominal examination should focus on tender areas (rebound, etc.), bowel sounds, and distension secondary to either bowel issues or urinary retention.

Genitourinary

Examine the genitourinary tract for evidence of intertriginous and perineal maceration or ulceration owing to either contracture or healing trauma. In addition, the penis and vulva should be examined for catheters, fistulas, or ulceration. A stool guiac examination is important if there is a history of gastrointestinal (GI) bleeding or if discontinuation of GI prophylaxis is being contemplated.

Musculoskeletal

A musculoskeletal examination may uncover unrecognized skeletal trauma or fractures. Observation focuses on bone or joint deformity (swelling, erythema), and absence and asymmetry of body parts (amputation, leg-length discrepancy, etc.). Because patients with TBI can have

Table 4
Upper Motor Neuron vs Lower Motor Neuron Injuries

	UMN acute/chronic	*LMN acute/chronic*	*Notes*
Weakness	+/+	+/+	Weakness is present in both
Bulk	Normal/normal	Normal/atrophic	
Tone	↓/↑	↓/↓	
Reflexes	↓/↑	↓/↓	
Babinski	+/+	–/–	Only distinguishing feature of acute UMN
Clonus	–/+	–/–	
Fasciculations	–/–	+/–	Only distinguishing feature of acute LMN

UMN, upper motor neurons; LMN, lower motor neurons.

extensive concomitant injuries, any abnormality observed should be palpated to ascertain not only stability, but also the structural origin of the deformity or tenderness. Muscle asymmetry or atrophy may indicate peripheral nerve damage.

Joints should be passively and actively ranged to assess weakness, contracture, spastic hypertonia and pain. Average ROM of commonly measured joints is readily available in standard textbooks. It is often difficult to determine if a fixed joint is limited by contracture or severe spastic hypertonia. The degree of improved ROM after a diagnostic block with a local anesthetic agent suggests the degree to which spastic hypertonia is the etiology.

Neurological

Because patients with TBI commonly experience neurological damage to both the central and peripheral nervous systems, differentiation between upper motor neuron (UMN) and lower motor neuron (LMN) lesions is critical during the neurological examination (*see* Table 4). In the trauma setting, weakness involving one side (hemiparesis), both legs (paraparesis), or both arms and both legs (tetraparesis) are most likely results of a UMN lesion. Conversely, LMN lesions involve a segment of a limb in a plexus, radicular, or peripheral nerve pattern.

The neurological examination begins with an assessment of LOC. Utilize the neurobehavioral criteria outlined in Table 5, which are based on recommendations of the American Congress of Rehabilitation Medicine.

Table 5
American Congress of Rehabilitation Medicine Guidelines for Level of Consciousness

Nomenclature	*Neurobehavioral criteria*
Coma	1. The patient's eyes do not open either spontaneously *or* to external stimulation. 2. The patient does not follow any commands. 3. The patient does not mouth or utter recognizable words. 4. The patient does not demonstrate intentional movement (may show reflexive movement, such as posturing, withdrawal from pain; or involuntary smiling). 5. The patient cannot *sustain* visual pursuit movements of the eyes through a 45° arc in any direction when the eyes are held open manually. 6. The above criteria are not secondary to use of paralytic agents.
Vegetative state	1. The patient's eyes open spontaneously or after stimulation. 2. Criteria 2–6 under "Coma" are met.
Minimally conscious state	1. A *meaningful* behavioral response has occurred after a specific command, question, or environmental prompt (e.g., attempt to shake examiner's outstretched hand). The response is considered to be unequivocally meaningful by the observer. 2. When the evidence for meaningful responsiveness is equivocal, the response can be shown to occur *significantly* less often when the specific command, question, or prompt associated with it is not present. 3. The response has been observed on at least one occasion during a period of formal assessment. (Formal assessment consists of regular, structured, or standardized evaluation procedures.)

Continued

Table 5 *(Continued)*
American Congress of Rehabilitation Medicine Guidelines for Level of Consciousness

Nomenclature	*Neurobehavioral criteria*
Locked-in syndrome	1. Eye opening is well sustained (bilateral ptosis should be ruled out as a complicating factor in patients who do not open their eyes but demonstrate eye movement to command when the eyes are opened manually). 2. Basic cognitive abilities are evident on examination. 3. There is clinical evidence of severe hypophonia or aphonia. 4. There is clinical evidence of quadriparesis or quadriplegia. 5. The primary mode of communication is through vertical or lateral eye movement or blinking of the upper eyelid.
Akinetic mutism	1. Eye opening is well maintained and occurs in association with spontaneous visual tracking of environmental stimuli. 2. Little to no spontaneous speech or movement is discernible. 3. Command-following and verbalization are elicited but occur infrequently. 4. The low frequency of movement and speech cannot be attributed to neuromuscular disturbance (e.g., spasticity, hypotonia) or arousal disorder (e.g., obtundation) as is typically noted in the minimally responsive state.

Determine if the patient demonstrates the characteristics of coma, vegetative state (VS), minimally conscious state (MCS), locked-in syndrome (rare following TBI), akinetic mutism, or wakefulness. Avoid the use of descriptors, such as "persistent" and "permanent" in favor of a statement of time (e.g., vegetative state of 7 months' duration).

The most common cognitive deficits associated with TBI are in attention, memory, and executive functioning ("metacognition"). Realize that there are significant limitations to the physician's bedside mental status examination. If needed, more detailed, standardized, and taxing assessment is provided by neuropsychology.

Orientation is determined by asking a patient his/her name (person), city and hospital (place), time (year, month, date, day, or season), and situation ("Why are you in the hospital?"); GOAT scores, as described under the Heading entitled, "Commonly Used Assessments in TBI Rehabilitation," can also be used. *Attention* is best assessed by asking the patient to repeat random digits both forward and backward. A normal performance is seven digits forward and five backward. *Memory* depends on accurate encoding and retrieval of information. Immediate (5 minutes) and delayed (15–30 minutes) memory can be assessed by asking the patient to recall a three- or four-word list (e.g., red ball, New York, freedom, rose). Make sure the patient can recite all items at least once before timing starts. Document how many items can be recalled spontaneously, with a clue (e.g., "it's a city" or "it's a type of flower"), from a list (e.g., "was the flower a tulip, a rose, or a lily?"), or not at all. Improved performance with clues or a list suggested retrieval rather than encoding problems.

Abstract reasoning is tested through interpretation of proverbs familiar to the patient (e.g., "people who live in glass houses should not throw stones" or "a rolling stone gathers no moss"), or interpretation of how objects are similar (e.g., how are the following two objects similar?: apple and orange; doctor and nurse; desk and bookcase; and happy and sad). *Judgment* can be tested by asking simple questions that reflect societal norms (e.g., "Why is it inappropriate to yell 'fire' in a crowded theater?" or "What would you do if you found a stamped, addressed envelope on the floor?"). A better functional assessment of judgment is safety awareness in a practical setting, such as the kitchen or on the street. Finally, assess disorders of *communication* falling into one or more of the following five categories: aphasia, apraxia, dysarthria, dysphonia, or cognitive–linguistic deficits, as outlined in Table 6.

Cranial nerves (CN) I, IV, VII, and VIII are the most commonly injured in persons with TBI, and are the focus here. CN IX and XI are the least commonly injured. Anosmia (CN I) occurs in 2–38% of patients with TBI,

Table 6
Disorders of Communication

Type	*Disorder of*	*Characteristics/Presentation*
Aphasia	Language	• CNS lesion • Deficits in: ▪ Comprehension • Verbal • Written ▪ Repetition ▪ Naming
Apraxia	Motor planning	• CNS lesion • Groping articulatory movements with efforts at self-correction, aprosody. • Extended periods of abnormal rhythm or intonation. • Occasionally difficulty initiating an utterance.
Dysphonia	Sound production	• Can be caused by damage to CNS or PNS (phrenic nerve lesion) • Voice may be low and breathy if one or both vocal cords are abducted or high pitched and strangulated if the vocal cords are adducted. • Phrenic nerve lesions may also lead to a low, breathy voice because the patient is unable to generate sufficient force to adequately phonate.
Dysarthria	Articulation	• Patient produces words that are slow, slurred, and difficult to understand.
Cognitive–linguistic deficits	Context and pragmatics	• Disorganized, tangential, wandering discourse. • Disinhibited, socially inappropriate speech. • Confabulation and pragmatic deficits. • Difficulty communicating in distracting environment.

CNS, central nervous system; PNS, peripheral nervous system.

and is associated with frontal skull fractures and in those with posttraumatic rhinorrhea. Have the patient identify distinctive, noncaustic smells one nostril at a time. Caustic agents, such as alcohol, will stimulate the sensory afferents of CN V and confuse the findings. CN IV is occasionally injured in TBI because of its long intracranial course. This causes a positional diplopia that is compensated for when the patient tilts his or her head up and toward the contralateral side—the so-called "head tilt" sign. A central CN VII injury, as in a cortical or subcortical injury, will result in weakness of the lower two-thirds of the face (recall that the frontalis muscle receives ipsilateral and contralateral innervation). Peripheral CN VII injury, associated with frontal bone fracture, will result in a complete droop on the ipsilateral side of the face, resulting in a wide-open eye unable to blink. Transverse temporal bone fractures result in an immediate, ipsilateral CN VII paralysis in 30–50% of cases. Patients with longitudinal temporal bone fracture can develop a delayed facial paralysis because of progressive swelling and edema that holds a better prognosis for at least partial recovery. CN VII is tested by observing asymmetry when asking a patient to smile, raise his or her forehead, frown, attempt a whistle, or puff their cheeks. Sensory testing of CN VII involves taste of the anterior two-thirds of the tongue. CN VIII injury is also seen with temporal bone fractures and presents with vestibular disorders (vertigo, dizziness, and tinnitus), hearing deficits, or both. The cochlear division can be tested using a tuning fork (512 Hz). Air conduction usually persists twice as long as bone conduction. In an abnormal or "positive" Rhinne test, bone conduction is better than air conduction, suggestive of conductive hearing loss. If the sound lateralizes to one ear on the Weber test, it indicates either ipsilateral conductive hearing loss or contralateral sensorineural hearing loss.

Manual muscle testing should be performed according to Kendall and McCreary's manual muscle testing technique, looking for patterns of weakness indicative of an LMN or UMN lesion. Until proven otherwise, the physician should assume a peripheral nerve lesion is present distal to any fracture site. The examiner should recognize the difference between a diagnostically significant degree of weakness (e.g., a subtle pronator drift) and a function degree of weakness (e.g., less than anti-gravity quadriceps weakness causing knee buckling with standing).

During reflex examination, note both the degree and asymmetry of the responses. Presence of pathological reflexes, such as Babinski (in the lower extremities) and Hoffman's sign (in the upper extremity), indicates UMN lesions.

Hypertonia is increased resistance to a passive stretch of a muscle, and is called "spastic hypertonia" if velocity-dependent, and "rigidity" if non-

Table 7
Common Patterns of Spastic Hypertonia

Location/Type		*Pattern*
Upper extremity		• Adduction and internal rotation of the shoulder • Flexion of the elbow and wrist • Pronation of the forearm • Flexion of the fingers and adduction of the thumb
Lower extremity patterns:	Flexor	• Hip adduction and flexion • Knee flexion • Ankle plantar flexion or equinovarus positioning
	Extensor	• Knee extension • Equinus and/or valgus ankle • Great toe dorsiflexion

velocity-dependent. Spastic hypertonia is graded using the Modified Ashworth Scale (*see* Table 3), with the most common patterns outlined in Table 7.

Sensory deficits to light touch (cotton tip applicator), temperature (hot or cold), and pinprick (disposable safety pin) should be noted, with attention to radicular and peripheral nerve distribution. Proprioception should be determined by holding the most distal joint of a digit by its sides and moving it slightly up or down. If the patient cannot accurately detect the distal movement, then progressively test a more proximal joint until they can identify the movement correctly. The Romberg test also tests proprioception. This test is performed by asking the patient to stand, feet together with eyes open, then with eyes closed. The patient with significant proprioceptive loss will be able to stand still with his or her eyes open because vision will compensate for the loss of position sense, but will sway or fall with their eyes closed because they are unable to keep their balance.

Coordination should be assessed using rapid alternating movements, finger-to-nose tests, or heel-to-shin tests bilaterally. Functional coordination is better assessed during occupational therapy. In addition, note any tremors either at rest or with intention. Both natural and tandem gait should be examined for any abnormalities, if possible.

If the patient is able to walk, gait should be examined using a gait aid, if necessary. Assess the speed, safety, and pattern of gait, noting any loss of balance or poor coordination. Always keep weight-bearing precautions and restrictions in mind. If the patient is unable to walk, assess transfers or wheelchair mobility.

Selected Physical Interventions

Several physical interventions are commonly used in conjunction with surgical and pharmacological treatment for the patient with TBI. Two will be discussed here: constraint-induced movement therapy (CIMT) and spastic hypertonia management.

Constraint-Induced Movement Therapy

CIMT is an approach to physical therapy that has been used in patients with arm weakness after stroke since the early 1990s. Although most research concerns patients who have suffered a stroke, the approach is commonly used in patients with TBI. Recall that function can be enhanced by either decreasing impairment in the affected arm (e.g., improving strength, coordination, etc.) or by developing compensatory strategies using the unaffected arm. Although compensation may be a faster approach to functional improvement, there may be long-term drawbacks. CIMT emphasizes use of the paralyzed arm by placing the "good" arm at a disadvantage, commonly by placing mittens on the unaffected arm for several hours a day. This results in "forced use" of the weak arm. In order to understand why CIMT might be beneficial, two concepts are essential. First, following a neurological insult, patients find the weak limb difficult to use and control. This frustration may lead to a theoretical shutdown of neuronal circuitry, so-called "learned nonuse." Second, after brain injury, the brain undergoes cortical reorganization based on use patterns. Repeated task-specific practice with the affected limb may help induce cortical reorganization and subsequent functional improvement. CIMT attempts to address both issues following TBI. As might be expected, patients frequently find CIMT extremely frustrating, and compliance is often poor. Because of this, modifications have been proposed to reduce both the intensity and length of treatment. Smaller studies in acute and chronic stroke have demonstrated encouraging initial results.

Management of Spastic Hypertonia

Spastic hypertonia is velocity-dependent resistance to passive ROM, as outlined under the Subheading entitled, "Neurological." It is likely the result of hyperactive α-motor neurons via a loss of suprasegmental influence on spinal cord interneurons. In addition to medication and injection management, physical interventions include positioning, splinting and other orthotics, and aggressive and frequent stretching. Goals in management of hypertonia include:

- Improved function (activities of daily living, mobility), sleep, or cosmesis.
- Improved ease of care for caregivers.
- Prevention of skin breakdown, orthopedic deformity, and need for corrective surgery by improved positioning in bed or wheelchair.
- Pain reduction.
- Facilitation of stretching for shortened agonist muscles and strengthening of antagonistic muscles.

Alleviation of nociceptive factors, such as pressure ulcers, infections (bladder, toenail, ear, and skin), deep venous thrombosis, constipation, bladder distention, fatigue, and excessively cold conditions precedes any other intervention. Physical interventions may be provided by physical therapists, occupational therapists, and nursing staff, and can include sustained stretching, massage, vibration, heat modalities, cryotherapy, functional electrical stimulation, biofeedback, strengthening of antagonistic muscle groups, and hydrotherapy. Therapists may also attempt optimal positioning to reduce synergy patterns (e.g., wheelchair seating, bed positioning). Orthotics (soft or hard, custom or prefabricated) or splints may help hold a limb in a functional position, reduce pain, and prevent contracture. Patients with variable leg swelling may require splint modification or new splints fairly often. Serial or inhibitive casting of the ankles, knees, fingers, wrists, and elbows may improve spastic hypertonia by lengthening muscle fibers and help maintain ROM. When using serial casting or splinting, frequent monitoring for skin breakdown is mandatory.

Principles of Medication Management in TBI

Basic Principles

Medication management in the brain-injured patient begins with an analysis of the current medications. Keeping in mind that not all cognitive deficits are organic, and that many are related to medications, the first principle of medication management is *minimalization*. This requires discontinuing *any* unnecessary medications, especially those which may be sedating or impairing neurological recovery (*see* section on detrimental medications and Table 8). The second principle is *substitution*. If a medication treatment is required, a medication (or class of medication) with the fewest side effects and least impact on neurological recovery should be chosen. The final principle is the addition of medications for the purpose of

Table 8
Medications Relatively Contraindicated Following TBI

1. First-generation neuroleptic medications including metoclopromide and possibly hydrochlorothiazide.
2. Benzodiazepines.
3. Selected antiepileptic drugs (phenytoin and phenobarbital).
4. Centrally acting antihypertensive drugs.

cognitive and functional augmentation. Examples of all three principles are also discussed.

Potentially Detrimental Medications

Detrimental side effects of medication in brain injury can be viewed in two categories: (1) medication-specific side effects that would manifest in any patient, regardless of recent brain injury (e.g., sedation is a common side effect of clonidine, regardless of brain injury); and (2) population-specific side effects of particular concern to individuals with acquired brain injury (e.g., benzodiazepines slow the rate of motor recovery after stroke). Excellent animal data and an emerging human literature indicate that medications in four classes can potentially impair neurological recovery after acquired brain injury.

Neuroleptic Agents

Older antipsychotic drugs, such as haloperidol, thiothixene, and chlorpromazine, block dopamine receptors in the brain and should be avoided. Recall the GI agent metoclopramide is chemically related to this medication class. The animal literature clearly implicates haloperidol as detrimental influence on neurological recovery. However, recent data in rats suggests the less antidopaminergic atypical antipsychotics, such as risperidone and olanzepine, may be less detrimental. These newer agents also have a lower risk of extrapyramidal symptoms and tardive dyskinesia. The very newest atypical agents (quetiapine, ziprasidone and aripiprazole) are reported to have even fewer side effects, but are also less studied and clinical experience in brain injury is quite limited.

Benzodiazepines

Benzodiazepines work at the γ-amino buteric acid receptor and readily cross the blood–brain barrier, leading to sedation and a decrease in learning and memory. Clinical data suggest that benzodiazepines delay motor recovery following a stroke. If the indication is anxiolysis, buspirone (a serotonergic agent) is a good substitute. If benzodiazepines are being used as a sleep aid, avoiding daytime naps and abstaining from coffee, tea, and other caffeinated foods close to bedtime might be helpful. If pharmacological intervention is required, either zolpidem or trazodone are acceptable substitutions.

Selected Anticonvulsants

Both phenobarbital and phenytoin have been shown to slow or alter neurological recovery in rats, and can potentially impair cognition in humans. Phenobarbital should be used only as a last resort for seizure prophylaxis or treatment. Phenytoin should not be continued beyond 7 days for seizure prophylaxis after TBI. Carbamazepine or valproic acid may be the preferred agents in partial and generalized seizure treatment, respectively. Experience is growing with newer anticonvulsant agents, such as lamotrigine and levetiracetam, and although they may have fewer cognitive side effects, sedation is still possible.

Centrally Acting Antihypertensive Agents

These medications alter the metabolism of norepinephrine and have been shown to retard neurological recovery in rats. Agents include methyldopa, clonidine, and prazosin. Reasonable substitutions to control blood pressure include calcium channel blockers, angiotensin-converting enzyme inhibitors, angiotensin receptor blockers, and hydrophilic β-blockers (atenolol). If rate control is desired, calcium channel blockers plus digoxin or atenolol can be used.

Medications for Cognitive and Functional Augmentation

Hypoarousal

Arousal is the most basic cognitive function, without which sensory information and motor responses can not be processed. The data on treatment of hypoarousal in patients with TBI are limited by the lack of controlled studies and detailed dosing regimens. Amantadine is a dopaminergic medication that was initially developed for patients with Parkinson's disease, and has been noted to improve arousal in patients with TBI. Although retrospective, the best current data on treatment of hypoarousal is for amantadine. Other dopaminergic medications, such as bromocriptine, levodopa/carbidopa, and selegeline, may also be helpful to promote arousal, although they are more useful in the treatment of attention deficits.

Likewise, modafinil was initially approved for treatment of narcolepsy but has been found to have positive effects on alertness as well. Ultimately, the efficacy of these medications in treating hypoarousal remains unclear without randomized, controlled trials.

Attention Deficits

Methylphenidate is a neurostimulant that has been used extensively to promote attentiveness in brain-injured patients. At doses of 0.3 mg/kg of body weight twice a day, controlled trials have shown that the agent improves attention and increases processing speed. Methlyphenidate has recently become available in sustained release formulations that may help reduce the peak and trough effects that some patients experience. There is a risk of abuse in patients with a prior substance abuse history, but addiction does not seem to be a common clinical occurrence. Dextroamphetamine, dexedrine, bromocriptine, and protriptyline have also been used to treat attention deficits following TBI and improve functional recovery.

Initiation Deficits

Dopaminergic agonists, such as amantadine, bromocriptine, and protriptyline, dextroamphetamine, and methylphenidate, may be useful in patients with TBI who have initiation deficits.

Memory Deficits

Hippocampal and frontal cortical cholinergic systems are believed to play a key role in attention, learning, storage, and retrieval of new information, and cholinergic dysfunction is believed to play a key role in memory impairment following TBI. Donepezil, an acetylcholinesterase inhibitor that was initially developed for Alzheimer's disease, has been shown, in small studies, to improve memory deficits in TBI. Reminyl, rivastigmine, and glantamine are newer medications in this class that have not yet been studied in TBI. Methylphenidate and bromocriptine may be helpful for memory deficits secondary to significant attention deficits.

Spastic Hypertonia

Some patients functionally utilize spastic hypertonia for transferring, standing, and walking. The physicians must determine not only the degree of spasticity using the Modified Ashworth Scale (impairment), but also the resultant functional deficit attributable to the tone (disability). Oral, injectable, and intrathecal medications all play a role in treatment. Among the oral agents, dantrolene sodium is a peripherally acting medication that prevents calcium release from sarcoplasmic reticulum, and may be the treatment of choice in patients with spasticity in TBI. The other available choices (e.g., baclofen, tizanidine, clonidine, and valium) frequently cause drowsiness and cognitive side effects in doses required to adequately control spasticity.

If oral medications are not tolerated well or are ineffective and spasticity is limited to a few, functionally significant muscle groups, phenol nerve, motor point injections, or muscular botulinum toxin injections may be appropriate. Serial casting following injections may enhance effectiveness and lengthen shortened muscle. Phenol is usually administered in a 5–6% aqueous concentration, and is injected near motor points in, or nerve branches going to, the affected muscle. It demyelinates γ nerve fibers immediately and lasts for about 6 months, resulting in a less-irritable muscle that can be stretched more easily. These injections can be uncomfortable for some patients, especially at the motor points. However, it is inexpensive and relatively long-acting. There is an approximate 10% risk of dysesthesias if phenol injections are performed near a nerve with sensory innervation. Nerves commonly treated with phenol injection include the musculocutaneous, obturator, femoral, and tibial nerves.

When botulinum toxin type A (Botox®) or B (Myobloc®) is injected into the muscle, it blocks presynaptic release of acetylcholine at the neuromuscular junction. Onset of action is usually 3–5 days after injection. Collateral sprouting of the axon occurs in about 3 months, corresponding to the return of hypertonia. These medications are quite expensive in comparison to phenol, but are simple to inject, fairly painless, and without risk of dysethesias. Owing to potential antibody formation, injections of the smallest effective amount at no less than 3-month intervals are encouraged.

If spasticity is too diffuse, severe, and too many muscle groups are affected, implantation of an intrathecal baclofen pump can effectively manage spastic hypertonia. A positive response to a small test dose of baclofen (via lumbar puncture) is required before implantation. The test dose predicts quantitatively, but not qualitatively, the response to baclofen eventually delivered through the pump. A catheter is attached to the pump and then subcutaneously tunneled posteriorly around the abdomen to the back, where it is placed into the intrathecal space. The rate of baclofen delivery can be adjusted by tiny amounts at either a continuous or variable rate during the course of a 24-hour period. Because only a small intrathecal dose is needed (50–1000 μg delivered in a few drops per day), the degree of sedation seen with oral baclofen is rare when delivered intrathecally. After the implantation, the dosage of baclofen is gradually titrated, using an external programmer, until the desired effect is obtained. The pump reservoir is percutaneously refilled every 1–6 months via a refill port. Because of limited battery life, the pump needs replacement every 5–7 years.

Medical Complications of TBI

Cardiovascular

In the rehabilitation setting, brain injury-associated hypertension is seen in 10–15% of patients. The mechanism is believed to be excessive catecholamine release from the adrenal glands, which leads to increased output and vasoconstriction. Also, there may be injury to the central blood pressure control centers in the brain. If hypertension first presents in the rehabilitation setting, a computed tomography scan might be considered to rule out new cerebral processes, such as normal pressure hydrocephalus. Treatment of hypertension should begin with the evaluation of the patients' medication, looking specifically for offending agents, such as steroids or nonsteroidal anti-inflammatory drugs. Atenolol (a hydrophilic β-blocker), calcium channel blockers, angiotensin-converting enzyme inhibitors, or angiotensin receptor blockers are all reasonable choices to control blood pressure.

Orthostatic hypotension is also frequent, and is associated with prolonged bed rest or medications. Antihypertensives should be discontinued, and anemia and dehydration should be ruled out before orthostasis is ascribed to prolonged bed rest. Reclining wheelchairs, abdominal binders, and support stockings can be used to reduce orthostasis. Pharmacological intervention is not often required, but options include salt tablets, midodrine, and florinef.

There is also some evidence that the massive release of catecholamines during the adrenergic surge following TBI also leads to myocardial injury, although dysrythmias are uncommon. If not part of the transfer records, a baseline electrocardiogram obtained on admission to the rehabilitation center can be a valuable tool for future cardiac management.

Gastrointestinal/Genitourinary

TBI often results in the elevation of liver function tests owing to either the trauma itself or medications (especially anticonvulsants). Severe brain injury (GCS < 9) can lead to stress ulcers and bleeding, particularly in the first 2 weeks after TBI, especially if mechanical ventilation is required. Prophylaxis with a proton pump inhibitor is recommended during the acute care phase, but may not be needed in rehabilitation if the patient has no GI history or symptoms nor any blood in the stool.

Oral phase dysphagia is common, and 30–45% will have some degree of aspiration. If aspiration is suspected, a formal swallow evaluation should be requested, with the addition of a Fiberoptic Endoscopic Evaluation of Swallowing with Sensory Testing (FEESST) or modified barium swallow. In vegetative or minimally conscious patients, the physician may wish to avoid agents that decrease stomach acidity (raise pH) because this may increase the incidence of Gram-negative pneumonia via aspiration.

Patients with TBI often demonstrate loss of control over urination and defecation because of injury to the frontal lobes. For urination, a timed voiding schedule should be initiated with frequent toileting (e.g., every 2 hours), followed by a gradual increase in interval length (every 4 hours) in order to retrain the bladder to empty at regular intervals. Urinary retention is uncommon and should prompt consideration of an unrecognized spinal cord injury. Male patients can be prescribed a condom catheter for hygiene and skin protection if a voiding program is unsuccessful. In addition, instrumentation with Foley catheters, fecal incontinence, and inadequate hydration can lead to urinary tract infections, which should be evaluated and treated appropriately.

A bowel program can be used to treat either constipation or incontinence, and should include adequate hydration, stool softeners, and stimulant suppositories. Also, use the gastrocolic reflex (approximately 30 minutes after a meal) and gravity (have the patients sit up when they defecate) to promote bowel movements. Diarrhea, especially in the setting of long-term antibiotic use, should prompt an evaluation for *Clostridium difficile* infection. Enteral feeding should be supplemented with fiber compounds, such as psyllium, or be changed to formulas high in fiber.

Endocrine

Approximately 20% of patients with TBI demonstrate endocrine complications. The most common endocrine complication after a TBI is syndrome of inappropriate antidiuretic hormone (SIADH). Less common endocrinopathies include diabetes insipidus (DI), anterior hypopituitarism (AH), cerebral salt-wasting (CSW), and primary adrenal insufficiency. The first three have central etiologies, whereas the latter two are peripheral in nature.

SIADH causes a dilutional (hypervolemic) hyponatremia because of inappropriate renal water conservation. The serum osmolality in patients with SIADH is less than 280 osm/kg, serum sodium is less than 135 mEq/L, and urine sodium is greater than 25 mEq/L. SIADH is associated with certain medications, such as carbamazepine, neuroleptics, and tricylic antidepressants. The treatment in most cases is fluid restriction (800–1000 mL/day). Demeclocycline is a tetracycline antibiotic that has been shown to help with SIADH.

Posttraumatic DI occurs in 2–4% of patients with TBI, but is rarely permanent. Most commonly, posttraumatic DI is associated with severe closed-head injury with a basilar skull fracture. DI is also frequently associated with CN injuries. The usual onset is 5–10 days following trauma. Clinical features of DI include polyuria and polydypsia. Lab tests reveal low urine osmolality and high serum osmolality (with normal serum glucose and sodium). DI can be treated with desmopressin acetate orally, subcutaneously, or intranasally.

Although most cases of hyponatremia resulting from brain injury are caused by SIADH, a less common etiology is cerebral CSW syndrome. CSW syndrome is caused by impaired renal tubular function, resulting in the inability of the kidneys to conserve salt. Clinically, patients manifesting CSW syndrome are dehydrated, lose weight, have orthostatic hypotension, and demonstrate a negative fluid balance. Lab findings are similar to those of DI, but elevated blood urea nitrogen and creatinine are noted. Treatment consists of intravenous normal saline.

AH, or panhypopituitarism, is a rare complication that presents weeks to months after a closed head injury, usually following severe craniocerebral trauma. The patient becomes progressively lethargic or anorexic and may demonstrate hypothermia, bradycardia, or hypotension with hyponatremia. The endocrine work-up for AH includes serum hormonal assays (e.g., cortisol, testosterone, and thyroid function tests). Treatment involves multiple hormonal replacement therapies and monitoring of serum levels, along with the clinical response of the patient. Primary adrenal insufficiency is also very rare and usually presents with psychiatric symptoms of depression, confusion, and apathy. Treatment by mineralocorticoid and glucocorticoid replacement therapy can result in a significant improvement of rehabilitation progress and outcome.

It is also common for menstruation to cease after TBI in female patients. It may take up to 1 year for normal menses to return. If resumption of menses are delayed beyond this period or menstrual characteristics are altered (metromenorrhagia) once menses resume, consider referral to a gynecologist for further evaluation.

Other

Central fevers may develop in patients with severe brain injury who have a damaged anterior hypothalamus. The diagnosis is one of exclusion. If infectious etiologies have been ruled out, dopamine agonists or nonsteroidal anti-inflammatory drugs can be used for treatment. Ulnar nerve entrapment at the cubital tunnel, brachial plexus injury, and common peroneal compression are the most common peripheral nerve injuries diagnosed in patients with TBI, and can be better evaluated with nerve conduction studies and electromyography. The clinician should have an extremely high index of suspicion for peripheral nerve lesions distal to any fracture site.

Cognitive Rehabilitation

In general, therapeutic strategies in cognitive rehabilitation can be divided into approaches that remediate cognitive abilities, and approaches that develop compensation for cognitive impairment. The rationale for recovery is that with extensive practice or exercise, it is possible to retrain and improve impaired cognitive function by reestablishing previously learned patterns of behavior. Example techniques include reinforced practice on auditory, visual and verbal tasks, number manipulation, computer-assisted stimulation, and video feedback. In contrast, compensatory interventions concede the unrecoverable loss of function, and instead, focus on adapting to the cognitive deficit. Examples of compensatory mechanisms include visual cues, memory books, mnemonics, self-monitoring techniques, and pagers that trigger behavior. The two approaches are not mutually exclusive, and in practice, most cognitive rehabilitation programs combine both restorative and compensatory strategies.

Selected Complications

Depression

Depression may occur in up to 50% of persons with TBI in the first year following injury. Psychotherapy, an important component of a comprehensive rehabilitation program, is used to treat depression and address both loss of self esteem associated with cognitive dysfunction and adjustment to physical disability. It should involve individuals with TBI, their family members, and significant others. Specific goals for this therapy emphasize emotional support, providing explanations of the injury and its effects, helping to achieve self esteem in the context of realistic self-assessment, reducing denial, and increasing ability to relate to family and society. Although the use of psychotherapy has not been studied systematically in patients with TBI, support for its use comes from demonstrated efficacy for similar disorders in other populations. The differential diagnosis of depression includes frontal lobe pathology, which can mimic mood disorders. Medication treatment can include selective serotonin reuptake inhibitors and neurostimulants, among others. Seizure risk is a concern when using tricyclic antidepressants or bupropion.

Agitation

Agitation should be considered a subtype of delirium characterized by excessive behaviors (aggression, akathesia, disinhibition, emotional lability), which occurs *during* the period of posttraumatic amnesia. It occurs in 11–50% of patients with TBI, and despite impressions to the contrary, it is quite short-lived in most cases. A recent study closely related agitation to impaired cognition, underscoring the need to eliminate any medication that may further undermine cognition. Agitation is a symptom, not a diagnosis, and it may be difficult or impossible for the patient to relate the underlying problem. Several etiologies should be explored, including pain, infection, hypoxia, metabolic abnormalities, urinary obstruction, drug withdrawal, or new intracranial lesion. The Agitated Behavioral Scale may be used to quantify agitation and measure response to treatment.

Nonpharmacological treatments should be attempted first, including reducing environmental stimulation and redirection. There is little research on which medications are most efficacious to treat agitation. Propranolol is probably the best studied, but hypotension and bradycardia are possible side effects. Other agents commonly used include amantadine, buspirone, valproic acid, first- and third-generation neuroleptics, carbamazepine, benzodiazepines, and neurostimulants. Recall that any agent can paradoxically *increase* agitation. Benzodiazepines should be used only temporarily at the lowest effective dose until trials of other agents are completed. In general, first-generation neuroleptics should be the last-resort treatment after all other agents have failed.

Heterotopic Ossification

Heterotopic ossification (HO) is the formation of normal, mature bone in the soft tissues around the large joints of the body (e.g., hips, elbows, shoulders, knees). The incidence of HO in TBI is variable (11–76%), but increases with spasticity, prolonged coma (>2 weeks), and fractures near a joint. It usually occurs 2 weeks to 4 months postinjury. However, functional limitation is only present in 10–20% of patients who develop HO. The affected limb may present with limited ROM, pain, local swelling, local warmth, erythema, increased spasticity, or the patient may develop a low-grade fever. The differential diagnosis of HO includes undiagnosed or new fracture, deep venous thrombosis, infection, tumor, or hematoma. Plain radiographs cannot identify HO for 3–4 weeks, but a triple-phase bone scan may be positive before then (phase I and II will show increased uptake). Alkaline phosphatase may also be increased, but is a nonspecific finding, especially in patients with multiple fractures. Disodium etidronate is a bisphosphonate that has been shown to prevent subsequent calcification of the osteoid matrix in patients with spinal cord injury. One small study suggests that this may apply to TBI as well. There is also some evidence that indomethacin, aspirin, and warfarin may help. However, no single agent can be considered as the standard of care in patients with TBI. Symptomatic treatment should be initiated with indomethacin, and acetaminophen and etidronate may help minimize the progression of HO. Short-term rest may be required if the joint is too painful to move, but ROM should be initiated as soon as possible. Most physicians recommend both passive and active ROM exercises in the pain-free range to minimize any functional limitations or ankylosis. If ankylosis is imminent, the joint should also be positioned in the most functional position. Other treatment options include surgery (once the HO is mature and alkaline phosphatase levels have returned to baseline) and low-dose radiation in extremely rare circumstances.

Hydrocephalus

Although ventriculomegaly is very common following severe TBI, overt hydrocephalus occurs less frequently, with an incidence of approximately 5%. Differentiation between hydrocephalus (too much cerebral spinal fluid) and hydrocephalus *ex vacuo* changes (too little or atrophied brain parenchyma) can be challenging. Risk factors include traumatic subarachnoid hemorrhage and meningitis. Acute hydrocephalus tends to be of the obstructive type treated with ventriculostomy. In the rehabilitation setting, hydrocephalus is more likely to be nonobstructive; that is, normal pressure hydrocephalus. The classic triad of gait instability, urinary incontinence, and dementia is of little use in the TBI population because these symptoms occur frequently as a result of the injury itself. Hydrocephalus should be considered in the setting of decrements in functional or mental status, even months to years after injury.

Seizure Disorder

Seizure occurrence following TBI is highly dependent on the severity of injury. In addition to the designation of partial or generalized, posttraumatic seizures are also classified on timing as immediate (within 24 hours of injury), early (days 1–7), or late (after day 7). Recent data indicates that biparietal contusions and dural penetration with bone or metal fragments carry a more than 60% seizure risk, whereas multiple intracranial operations, multiple subcortical contusions, subdural hematoma, and midline shift greater than 5mm carry a more than 25% risk. *Standard of care is that seizure prophylaxis with any agent should not continue beyond 1 week postinjury.* Either phenytoin or valproate are effective prophylaxis for early seizures; however, the latter may be associated with more side effects. Both phenobarbital and phenytoin should be avoided in the treatment of established seizures because of the potential detrimental impact on the rate of neurological recovery, as discussed in the Subheading entitled "Selected Anticonvulsants."

VS and MCS

The definition of VS and MCS are discussed under the Subheading entitled, "Neurological" and outlined in Table 5. In general, the care for this subpopulation consists of superb medical and nursing care, physical management and positioning, pharmacological trials, and sensory assessment using a standardized scale. Patients at this level often require a gastostomy tube and tracheostomy, and are at risk for multiple medical complications. A complete evaluation of neuromedical causes of impaired consciousness should include assessment for occult infections, such as retroperitoneal abscess, sinusitis, and osteomyelitis (in the appropriate clinical circumstances), endocrine abnormalities, and hydrocephalus. Nursing care should focus on the establishment of a bowel program, skin maintenance, and, in conjunction with therapists, a seating/positioning schedule. Aggressive management of spastic hypertonia (as described under the Subheading entitled "Medications for Cognitive and Functional Augmentation") may be mandatory to achieve acceptable seating and positioning goals. Many medications (most neurostimulant or dopaminergic agents) have been used in an attempt to improve arousal in severely injured patients. There are no randomized, controlled trials establishing efficacy for any specific agent, but recent observational data from a multicenter cohort suggest that amantadine may be effective. Finally, assessment of the severely injured patient using a standardized assessment tool with well-trained staff is critical to quantify clinical changes as a result of either natural recovery or clinical interventions. The Coma Recovery Scale, Coma–Near Coma Scale, and Western Neurosensory Stimulation Profile are probably the most frequently used. It is unclear whether "sensory stimulation" or "coma stimulation" is effective or not, and using the standardized scales might be best viewed as an assessment rather than a therapeutic intervention.

Mild TBI

At the other end of the TBI spectrum is mild TBI (MTBI), which accounts for at least 80% of all TBI. The American Congress of

Table 9
American Congress of Rehabilitation Medicine Definition of Mild Traumatic Brain Injury

Inclusion criteria (more than one must be present)

1. Any period of loss of consciousness for up to 30 minutes.
2. Any loss of memory of events immediately before or after the incident as far back as 24 hours.
3. Any alteration of mental state at the time of accident (dazed, disoriented, or confused).
4. Focal neurological deficit(s) that may or may note be transient.

Exclusion criteria (one or more must be manifest)

1. Loss of consciousness exceeding 30 minutes.
2. Posttraumatic amnesia persisting longer than 24 hours.
3. After 30 minutes, the GCS falls below 13.

Rehabilitation Medicine definition of MTBI is presented in Table 9. It should be noted that the diagnosis of MTBI may still be made in the absence of LOC. In addition, those patients with an initial GCS score of 13–15 with positive finding on brain magnetic resonance imaging or computed tomography scan more closely resemble moderate TBI on neuropsychological testing 6 months following injury. Approximately 10–20% of persons with MTBI will develop postconcussive disorder. Although headache, dizziness, memory, and attention deficits are common, there is no symptom constellation to constitute a "syndrome." The etiology of postconcussive disorder is somewhat debatable, but may have components of organic neurological injury, underlying psychopathology, and malingering depending on the patient. Treatment includes medical interventions for cognitive and mood deficits, physical treatments for headache and pain, and psychotherapy to address issues of depression, self-confidence, and somatization.

Prognosis

Predicting the outcome following TBI is difficult. Prognostication is limited by relatively poor assessment and outcome measures. The Glasgow Outcome Scale has been used in many outcome studies, but is limited in its clinical usefulness because of the extremely broad categories of classification. Premorbid factors, such as age, prior brain injury, general and psychiatric health, and a history of drug or alcohol use, come into play. Outcome is associated with the severity of injury as measured by GCS, length of unconsciouness, or posttraumatic amnesia. Patients with acute complications of hypoxia, mass lesions on initial neuroimaging, and cardiopulmonary problems tend to do more poorly. Assessment of outcome becomes easier the farther removed the patient is from time of injury. The trajectory of recovery may be much more apparent several weeks, rather than several days, after injury. When addressing the issue of prognosis, one must clarify, "Prognosis for what?" Assessing the chances for independent ambulation with or without an assistive device or independence in activities of daily living is much different that of return to work or life or death. Particularly among patients with higher level professional jobs, even a small decrement in intellectual ability can be devastating to job performance. On the other hand, persons employed in more physical labor (i.e., construction) may be far more impacted by a physical rather than a cognitive disability.

Key References and Suggested Additional Reading

American Congress of Rehabilitation Medicine. Definition of Mild Traumatic Brain Injury. J Head Trauma Rehabil 1993; 8:86–87.

American Congress of Rehabilitation Medicine. Recommendations for use of uniform nomenclature pertinent to patients with severe alterations in consciousness. Arch Phys Med Rehabil 1995; 76: 205–209.

Bickley LS, Hoekelman RA. Bates' Guide to Physical Examination and History Taking. Baltimore, Lippincott Williams & Wilkins; 7th ed., 1999.

Braddom RL, Buschbacher RM. Physical Medicine and Rehabilitation. Philadelphia, W.B. Saunders; 2nd ed., 2000.

Cicerone KD Dahlberg C, Kalmar K, et al. Evidence-based cognitive rehabilitation: recommendations for clinical practice. Arch Phys Med Rehabil 2000; 81: 1596–1615.

Dobkin BH. The Clinical Science of Neurological Rehabilitation, 2nd ed. Contemporary Neurological Series. Oxford, Oxford University Press, 2003.

Glen MB, Wroblewski B. Twenty Years of Pharmacology. J Head Trauma Rehabil 2005; 20:55–61.

Horn L and Zasler N. Medical Rehabilitation of Traumatic Brain Injury. Philadephia, Mosby, 1996.

Kendall FP, McCreary EK, Provance PG. Muscles: Testing and Function. Baltimore, Lippincott, Williams & Wilkins; 5th ed., 2005.

Mark VW, Taub E. Constraint-induced movement therapy for chronic stroke hemiparesis and other disabilities. Restorative Neurol Neurosci 2004; 24:317–336.

NIH Consensus Development Panel on Rehabilitation of Persons with Traumatic Brain Injury. JAMA 1999; 282:974–983.

Rosenthal M. Rehabilitation of the Adult and Child with Traumatc Brain Injury. Philadelphia, F.A. Davis, 1999.

2 Stroke

Brenda S. Mallory

Background

Strokes (also called cerebrovascular accidents) occur suddenly and are clinically defined as a focal vascular lesion, which causes an abrupt onset of a neurological deficit that lasts longer than 24 hours. The deficit depends on the area of brain affected. In a transient ischemic attack (TIA), the neurological deficits last less than 24 hours but are usually 5 to 15 minutes.

Stroke Statistics

Approximately 700,000 strokes occur annually in the United States (200,000 are recurrent strokes).

- Stroke is the third leading cause of death in the United States, behind heart disease and cancer.
- There are 4.7 million stroke survivors in the United States.
- The first-stroke incident rate (per 100,000) is 167 for white males and 323 for black males.
- Stroke is the leading cause of disability in the United States.
- Approximately 25% of stroke survivors die within 1 year, and about 50% die within 8 years.
- Approximately 50–70% of stroke survivors obtain functional independence.
- Approximately 15–30% of stroke survivors remain permanently disabled.
- About 20% of stroke survivors require institutional care.

From: *Essential Physical Medicine and Rehabilitation*
Edited by: G. Cooper © Humana Press Inc., Totowa, NJ

Etiology

Strokes are caused by ischemic infarction or hemorrhagic disruption of the brain. Ischemic strokes are the result of decreased blood flow and are caused by thrombosis, embolism, or other disorders of the blood or blood vessel walls.

Ischemic Stroke (88% of All Strokes)

Arterial Thrombosis (Atherosclerosis)

- A thrombus is an aggregation of primarily platelets and fibrin (that may have other cellular elements) within a blood vessel.
- Platelets stick to an ulcerated atherosclerotic plaque, forming a white thrombus (thrombogenesis).
- A red thrombus of fibrin and red blood cells forms and propagates on top of the white thrombus, especially in areas of slow-moving blood flow.
- Primary atherosclerotic thrombus fills the arterial lumen, partially or completely occluding the lumen.
- Secondary thrombi propagate retrogradely and anterogradely.
- A lacunar infarction results from thrombosis in small brain arteries (30–300 μm) and leaves a lacune of about 3 mm to 2 cm.
- Arterial thrombosis may also be caused by other disorders of the vessels or blood.

Embolism

- Emboli plug downstream arteries and consist of pieces of thrombus or other material that originate from proximal arteries, the heart, or are paradoxical via a patent foramen ovale.
- Atrial fibrillation is the most common cause of cerebral embolism.
- The average annual stroke risk in patients with atrial fibrillation ranges from 0.5 to 15%, depending on the number of risk factors (older age, hypertension, poor left ventricular function, prior cardioembolism, diabetes, and thyrotoxicosis)
- The most common cause of artery-to-artery cerebral embolism is carotid bifurcation atherosclerosis.

Other

- Collagen vascular diseases.
- Vasculitis.
- Hypercoaguable states.

- Fibromuscular dysplasia.
- Temporal arteritis.
- Granulomatous arteritis.
- Moyamoya disease.
- Venous thrombosis.
- Carotid and vertebral artery dissection.
- Cerebral autosomal-dominant arteriopathy with subcortical infarcts and leukoencephalopathy (CADASIL).
- Mitochondrial encephalopathy, lactic acidosis, and stroke-like syndrome (MELAS).

Hemorrhage (12% of All Strokes)

Intracerebral Hemorrhage (9% of All Strokes)

- Has a mortality rate of 50%.
- Main causes are hypertension (HTN), trauma, and cerebral amyloid angiopathy.
- Also caused by drug abuse (amphetamines and cocaine), tumors, vascular malformations, coagulation disorders, use of anticoagulants and/or thrombolytic agents, and hemorrhage into a cerebral infarct.

Subarachnoid Hemorrhage (3% of All Strokes)

- Main causes are trauma and rupture of a saccular aneurysm.
- Other causes are vascular malformations and the extension of an intracerebral hemorrhage.
- About 30,000 aneurysms rupture annually in the United States.
- The re-bleeding rate of a ruptured aneurysm is 20% in the first 2 weeks, and 3% per year afterward.

Pathogenesis

Ischemic Stroke

Following a critical loss of blood flow, brain cells are reversibly or irreversibly injured, depending on the severity and duration of ischemia. After a stroke, there is a core area of severe injury and cell death surrounded by an area of less severely damaged cells called the *ischemic penumbra*. Cells in the ischemic penumbra are electrically silent but are able to maintain their membrane potentials, and can recover if reperfused. If blood flow is restored promptly, no or few cells die, and the patient experiences a TIA.

The following three major mechanisms promote cell death after a stroke:

1. Excitotoxicity.
   a. There is failure to generate adenosine triphosphate.
   b. There is electrical failure.

c. There is ionic pump failure with an inability to maintain ionic gradients.
d. There is a release of the excitatory amino acid glutamate.
e. There is failure of glutamate reuptake.
f. Glutamate binds to postsynaptic membranes causing excessive Ca^{++} entry into damaged brain cells.
g. Calcium-dependent synthases and proteases break down cytoskeletal and enzymatic proteins and generate nitric oxide-free radicals and peroxynitrite anion.

2 Oxidative stress.
a. Mitochondrial functions, such as oxidative phosphorylation, fail, and reactive oxygen radicals are released that attack proteins, lipids, and nucleic acids.

3. Apoptosis.
a. Molecules promote cell death by mechanisms resembling apoptosis (programmed cell death).

Hypertensive Intracerebral Hemorrhage

The rupture of a small penetrating artery, weakened by lipohyalinosis, deep in the brain results in hypertensive intracerebral hemorrhage. The areas most commonly involved are the putamen and internal capsule, caudate nucleus, thalamus, cerebral lobes, pons, and cerebellum.

Cerebral Amyloid Angiopathy

This results from the deposition of amyloid in the walls of cerebral arterioles, which causes the arterioles to degenerate. It is thought to be a common cause of lobar hemorrhage in the elderly and has no specific treatment.

Saccular Aneurysms

These occur at the bifurcation of large-to-medium-sized intracranial arteries, and rupture results from thinning of the arterial wall.

Risk Factors for Stroke

Many risk factors can be modified by medical or surgical interventions or changes in lifestyle, but some are not modifiable. Primary and secondary prevention of stroke can be determined by the identification of modifiable risk factors.

The following risk factors for stroke can be treated:

1. HTN.
a. High blood pressure (140/90 mmHg or higher) is the most important risk factor for stroke.

   b. Persons with blood pressure lower than 120/80 mmHg have about half the lifetime risk of stroke compared with those who have HTN.
2. Atrial fibrillation.
   a. The use of anticoagulation medications depends on risk factors, such as age, previous TIA or stroke, HTN, heart failure, diabetes, clinical coronary artery disease, mitral stenosis, prosthetic heart valves, or thyrotoxicosis.
3. Diabetes.
   a. Treatment of diabetes can delay complications that increase the risk of stroke.
4. Cigarette smoking.
   a. Risk returns to baseline risk 5 years after quitting.
5. High blood cholesterol.
   a. High levels of low-density lipoprotein (>100 mg/dL) and triglycerides (≥150 mg/dL) increase the risk of stroke in people with previous coronary heart disease, ischemic stroke, or TIA. Low levels (<40 mg/dL) of high-density lipoprotein also may increase stroke risk.
6. Carotid stenosis.
   a. The risk of stroke in patients with asymptomatic carotid artery stenosis (≥60%) is approximately 2% per year, whereas symptomatic patients have a 13%-per-year risk of stroke.
7. Transient ischemic attacks.
   a. Following a TIA, 10% of patients will develop a stroke in 90 days, and 5% in 2 days. Patients at risk for stroke should be counseled to call 911 if they experience symptoms of sudden hemiplegia or hemianesthesia, gait disturbance, visual changes, difficulty with speech, or severe headache.
   b. One type of TIA, amaurosis fugax, is transient monocular blindness resulting from emboli to the central retinal artery.
8. Other heart disease.
   a. People with coronary heart disease or heart failure have a higher risk of stroke than those with hearts that work normally. Dilated cardiomyopathy, heart valve disease, and some types of congenital heart defects also raise the risk of stroke.
9. Physical inactivity.
   a. There is a lower relative risk of stroke (0.86 in men and up to 0.66 in women) associated with vigorous exercise.
10. Excessive alcohol.
   a. Drinking an average of more than one alcoholic drink a day for women or more than two drinks a day for men can raise blood pressure, and may increase the risk for stroke.
11. Illegal drugs.
   a. Intravenous drug abuse carries a high risk of stroke. Cocaine use has been linked to strokes and heart attacks.

The following risk factors for stroke that cannot be treated:

1. Increasing age.
2. Gender.
   a. Stroke is more common in men than in women. Women who are pregnant have a higher risk of stroke, as do women taking birth control pills who also smoke or have high blood pressure or other risk factors.
3. Heredity and race.
   a. Stroke risk is greater if a parent, grandparent, sister, or brother has had a stroke.
   b. African Americans have a much higher risk of death from a stroke than Caucasians, partly because blacks are more at risk for high blood pressure, diabetes, and obesity.
4. Prior stroke or heart attack.

History

Patients with an acute stroke need to be evaluated urgently to determine if the stroke is ischemic, and whether the patient can be treated with intravenous recombinant tissue plasminogen activator (rtPA).

Ischemic Stroke

- Most patients will have a history of a sudden onset of a focal neurological symptom.
- Some will have a step-wise, gradual worsening or waxing and waning of symptoms.
- Most are alert.
- Some are lethargic. Try to get history from friends, family, or bystanders.
- Approximately 25% will have headaches.
- Nausea and vomiting can occur in brain stem or cerebellar strokes.
- Neurological symptoms depend on the arterial territory involved (*see* Table 1).
- Ask patients about medications, especially anticoagulants and antiplatelet agents.
- Symptom onset from the time that the patient was last known to be symptom free is needed to guide thrombolytic therapy.
- A history of recent medical or neurological events should include the following:
  - Epilepsy.
  - Migraines.
  - Previous stroke or myocardial infarction.
  - Surgery.
  - Trauma.
  - Hemorrhage.

Table 1
Stroke Syndromes

Artery	*Anatomy supplied*	*Stroke syndrome*
Common carotid	Forebrain except occipital lobe	Asymptomatic or MCA syndrome
Internal carotid	Forebrain except occipital lobe	Asymptomatic or MCA syndrome
Middle cerebral	Surface cortical branches • Most of the convexity of the hemisphere including: ▪ Lateral orbital surface of frontal lobe ▪ Insula ▪ Middle and inferior frontal gyri ▪ Precentral gyrus ▪ Postcentral gyrus ▪ Inferior parietal lobule ▪ Superior parietal lobule (inferior part) ▪ Lateral surface of temporal lobe Deep branches • Internal capsule (superior half) • Basal ganglia • Optic radiation	Contralateral hemiplegia • Arm/face > leg (surface branches) • Proportional (deep branches) Contralateral sensory loss • Arm/face > leg Homonomous hemianopsia Homonymous quadrantanopia • Lower (parietal lobe) • Upper (temporal lobe) Dominant • Motor aphasia • Sensory aphasia • Global aphasia • Apraxia • Gerstmann's syndrome Nondominant • Anosognosia • Unilateral asomatognosia

Continued

Table 1 ***(Continued)***

Artery	*Anatomy supplied*	*Stroke syndrome*
Anterior cerebral	Surface cortical branches • Frontal pole • Part of orbital surface of frontal lobe • Anterior medial surface of frontal and parietal lobes including: ▪ Paracentral lobule ▪ Cingulate gyrus ▪ Medial frontal gyrus ▪ Corpus callosum (except splenum) Heubner's artery (deep branch) • Anterior putamen • Inferior head of the caudate nucleus • Anterior limb of the internal capsule (inferior half)	Contralateral leg weakness Contralateral leg sensory loss Contralateral hemiplegia • Leg > arm/face • Arm/face > leg (Heubner's artery) Mutism Abulia (akinetic mutism) Urinary incontinence Head and eyes deviate to side of lesion Gegenhalten rigidity Forced grasping Ideomotor apraxia Alien arm or hand Acute confusion Dominant • Transcortical motor aphasia • Transcortical mixed aphasia
Posterior cerebral	Surface cortical branches • Uncus • Parahippocampal gyrus • Medial and lateral occipitotemporal gyri • Cuneus • Lingual gyrus • Precuneus • Posterolateral occipital lobe	Hemispheric territory • Contralateral homonomous hemianopsia • Alexia without agraphia • Color anomia • Amnesia • Prosopagnosia • Visual object agnosia

Continued

Table 1 *(Continued)*

Artery	*Anatomy supplied*	*Stroke syndrome*
Posterior cerebral *(Continued)*	Interpeduncular branches • Midbrain Perforating branches • Hypothalamus • Pituitary • Anterior medial thalamus • Mammillary bodies • Subthalamus • Globus pallidus • Lateral geniculate body	Thalamic syndrome • Contralateral sensory loss • Choreoathetosis • Ataxia • Tremor • Dejerine-Roussy syndrome Weber syndrome • Contralateral hemiplegia • Third nerve palsy
Basilar	Brainstem Cerebellum	Locked-in syndrome (paramedian branch occlusion at level of ventral basal pons) • Quadriplegia • Bilateral cranial nerve palsy • Preservation of spinothalamic sensation and upgaze
Posterior inferior cerebellar	Medulla oblongata Inferior surface of cerebellum Dentate nucleus	Lateral medullary syndrome (Wallenberg's syndrome; may be caused by other artery occlusion) • Dysarthria • Ipsilateral limb ataxia • Vertigo • Nystagmus

Continued

Table 1 *(Continued)*

Artery	*Anatomy supplied*	*Stroke syndrome*
Posterior inferior cerebellar *(continued)*		• Ipsilateral Horner's syndrome • Ipsilateral sensory loss face • Contralateral sensory loss in limbs and trunk • Dysphagia • Vocal cord paralysis • Hiccup
Lacunar syndromes	Posterior limb of the internal capsule or ventral pons	Pure motor hemiparesis
	Ventrolateral thalamus	Pure sensory stroke
	Ventral pons	Ataxic hemiparesis
	Ventral pons or genu of the internal capsule	Dysarthria and clumsy hand or arm
	Genu and anterior limb of the internal capsule	Pure motor hemiparesis with motor
Aphasia		

Stroke syndromes are variable due to arterial anatomic variation and collateral circulation.
MCA, middle cerebral artery.

- The presence of one of the following symptoms double the chance of an individual having an intracranial hemorrhage:
  - Coma on arrival.
  - Vomiting.
  - Severe headache.
  - Current warfarin therapy.
  - Systolic blood pressure higher than 220 mmHg.
  - Glucose level higher than 170 mg/dL in a nondiabetic patient.

Intracerebral Hemorrhage

- The usual presentation is sudden onset of a focal neurological deficit that progresses over minutes to hours.
- Many patients will have maximum symptoms at onset.
- Associated symptoms are elevated blood pressure, depressed level of consciousness, headache, nausea, and vomiting.
- Approximately 6% will have seizures.
- No set of clinical features can reliably distinguish hemorrhagic from ischemic stroke.

Subarachnoid Hemorrhage

- The usual presentation is the sudden onset of a severe headache.
- The headache is often called "the worst headache of my life." It is also described as a "thunderclap" headache.
- Associated symptoms may be a brief loss of consciousness, nausea or vomiting, focal neurological deficits, or a stiff neck.
- It is a medical emergency.

Definitions

Abulia is lacking will, initiative, or drive.

Agnosia is the inability to recognize a previously known stimulus via a sensory modality, and is variously defined to include disorders at both the discriminative sensory level and the associative sensory level, or at the associative sensory level alone.

Anosognosia is the unawareness of left hemiparesis following a nondominant parietal lesion.

Aphasia is the loss or impairment (dysphasia) of language owing to a cerebral lesion.

Apraxia is the inability to produce a purposeful movement in the absence of a severe disorder of sensation, strength, coordination, cognition, perception, or language.

Asomatognosia is the loss of awareness of one's body schema and its relation to extrapersonal space, and is anatomically localized in the parietal lobes. Unilateral asomatognosias are usually related to a lesion in the nondominant parietal lobe, and include neglect of one side of the body, dressing apraxia, sensory extinction, and constructional apraxia.

Associative level of perception is multimodal sensory integration (visual, tactile, auditory, language, and memory) resulting in the recognition of a previously known sensory stimulus.

Astereognosis is the inability to identify an object by palpation despite intact primary sensory modalities, and is usually caused by a lesion of the opposite sensory cortex.

Dejerine-Roussy syndrome is a pain syndrome that is often delayed in onset after a posterolateral thalamic lesion, and affects all or part of the contralateral body.

Discriminative level of perception is the awareness of the characteristics of a unimodal sensory stimulus, such as shape, weight, color, and movement, and can be tested by two-point discrimination, cutaneous localization, figure writing (graphesthesia), and stereognosis.

Dyspraxia is difficulty in producing a purposeful movement in the absence of a severe disorder of sensation, strength, coordination, cognition, perception, or language.

Gerstmann's syndrome is a bilateral asomatognosia resulting from a dominant parietal lesion, and is characterized by finger agnosia, acalculia, agraphia, and left–right confusion.

Ideational apraxia is the inability to produce a purposeful movement because of loss of the plan of action; it is identified when a patient cannot correctly utilize a familiar object, and is thought to be produced by a lesion of the left angular gyrus, which affects the limbs bilaterally. (It has been likened to sensory aphasia.)

Ideomotor apraxia is the inability to produce a purposeful movement when commanded, and can be produced by a lesion in the region of the supramarginal gyrus involving the fibers of the left arcuate fasciculus, in the left premotor cortex (both with bilateral effects), in the corpus callosum, or in the right premotor area causing left limb apraxia. (It has been likened to conduction aphasia.)

Impersistence is the failure to continue a voluntary action, such as eye closure or hand gripping, for more than a few seconds, and is thought to be a disorder of attention that is usually the result of a right frontal lesion.

Motor aphasia (Broca's aphasia) is nonfluent, effortful speech with good comprehension and the inability to repeat.

Primary sensory modalities are touch, pain, temperature, and vibration.

Prosopagnosia is a type of visual agnosia characterized by the inability to recognize individual faces, and is usually the result of a lesion in the bilateral inferior parieto-occipital area or, rarely, with a right inferior parieto-occipital lesion.

Sensory aphasia (Wernicke's aphasia) is fluent, nonsensical speech (jargon speech) with impaired comprehension and the inability to repeat.

Transcortical aphasias are similar to motor and sensory aphasias, but with preserved repetition.

Visual object agnosia is the inability to recognize any object, and is usually caused by a more extensive lesion in the bilateral inferior parieto-occipital area or, rarely, with a left inferior parieto-occipital lesion.

Clinical Examination

- Vital signs.
- Signs of trauma.
- Cardiovascular exam.
- Skin.
- Evidence of active bleeding.
- Neurological exam.
- Level of consciousness.
  - Glasgow Coma Scale (eye opening, verbal response, motor response).
- Cognition.
  - Speech (fluency and repletion).
  - Comprehension.
  - Naming.
  - Reading.
  - Writing.
  - Calculation.
  - Object recognition.
  - Copying a geometric pattern.
  - Memory.
  - Reasoning.
  - Emotional state.
- Cranial nerves.
  - Assess swallowing ability before the patient drinks.
- Motor system.
  - Inspection.
  - Strength.
  - Tone.
  - Reflexes.
  - Coordination.
- Sensation.
- National Institutes of Health Stroke Scale (NIHSS).
  - The NIHSS provides prognostic information and helps identify patients at greatest risk for intracranial hemorrhage associated with thrombolytic therapy. The NIHSS is available on the National Institute of Neurological Disorders and Stroke website at http://www.ninds.nih.gov/doctors.

Diagnostic Evaluation

The emergency diagnostic evaluation for acute stroke includes the following:

- Brain computed tomography (CT) scan.
  - Because clinical features alone cannot differentiate ischemic from hemorrhagic stroke, brain imaging is needed.
  - The usual initial brain imaging test is noncontrast-enhanced CT.
  - For rtPA candidates, the goal time from arrival to CT interpretation is 45 minutes.
- Electrocardiogram.
  - Acute myocardial infarction can lead to stroke.
  - Acute stroke can lead to myocardial ischemia.
  - Atrial fibrillation can be detected.
- Blood glucose.
- Serum electrolytes.
- Renal function tests.
- Complete blood count, including platelet count.
- Prothrombin time:international normalized ratio.
- Activated partial thromboplastin time.
- Others as indicated.
  - Hepatic function study.
  - Toxicology screen.
  - Blood alcohol level.
  - Pregnancy test.
  - Arterial blood gas.
  - Lumbar puncture.
  - Electroencephalography.
  - Chest X-ray.

Other diagnostic studies can be obtained after the patient receives initial treatment.

Doppler ultrasonography can identify stenosis at the origin of the internal carotid artery. *Transcranial doppler* can asses anterior and posterior brain circulation, including stenotic lesions in the large intracranial arteries.

Angiography

- If the cause of an intracerebral hemorrhage is uncertain, angiography should be considered.
- Magnetic resonance angiography, CT angiography, and catheter angiography are used.
- Catheter cerebral angiography is the standard for diagnosing cerebral aneurysms as the cause for subarachnoid hemorrhage (SAH).
- Timing of cerebral angiography depends on the patient's clinical state.

Multimodal Magnetic Resonance Imaging

- *Diffusion-weighted* magnetic resonance imaging allows for early identification of ischemic regions within minutes of stroke onset because of early changes of decreased water diffusion within ischemic brain tissue. The diffusion-weighted imaging lesion contains irreversibly damaged brain, as well as the ischemic penumbra.
- *Gradient-recalled echo* magnetic resonance imaging sequences have recently been shown to be superior to CT for detecting any hemorrhage and equivalent to CT for acute hemorrhage.
- *Oxygen-15 positron-emission tomography* can identify the penumbra in stroke patients.

Differential Diagnosis

- Unrecognized seizures.
- Confusional states.
- Syncope.
- Toxic or metabolic disorders, including hypoglycemia.
- Brain tumors.
- Subdural hematoma.
- Migraine.

Treatment

Treatment of Ischemic Stroke

General Supportive Care

Hospitalization

- Most patients should be admitted to the hospital.
- Treatment is best accomplished in comprehensive stroke units, which also incorporate comprehensive rehabilitation.
- Stoke units decrease mortality and morbidity from stroke.
- The American Stroke Association (ASA; a division of the American Heart Association) recommends early mobilization and prevention of subacute complications of stroke.
- Subcutaneous administration of heparin or low-molecular-weight heparin or heparinoids, the use of intermittent external compression stocking, or aspirin for patients who cannot receive anticoagulants is strongly recommended by the ASA to prevent deep vein thrombosis among immobilized patients.

Maintain Adequate Tissue Oxygenation

- Monitor with pulse oximetry with target oxygen saturation level of 95% or higher.

Lower Elevated Body Temperature

- Treat fever with antipyretic agents and cooling devices.
- Treat the source of fever.

Monitor and Manage Blood Pressure

- In most patients, a decline in blood pressure occurs spontaneously.
- Withhold antihypertensive agents, unless the diastolic blood pressure is higher than 120 mmHg or the systolic blood pressure is higher than 220 mmHg (unless there is end-organ involvement or the patient is eligible for thrombolytic therapy).
- Intravenous labetalol is a good choice of drug to treat hypertension in acute ischemic stroke.
- Thrombolytic therapy is not given to patients with a diastolic blood pressure higher than 110 mmHg or a systolic blood pressure higher than 185 mmHg at the time of treatment.
- Before, during, and 24 hours following rtPA therapy, the blood pressure needs careful management.

Control Hyperglycemia or Hyperglycemia

- Lower elevated glucose levels to less than 300 mg/dL.

Save the Penumbra (Restore or Improve Perfusion)

The desired result of thrombolytic therapy is clot lysis with resulting recanalization and restoration of obstructed cerebral blood flow.

Intravenous rtPA

- Intravenous rtPA (a thrombolytic agent) is strongly recommended by the ASA for carefully selected patients who can be treated within 3 hours of onset of ischemic stroke.
- The major risk is symptomatic brain hemorrhage (6.4%).
- Intravenous rtPA leads to a complete or near-complete reversal of a stroke in about one of every three patients treated.
- Bleeding in the brain occurs in about 5.2% of patients.
- Intra-arterial rtPA is a treatment option for selected patients.
- Intra-arterial rtPA requires immediate cerebral angiography and interventional neuroradiology at an experienced stroke center.

Anticoagulants

ASA recommendations include the following:

- Urgent, routine anticoagulation is not recommended for the purpose of improving neurological outcome or preventing recurrent stroke in most patients.

- Initiation of anticoagulant therapy within 24 hours of treatment with intravenous rtPA is not recommended.
- Anticoagulants are associated with an increased risk of serious bleeding complications, including the risk of symptomatic, hemorrhagic transformation of ischemic strokes.
- Warfarin benefits patients with atrial fibrillation; however, the best time to start after an acute ischemic stroke is unclear.

Antiplatelet Agents

ASA guidelines include the following:

- The primary benefit of aspirin seems to be in preventing a subsequent stroke.
- Aspirin should be given within 24 to 48 hours of ischemic stoke onset in most patients.
- Aspirin should not be given within 24 hours of the use of a thrombolytic agent.
- Aspirin should not be used as a substitute for intravenous rtPA or other acute therapies for the treatment of acute ischemic stroke.

Other Antiplatelet Regimens

Common antiplatelet regimens include clopidogrel and the combination of aspirin and dipyridamole.

Surgery

Carotid Endarterectomy

- Although not currently recommended by the ASA for the treatment of patients with an acute ischemic stroke, studies of emergency carotid endarterectomy (CEA) have shown successful recanalization of the internal carotid artery.
- CEA reduces the risk of stroke in patients with recently symptomatic stenosis.
- The benefit of CEA is greater in men than in women, for those with stroke compared with those with a TIA, and those with hemispheric symptoms compared with those with retinal symptoms.

Extracranial–Intracranial Bypass

It is not recommended by the ASA for the treatment of patients with an acute ischemic stroke.

Endovascular Treatment

Carotid stenting may be a reasonable alternative to CEA in patients at high risk of perioperative complications of CEA.

ENDOVASCULAR MECHANICAL THROMBOLYSIS

- A variety of devices are available to break up and remove clots, but their efficacy is unclear.

Treatment of Intracerebral Hemorrhage

Reverse the Effects of Anticoagulation

GENERAL SUPPORTIVE CARE

- Intubate.
  - Intubate for hypoxia (PO_2 < 60 mmHg or PCO_2 > 50 mmHg) or obvious risk of aspiration.
- Monitor and manage blood pressure.
  - Severe hypertension should be treated (>180/105 mmHg).
  - If the patient has an intracerebral pressure (ICP) monitor; the cerebral perfusion pressure should be kept at more than 70 mmHg.
- Manage increased ICP.
  - Increased ICP is defined as 20 mmHg or more for longer than 5 minutes.
  - The goal of treatment is to have an ICP of less than 20 mmHg and cerebral perfusion pressure higher than 70 mmHg.
  - ICP monitoring is recommended by the American Heart Association in patients with a Glasgow Coma Scale score of lower than 9 and other patients thought to be deteriorating owing to an increased ICP.
  - Treatment of elevated ICP includes ventricular drains (for secondary hydrocephalus), osmotherapy, hyperventilation, and muscle relaxants.

SURGERY

- Patients with cerebellar hemorrhage more than 3 cm in diameter with brainstem compression or hydrocephalus are surgical candidates.
- Patients with small hemorrhages (<10 cm^3) are nonsurgical candidates.

Treatment of Subarachnoid Hemorrhage

- Patients with SAH should have an early referral to a treatment center.
- Treatment includes intraluminal thrombosis of an aneurysm, with coils that are delivered via a catheter or direct surgical repair, with either clipping or wrapping of the aneurysm.
- Oral nimodipine reduces poor outcome.
- Hypertension/hypervolemia/hemodilution (triple-H therapy) prevents complications of vasospasm.
- Vasospasm that is not responsive to medical therapy can be treated with transluminal angioplasty.

Rehabilitation

Goals

- Prevent, recognize, and manage comorbid illnesses.
- Prevent, recognize, and manage complications.
- Reduce activity restrictions (disabilities) that result from impairments.
- Reduce participation limitations (handicaps) that limit involvement in life situations.
- Maximize psychosocial adjustment to disease and disability for the patient and the family.
- Prevent recurrent stroke.

When

- Start rehabilitation in the acute care hospital after the patient's medical condition has been stabilized.
- This is often within 24 to 48 hours of the stroke.
- Post-acute stroke rehabilitation is started when the stroke patient is medically stable.

Where

Some patients will recover from the acute stroke and not need rehabilitation services, but those who do need rehabilitation services can receive them in a setting determined primarily by functional status and availability of social support. The settings for post-acute stroke rehabilitation include acute inpatient rehabilitation hospitals or units, subacute inpatient rehabilitation facilities, outpatient rehabilitation facilities, and home-based rehabilitation. General criteria for rehabilitation are as follows:

- Acute inpatient rehabilitation.
  - The patient has endurance sufficient to tolerate 3 hours of therapy daily.
  - The patient is medically stable but needs close medical supervision and rehabilitation nursing services.
  - The patient has significant activity restrictions in mobility and self-care.
  - The patient has the ability to learn.
- Subacute inpatient rehabilitation.
  - The patient has endurance sufficient to tolerate less intense treatment.
  - The patient is medically stable and needs general medical supervision and skilled nursing services.
  - The patient has significant activity restrictions in mobility and self-care.
  - The patient has the ability to learn.

- Outpatient-based rehabilitation.
  - The patient has sufficient function and social support to travel to an outpatient facility.
- Home-based rehabilitation.
  - This is for patients that cannot readily travel to outpatient services.

How

Although stroke care in the United States is often fragmented, the importance of improving stroke care is receiving increasing emphasis. The Joint Commission on Accreditation of Healthcare Organizations awards certificates for primary stroke centers, and a list of centers can be found at http://www.jcaho.org/dscc/dsc/certified+organizations/certified+organizations-disease.htm. The ASA (http://www.strokeassociation.org/) has developed recommendations for the establishment of stroke systems of care. The Department of Veterans Affairs and Department of Defense has published a clinical practice guideline for the management of stroke rehabilitation in the primary care setting that can be accessed at http://www.guideline.gov/summary/summary.aspx?view_id=1&doc_id=3846. Patients with acute stroke should receive organized and coordinated care, which includes acute stroke treatment, secondary prevention of stroke, and rehabilitation by a multidisciplinary team. Rehabilitation involves the following assessments and interventions.

- Basic assessment.
  - Basic assessment includes an assessment of cognitive skills, severity of disability, depression, sensory deficits, communication, and swallowing deficits.
  - Tools for the measurement of disability include the Barthal Index, Functional Independence Measure, and Modified Rankin Scale.
  - Tools for the assessment of depression in the rehabilitation setting include the hospital anxiety and depression scale, the general health questionnaire-12, and for those with communication problems, the visual analog mood scale or hospital stroke aphasic depression questionnaire.
- Psychosocial assessment.
  - The patient should receive a referral to a social worker for comprehensive assessment and intervention.
- Bladder and bowel assessment and intervention.
  - Interventions include prompted voiding, bladder training (includes patient education, scheduled voiding, and positive reinforcement), and bowel management programs.
- Nutrition assessment.
  - Nutritional assessment and correction of major nutritional problems are recommended by the ASA.

- Patient and family education.
  - The rehabilitation team, the patient, and the family should develop the rehabilitation plan jointly.
  - It is important that the patient's caregivers have adequate support and training for their role.
- Secondary stroke prevention.
  - Secondary prevention of stroke includes the treatment of underlying disease, lowering blood pressure, lowering blood cholesterol with statins, management of other risk factors, CEA, carotid stenting, and antiplatelet therapy.
- Prevent and manage complications.
- Initiate rehabilitation interventions.
  - Exercise therapy includes strengthening, aerobics, stretching, and coordination and balance training.
  - Task-specific therapy seems to be the most efficacious therapy for motor function.
  - Robotic therapy can increase the intensity of therapy that involves repetitive movement and allow for the precise control and measurement of therapy that may ultimately determine the optimal dosage.
  - Consider use of partial body-weight support with treadmill training, which may improve gait.
  - Consider constraint-induced therapy (constraining the uninvolved limb and forcing use of the involved limb) for select patients.
  - Functional electrical stimulation may decrease shoulder subluxation, strengthen select muscles, and facilitate gait training.
  - Treat spasticity with nonpharmacological (remove painful stimuli, positioning, stretching, splinting, and surgery) and pharmacological (oral tizanidine, dantrolene, baclofen, injection of botulinum toxin or phenol, and intrathecal baclofen) means.
  - Consider biofeedback for select patients.
  - Prevent and manage shoulder pain.
  - Provide cognitive retraining, if needed.
  - Virtual reality and motor imagery are therapies under study.
  - Treat dysphagia.
  - Treat language and communication disorders. Higher intensity of speech therapy seems to improve speech outcome.
  - Extending therapy into the community after the initial rehabilitation can allow for continued improvement in endurance and function.

Complications

Pneumonia

- Risk factors for aspiration pneumonia are a wet-sounding quality to the voice after swallowing, incomplete mouth closure, or a high NIHSS.

- The presence of a gag reflex does not always predict protection from aspiration.
- Having the patient drink a glass of water is a useful screen for aspiration.
- A fiberoptic endoscopic evaluation of swallowing test or a videofluoroscopic modified barium swallow examination can objectively evaluate swallowing function.

Deep Venous Thrombosis

- A deep venous thrombosis can be detected in approximately one-third to one-half of patients who have a moderately severe stroke.

Pulmonary Embolism

- This accounts for approximately 10% of deaths after a stroke.
- A pulmonary embolism can be detected in about 1% of persons who have had a stroke.

Pressure Sores and Palsies

- Pressure sores usually occur over the sacrum of immobile patients, and prevention includes frequent turning, minimizing bed rest, and the use of pressure-relieving surfaces for bed and chair, as well as controlling incontinence.
- Pressure palsies can occur with the ulnar nerve in the cubital tunnel, the radial nerve as its exits the spiral groove, and the peroneal nerve at the fibular head.

Contractures

- Limitation in joint motion can usually be prevented by active or passive range of movement exercises daily, controlling spasticity, and splints, especially for the hand and ankle.

Shoulder Pain

- Shoulder pain in the involved limb is common following a stroke, and its cause is multifactorial.
- Prevention strategies include careful attention to correct handling of the paretic arm, avoiding impingement associated with overhead use of the arm, and maintaining shoulder range of movement.

Neurological Complications

- Cerebral edema and increased ICP can be seen with ischemic stroke, and are usually related to large vessel occlusions with multilobar infarctions, with brain edema peaking 3 to 5 days post-stroke.

- Seizures are more common with hemorrhagic stroke. Following ischemic stroke, seizures usually occur within 24 hours and are usually partial.
- Recurrent stroke is frequent; approximately 25% of people who recover from their first stroke will have another stroke within 5 years.
- Complications of SAH include re-bleeding, cerebral vasospasm, hydrocephalus, and hyponatremia.

Depression

- The peak incidence of depression is between 6 months and 2 years post-stroke, with prevalence between 10 and 34%.
- Lesions of the left frontal pole and the pallidus are related to post-stroke depression.
- The role of antidepressant drugs or psychotherapy in the prophylaxis of depression is not clear.

The University of Massachusetts Medical School and the ASA have developed a program called "StrokeSTOP" that encourages the active prevention and treatment of stroke by future physicians. The StrokeSTOP program can be accessed online at www.umassmed.edu/strokestop. Information for clinicians treating acute stroke is also available from the Brain Attack Coalition website, found at http://www.stroke-site.org/index.html.

Key References and Suggested Additional Reading

Organized inpatient (stroke unit) care for stroke, Cochrane Database Syst Rev 2002; 1: CD000197.

Adams HP, Jr, Adams RJ, Brott T, et al. Guidelines for the early management of patients with ischemic stroke: a scientific statement from the Stroke Council of the American Stroke Association. Stroke 2003;34: 1056–1083.

Adams H, Adams R, Del Zoppo G, Goldstein LB. Guidelines for the early management of patients with ischemic stroke: 2005 guidelines update a scientific statement from the Stroke Council of the American Heart Association/American Stroke Association. Stroke 2005;36: 916–923.

American Heart Association. Heart Disease and Stroke Statistics—2005 Update. http://www.americanheart.org/presenter.jhtml?identifier=1928. American Heart Association. Last accessed April 24, 2005.

Barnett HJ, Taylor DW, Eliasziw M, et al. Benefit of carotid endarterectomy in patients with symptomatic moderate or severe stenosis. North American Symptomatic Carotid Endarterectomy Trial Collaborators. N Engl J Med 1998;339: 1415–1425.

Baron JC, Cohen LG, Cramer SC, et al. Neuroimaging in stroke recovery: a position paper from the First International Workshop on Neuroimaging and Stroke Recovery. Cerebrovasc Dis 2004;18: 260–267.

Baron JC, Warach S. Imaging. Stroke 2005; 36: 196–199.

Bartels MN. Pathophysiology and medical management of stroke, In: Gillen G, Burkhardt A, eds, Stroke Rehabilitation: A Function-Based Approach, 2nd ed. St. Louis, MO: Mosby. 2004, pp. 1–30.

Bogey RA, Geis CC, Bryant PR, Moroz A, O'Neill BJ. Stroke and neurodegenerative disorders. 3. Stroke: rehabilitation management. Arch Phys Med Rehabil 2004; 85(Suppl 1): S15–S20.

Broderick JP, Adams HP, Jr, Barsan W, et al. Guidelines for the management of spontaneous intracerebral hemorrhage: a statement for healthcare professionals from a special writing group of the Stroke Council, American Heart Association. Stroke 1999;30: 905–915.

Glanz M, Klawansky S, Stason W, Berkey C, Chalmers TC. Functional electrostimulation in poststroke rehabilitation: a meta-analysis of the randomized controlled trials. Arch Phys Med Rehabil 1996; 77:549–553.

Gordon NF, Gulanick M, Costa F, et al. Physical activity and exercise recommendations for stroke survivors: an American Heart Association scientific statement from the Council on Clinical Cardiology, Subcommittee on Exercise, Cardiac Rehabilitation, and Prevention; the Council on Cardiovascular Nursing; the Council on Nutrition, Physical Activity, and Metabolism; and the Stroke Council. Stroke 2004; 35:1230–1240.

Gresham GE, Alexander D, Bishop DS, et al. American Heart Association Prevention Conference. IV. Prevention and Rehabilitation of Stroke. Rehabilitation. Stroke 1997;28: 1522–1526.

Ingall TJ, O'Fallon WM, Asplund K, et al. Findings from the reanalysis of the NINDS tissue plasminogen activator for acute ischemic stroke treatment trial. Stroke 2004;35: 2418–2424.

Kumral E, Bayulkem G, Evyapan D, Yunten N. Spectrum of anterior cerebral artery territory infarction: clinical and MRI findings. Eur J Neurol 2002;9: 615–624.

Lindsay KW, Bone I. Neurology and Neurosurgery Illustrated, 4th ed, Edinburgh: Churchill Livingstone, 2004.

Lo EH, Moskowitz MA, Jacobs TP. Exciting, radical, suicidal: how brain cells die after stroke. Stroke 2005; 36:189–192.

Markus HS. Current treatments in neurology: Stroke J Neurol 2005;252: 260–267.

Mayberg MR, Batjer HH, Dacey R, et al. Guidelines for the management of aneurysmal subarachnoid hemorrhage. A statement for healthcare professionals from a special writing group of the Stroke Council, American Heart Association. Stroke 1994; 25: 2315–2328.

Mohr JP, Gautier JC. Ischemic stroke. In: Mohr JP, Gautier JC, eds, Guide to Clinical Neurology. New York: Churchill Livingstone, 1995, pp. 543–593.

Moroz A, Bogey RA, Bryant PR, Geis CC, O'Neill BJ. Stroke and neurodegenerative disorders. 2. Stroke: comorbidities and complications. Arch Phys Med Rehabil 2004;85(Suppl 1): S11–S14.

National Institute of Neurological Disorders and Stroke rt-PA Stroke Study Group Tissue plasminogen activator for acute ischemic stroke. N Engl J Med 1995;333: 1581–1587.

National Institute of Neurological Disorders and Stroke, Stroke Information Page. http://www.ninds.nih.gov/disorders/stroke/stroke.htm. Last accessed April 24, 2005.

O'Neill BJ, Geis CC, Bogey RA, Moroz A, Bryant PR. Stroke and neurodegenerative disorders. 1. Acute stroke evaluation, management, risks, prevention, and prognosis. Arch Phys Med Rehabil 2004; 85(Suppl 1):S3–S10.

Parent A, Carpenter MB. Carpenter's Human Neuroanatomy, 9th ed. Baltimore: Williams & Wilkins, 1995.

Rickards H. Depression in neurological disorders: Parkinson's disease, multiple sclerosis, and stroke. J Neurol Neurosurg Psychiatry 2005;76(Suppl 1): i48–i52.

Schwamm LH, Pancioli A, Acker JE, III, et al. Recommendations for the establishment of stroke systems of care: recommendations from the American Stroke Association's Task Force on the Development of Stroke Systems. Stroke 2005;36:690–703.

Smith WS, Johnston SC, Easton JD. Part 15. Neurologic Disorders, Section 2. Diseases of the Central Nervous System. In: Kasper, D. L., Braunwald E., Fauci A. S., et al, eds. Cerebrovascular Diseases. Harrison's Online, McGraw-Hill. http://www.accessmedicine.com. Last accessed March 27, 2005.

Teasell R. Stroke recovery and rehabilitation. Stroke 2003;34:365–366.

Teasell RW, Kalra L. What's new in stroke rehabilitation. Stroke 2004;35: 383–385.

Teasell RW, Kalra L. What's new in stroke rehabilitation: back to basics. Stroke 2005;36:215–217.

University of Massachusetts Medical School and the American Stroke Association. http://www.umassmed.edu/strokestop/. 2003, Last accessed April 24, 2005.

Veterans Health Administration, DoD. VA/DoD clinical practice guideline for the management of stroke rehabilitation in the primary care setting. http://www.guideline.gov/summary/summary.aspx?view_id=1&doc_id=3846. Washington, DC: Department of Veteran Affairs, 2003. Last accessed April 24, 2005.

Victor RD, Ropper AH. Principles of Neurology, 7th ed. New York: McGraw-Hill, 2000.

3 Spinal Cord Injury

Monifa Brooks and Steven Kirshblum

Introduction

Spinal cord injury (SCI) is a devastating event that may affect every aspect of an individual's life. There are approximately 10,000 new traumatic SCIs each year, a figure that has been relatively stable over the past 20 years, with an estimated 200,000 people living with SCI in the United States. Patients with SCI utilize a tremendous amount of health care resources. The direct costs alone are estimated at $10 billion. When one considers that the average age at the time of injury is 37.7 years, one can only imagine the magnitude of the indirect costs associated with lost income potential. The psychological impact on patients and their families is even more difficult to measure.

Epidemiology

Data from the SCI National Model Systems indicate that motor vehicle crashes continue to be the most common cause of newly acquired SCIs in the United States. Falls are the second leading cause of SCI, although this is far more common among the elderly. Violence is the third leading cause of SCI and is more common in urban areas, now representing the second leading etiology of SCI among young African-American males. Sports injuries account for approximately 7.5% of SCIs and are more common in the younger age groups. Of those who sustain sports-related injuries, diving remains the most frequent activity responsible for injuries to the spinal cord, followed by skiing, football, and horseback riding, respectively.

From: *Essential Physical Medicine and Rehabilitation*
Edited by: G. Cooper © Humana Press Inc., Totowa, NJ

Table 1
Life Expectancy (in Years) Post-Injury by Severity of Injury and Age at Injury

		For persons surviving at least 1 year post-injury				
Age at injury	*No SCI*	*Motor functional at any level*	*Para*	*Low tetra (C5–C8)*	*High tetra (C1–C4)*	*Ventilator-dependent at any level*
20	58.2	53.2	45.9	41.4	37.8	23.1
40	39.3	34.7	28.3	24.4	21.5	10.9
60	22	18.1	13.2	10.6	8.7	3.0

Adapted from National Spinal Cord Injury Statistical Center: Spinal Cord Injury: Facts and Figures at a Glance 2005. Birmingham: University of Alabama at Birmingham, 2005.

Men remain nearly four times more likely to suffer an SCI than women, accounting for 78.2% of newly injured patients. There is a bimodal distribution of SCI, with young adults and the elderly more commonly affected. The mean and median ages at the time of injury are 32.6 and 37.7 years, respectively. Cervical spine injuries account for 52.9% of all new, traumatic SCIs. Nearly half (41.5%) of all injuries are classified as neurologically complete. The percentage of patients who require chronic ventilator support has increased threefold since the 1970s. This is likely the result of improved medical management of patients with high cervical level injuries. Still only 6.8% of patients with SCI require prolonged mechanical ventilation.

Life expectancy for patients with new SCIs across all levels and American Spinal Injury Association (ASIA) classifications is lower than age-matched controls (Table 1). In general, patients with high cervical injuries and those at the extremes of age have significantly shorter life expectancies. Pulmonary diseases are the leading cause of mortality within the first year following injury. The role of the physiatrist is to address both quantity and quality of life for individuals with SCIs.

Evaluation and Classification of Injuries

Before the 1970s, there was no standardized method of examining spinal cord injured patients. In 1972 the ASIA was formed with the goal of unifying the way that patients with SCI are examined, as well as how the exam results are communicated to fellow health care professionals. The most accurate way to assess an SCI is to perform a standardized physical examination called the International Standards for Neurological Classification of Spinal Cord Injury Patients, also commonly called the ASIA guidelines.

The ASIA exam forms the basis for classification of SCIs—the ASIA Impairment Scale (AIS). The importance of this classification lies in its ability to provide insight to functional outcomes, including recovery of ambulation.

The term *tetraplegia* is used to designate patients with neurological levels within the cervical region, whereas paraplegia refers to neurological levels below the cervical region. The ASIA exam broadly allows for classification of persons with SCI into two broad categories: neurological complete and incomplete injuries. Complete injuries are those without any sparing of the lowest sacral segments. Patients are classified by their neurological level of injury, defined as the last level with both normal sensory and motor function (key definitions are found in Table 2).

The ASIA exam is composed of both a sensory and motor examination. For standardization, the exam is performed with the patient in the supine position. The sensory exam is performed separately for light touch and pin-prick modalities. Each of 28 dermatomes (Fig. 1) is tested and graded 0 for absent, 1 for impaired, 2 for normal, or NT for not testable. The face is used as the reference point in testing sensation in each dermatome. A grade of 2 indicates the sensation is equal to that of the face. For the pin-prick examination, a grade of 1 indicates the ability to distinguish sharp from dull; however, the sensation is qualitatively different as compared with the face. If the patient cannot distinguish the pin form the dull aspect of the safety pin used for testing, then the score is 0. One also scores a 0 if there is no sensation at all. For the light touch exam, a cotton tip applicator is used. A score of 1 is recorded if the sensation is less than on the face, and a 0 if there is no sensation at all. The lowest sacral segment, S4–S5, should be tested with a pin and cotton swab as well. It is important to document the different modalities of sensation spared because preservation of pin-prick sensation in the lowest sacral segments yields a better prognosis for neurological recovery. This may be secondary to the proximity of the spinothalamic tract, which conveys pin-prick sensation, to the corticospinal tract, which conveys motor fibers. As part of the rectal examination, anal sensation should be tested and graded as either present or absent.

The maximum sensory score is 112 (56 for each side of the body) for light touch and pin sensation. The *sensory level* is the most caudal level, where sensation for light touch and pin-prick are both graded as 2 (normal) for both sides of the body.

The motor exam is conducted using conventional manual muscle testing techniques in 10 key muscle groups in the supine position. Muscles are graded from 0 to 5 (Table 3). The maximum Motor Index Score is 100 (50

Table 2
Key Terms in the ASIA Classification

Glossary of key terms

Key muscle groups:

Ten muscle groups that are tested as part of the standardized spinal cord examination.

Root level	*Muscle group*	*Root level*	*Muscle group*
C5	Elbow flexors	L2	Hip flexors
C6	Wrist extensors	L3	Knee extensors
C7	Elbow extensors	L4	Ankle dorsiflexors
C8	Long finger flexors	L5	Long toe extensor
T1	Small finger abductors	S1	Ankle plantarflexors

Motor level:

The most caudal key muscle group that is graded 3/5 or greater with the segments cephalad graded normal (5/5) strength.

Motor index score:

Calculated by adding the muscle scores of each key muscle group; a total score of 100 is possible.

Sensory level:

The most caudal dermatome to have normal sensation for both pin-prick/dull and light touch on both sides.

Sensory index score:

Calculated by adding the scores for each dermatome; a total score of 112 is possible for each pin-prick and light touch.

Neurological level of injury:

The most caudal level at which both motor and sensory modalities are intact.

Complete injury:

The absence of sensory and motor function in the lowest sacral segments.

Incomplete injury:

Preservation of motor and/or sensory function below the neurological level that includes the lowest sacral segments.

Skeletal level:

The level at which, by radiological examination, the greatest vertebral damage is found.

Zone of partial preservation (ZPP):

Used only with complete injuries; refers to the dermatomes and myotomes caudal to the neurological level that remain partially innervated. The most caudal segment with some sensory and/or motor function defines the extent of the ZPP.

Adapted from Kirshblum SC, Donovan WH. Neurologic assessment and classification of traumatic spinal cord injury. In: Kirschblum SC, Campagnolo D, DeLisa JE, eds. Spinal Cord Medicine. Philadelphhhia: Lippincott, Williams & Wilkins, 2002:82–95.

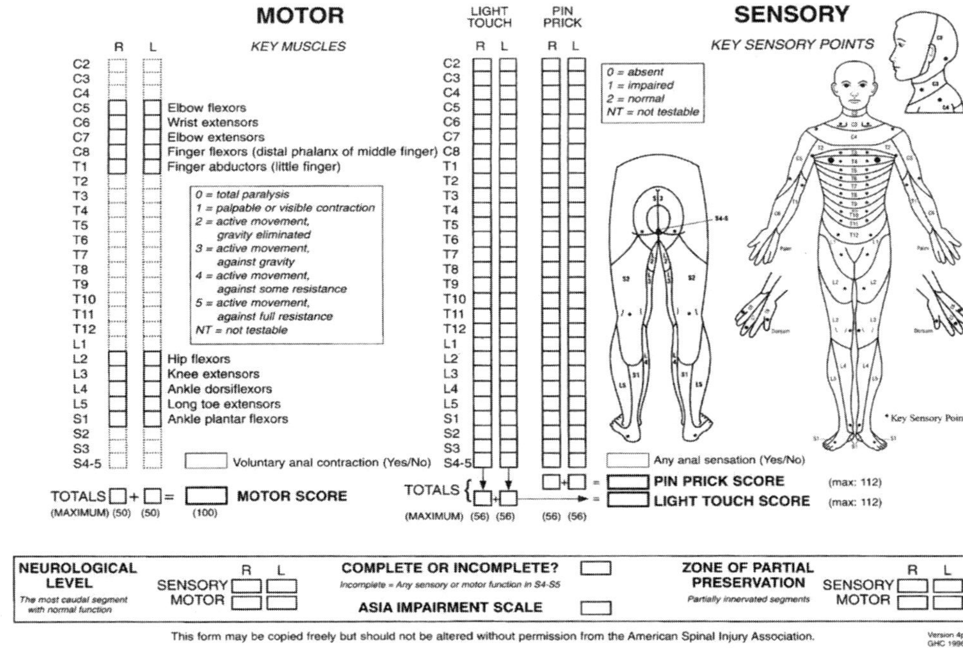

STANDARD NEUROLOGICAL CLASSIFICATION OF SPINAL CORD INJURY

MOTOR

KEY MUSCLES

	R	L	
C2			
C3			
C4			
C5			Elbow flexors
C6			Wrist extensors
C7			Elbow extensors
C8			Finger flexors (distal phalanx of middle finger)
T1			Finger abductors (little finger)
T2			
T3			
T4			
T5			
T6			
T7			
T8			
T9			
T10			
T11			
T12			
L1			
L2			Hip flexors
L3			Knee extensors
L4			Ankle dorsiflexors
L5			Long toe extensors
S1			Ankle plantar flexors
S2			
S3			
S4-5			

0 = total paralysis
1 = palpable or visible contraction
2 = active movement, gravity eliminated
3 = active movement, against gravity
4 = active movement, against some resistance
5 = active movement, against full resistance
NT = not testable

Voluntary anal contraction (Yes/No)

TOTALS ☐ + ☐ = ☐ MOTOR SCORE
(MAXIMUM) (50) (50) (100)

LIGHT TOUCH R L — PIN PRICK R L

C2, C3, C4, C5, C6, C7, C8, T1, T2, T3, T4, T5, T6, T7, T8, T9, T10, T11, T12, L1, L2, L3, L4, L5, S1, S2, S3, S4-5

TOTALS { ☐ + ☐ → = LIGHT TOUCH SCORE (max: 112)
☐ + ☐ = PIN PRICK SCORE (max: 112)
(MAXIMUM) (56) (56) (56) (56)

SENSORY

KEY SENSORY POINTS

0 = absent
1 = impaired
2 = normal
NT = not testable

Any anal sensation (Yes/No)

* Key Sensory Points

NEUROLOGICAL LEVEL
The most caudal segment with normal function
R L
SENSORY ☐ ☐
MOTOR ☐ ☐

COMPLETE OR INCOMPLETE? ☐
Incomplete = Any sensory or motor function in S4-S5

ASIA IMPAIRMENT SCALE ☐

ZONE OF PARTIAL PRESERVATION
Partially innervated segments
R L
SENSORY ☐ ☐
MOTOR ☐ ☐

This form may be copied freely but should not be altered without permission from the American Spinal Injury Association.

Version 4p
GHC 1996

Fig. 1. Reprinted from the International Standards for Classification of Spinal Injuries, 2000.

Table 3
Manual Muscle Test Scoring

Muscle grade	
0	No movement
1	Trace or palpable contraction
2	Full range of motion with gravity eliminated
3	Full range of motion against gravity
4	Capable of providing some resistance against passive range of motion
5	Provides full resistance against passive range of motion

for each side of the body). Examination of voluntary anal sphincter contraction is included with the motor exam and is graded as either present or absent. The *motor level* is defined as the most caudal level with a score of 3 or higher, with the more cephalad levels having a score of 5 (normal). For injuries with no corresponding motor level (i.e., above C4, T2–L1), the last normal sensory level is used. For example, a person with normal strength in all key muscles of the upper extremities, 0/5 strength in the key muscles of the lower extremities, normal sensation in the C2–T4 dermatomes, and absent sensation in the T5–S5 dermatomes would be assigned a motor level of T4.

The *neurological level of injury* is the level where both the motor and sensory levels are considered normal. Once this is determined, the patient's injury can be classified using the AIS, separating the patient's injury into a neurologically complete versus incomplete injury (Table 4). A neurologically complete injury is defined as the individual having no *sacral sparing*, which refers to having any of the following residual findings: light touch or pin-prick in the S4–S5 dermatome (can be on either side, impaired or intact), anal sensation, or voluntary anal contraction preserved. Patients who have an incomplete injury, i.e., presence of sacral sparing, have a significantly better prognosis for motor recovery than those without preservation of the lower sacral segments.

Steps in classifying the injury are outlined in Table 5.

Acute Medical Management

The care of a patient with SCI begins as soon as an injury to the spinal cord is suspected. In the field, any patient with a potential SCI should be immobilized with a back and neck brace before transport. Upon presentation to the hospital, routine imaging of the spine is necessary to identify spine instability. Patients must remain immobilized until the spine is "cleared"—that is, when instability has been ruled out, is properly immo-

Table 4
ASIA Impairment Scale

A Complete	No motor or sensory function is preserved in the sacral segments S4–S5.
B Incomplete	Sensory but not motor function is preserved below the neurological level and includes the sacral segments S4–S5.
C Incomplete	Motor function is preserved below the neurological level, and more than half the key muscles below the neurological level have a muscle grade of less than 3.
D Incomplete	Motor function is preserved below the neurological level, and at least half of key muscles below the neurological level have a muscle grade of 3 or more.
E Normal	Motor and sensory function are normal.

Adapted from International Standards for Classification of Spinal Injuries, 2000.

Table 5
Summary of the Steps in Classifying an Individual With a Spinal Cord Injury

1. Perform sensory exam in 28 dermatomes bilaterally for pin-prick and light touch, including the S4–S5 dermatome and test for anal sensation on rectal examination.
2. Determine sensory level (right and left) and total sensory score.
3. Perform motor exam in the 10 key muscle groups, including voluntary anal contraction on rectal examination.
4. Determine motor level (right and left) and motor index score.
5. Determine the neurological level of injury.
6. Classify injury as complete or incomplete.
7. Categorize ASIA Impairment Scale (AIS) (A through E).
8. Determine zone of partial preservation if AIS A.

Adapted from Kirshblum SC, Donovan WH. Neurologic assessment and classification of traumatic spinal cord injury. In Kirshblum SC, Campagnolo D, DeLisa JE, eds. Spinal Cord Medicine. Philadelphia: Lippincott Williams & Wilkins, 2002:82–95.

bilized by an orthosis (i.e., HALO or thoraco-lumbar sacral orthosis), or surgically stabilized. Most acutely injured patients receive intravenous steroids given as a one-time bolus, followed by a continuous infusion over 24 hours as per the National Acute Spinal Cord Injury Studies. Although the benefit of administering steroids has been questioned, many physicians continue to prescribe methylprednisolone given as a 30 mg/kg bolus followed by 5.4 mg/kg given over the next 23 hours.

Postacute Medical Managment

The newly injured patient with SCI is at tremendous risk for morbidity during the postacute period. When devising a treatment plan, it is helpful to consider the effect of an SCI on each individual organ system. The following sections will demonstrate the myriad of medical challenges patients with SCI present.

Integumentary System

The combination of immobility and decreased sensation make patients with SCI especially prone to the development of pressure ulcers. The incidence of pressure ulcers in the SCI population ranges from 25 to 66%. There are three primary causes of pressure ulcer development: pressure, shear, and friction. Secondary causes include decreased mobility, sensory-motor dysfunction, poor nutrition status, vascular disease, urinary and fecal incontinence, prolonged sedation, and impaired cognition.

The first line of treatment is prevention. It is essential that all persons with sensory and/or motor deficits be turned and repositioned at least every two hours. Studies have shown that significant tissue damage occurs after constant pressure of at least 70 mmHg is applied (usually over a bony prominence) for more than 2 hours. In cases where patients can not be turned, a special pressure-relieving bed is indicated. Pressure-relieving boots are helpful in preventing the development of pressure ulcers on the heels. Although specialty beds and protective footwear are valuable adjuncts, they are in no way a substitute for repositioning the patient.

Patients should be taught to inspect their skin using appropriate adaptive mirrors to assess for early signs of skin breakdown, specifically erythema, as early as possible. Additionally, persons with SCI and their caregivers should be educated as to the different areas of potential breakdown in the sitting versus supine position. Acutely after injury, while the patient is mostly supine, the sacrum, heels, occiput, and elbows are most prone to ulceration. While seated, the ischial tuberosities, distal thighs, and scapular spines are areas prone to developing pressure ulcers. Figure 2 illustrates areas of increased pressure in the supine, side-lying, and seated patient.

Once a pressure ulcer has developed, appropriate staging is important to document effectiveness of the wound treatment regimen. Wounds are classified by depth of tissue compromise. The National Pressure Ulcer Advisory Panel classification divides pressure ulcers into four stages based on the depth of the wound (Table 6).

Treatment of stage I ulcers is generally maintaining pressure relief from the area by adhering to a turning schedule and/or use of a pressure-reliev-

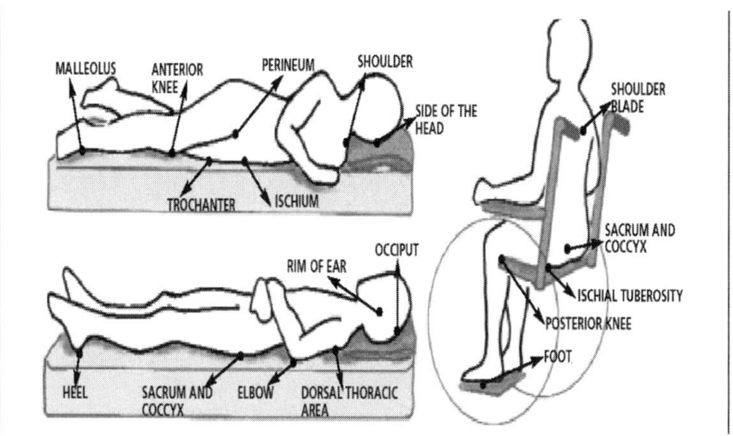

Fig. 2. Sites of potential pressure ulcers.

Table 6
NPUAP Staging of Pressure Ulcers

Stage I	Non-blanchable erythema lasting more than 30 minutes
Stage II	Partial thickness loss of skin involving the epidermis and possibly extending to the dermis
Stage III	Full thickness destruction into subcutaneous tissue
Stage IV	Deep-tissue destruction extending into the fascia, muscle, bone or joint

Adapted from National Pressure Ulcer Advisory Panel (NPUAP). Pressure ulcers prevalence, costs, and risk assessment; consensus development conference statement. Decubitus 1989; 2:24–28.

ing mattress. Stage II and III wounds can be treated with a variety of topical agents. Wound care should include cleansing the area with normal saline or sterile water. Solutions such as acetic acid, betadine, and hydrogen peroxide should be avoided because they may impede tissue granulation. Mechanical debridement with wet-to-dry dressings must be used cautiously because they will remove viable, as well as nonviable, tissue. Enzymatic debridement (i.e., papain) has been shown to decrease healing time and can be applied selectively to areas of necrotic tissue. Sharp debridement is recommended for wounds with necrotic tissue that is clearly delineated and easily grasped. Finally, surgery should be considered for deep stage III and IV wounds. In appropriately selected cases, surgery can lead to earlier mobilization by significantly decreasing healing time.

Thromboembolic Disease

Virchow's triad, which describes three predisposing factors to the development of deep venous thrombus (DVT), includes stasis, endothelial injury, and presence of a hypercoaguable state. Newly injured patients with SCI satisfy all of these conditions and are at increased risk of developing a DVT. Pulmonary embolism (PE) is the third leading cause of mortality in the first year following injury. The reported incidence of DVT during the acute post-injury period varies depending on the method of detection used to screen for the thrombus, but has been reported in approximately 64% of patients not on proper prophylaxis. Model System data reported an incidence of 9.8% for DVT and 2.6% for PE during acute rehabilitation, and an incidence of 2.1 and 1% at 1 year and 2 year follow-up, respectively. The incidence is highest during the first 7 to 10 days after injury. Patients with neurologically complete injuries are at higher risk than those with incomplete injuries. There is ample literature demonstrating the efficacy of chemoprophylaxis in decreasing the incidence of DVT and PE in the acutely injured patient. Current recommendations include the use of low-molecular-weight heparin during the acute injury period—at least the first 8 weeks following injury for the uncomplicated patient with SCI. For patients at higher risk, prophylaxis should continue for at least 12 weeks. Indications for inferior vena cava filters include recent cerebral hemorrhage, thrombocytopenia, very high cervical level of injury, failed prophylaxis, or other contraindications to anticoagulation. Treatment of a DVT or PE is similar to that of the general population and includes anticoagulation (unless contraindicated) that should continue for 6 months.

Pulmonary System

Respiratory failure remains the leading cause of death in acute SCI. Although most patients with SCI have no intrinsic lung disease, the effect of paralysis on the respiratory mechanism can be devastating. Approximately two-thirds of all patients with SCI will experience a complication of the pulmonary system including respiratory failure requiring mechanical ventilation, pneumonia, and/or atelectasis. Careful monitoring of the acutely injured patient is required to decrease morbidity and mortality associated with respiratory dysfunction.

The primary muscle for inspiration is the diaphragm, which receives its innervation from the C3–C5 nerve roots. Accessory muscles of inspiration include the scalenes, intercostals, pectoralis, and serratus anterior muscles; however, these alone are insufficient to maintain adequate ventilation. SCIs in the high cervical region (above C5) may render patients initially ventilator dependent. Although patients with injuries at the C4 or C5 level may initially require mechanical ventilation, most of these patients will be successfully weaned from the ventilator. Expiration is largely a passive activity caused by recoil of the chest wall. However, forceful expiration, such as that required for effective cough, does require contraction of the abdominal and thoracic musculature, innervated by the thoracic level nerve roots. Thus, the pattern of pulmonary dysfunction most commonly seen in spinal cord patients is one of restriction rather than obstruction. A mixed pattern may be present in patients with a premorbid history of obstructive lung disease.

Epidemiological studies indicate that 20 to 25% of acutely injured patients with SCI will experience respiratory failure requiring mechanical ventilation during the acute injury phase. Indications for intubation include respiratory rate greater than 30, severe atelectasis, vital capacity less than 15 mg/kg (approximately 1 L), respiratory distress with pending muscle fatigue, pO2 less than 60, or pCO2 more than 40. Once patients are intubated, vital capacity is a key parameter to follow. A vital capacity of approximately 15 to 20 mg/kg is a good predictor of successful weaning .

In the cervical- and high-thoracic-level-injured patients, the effective management of pulmonary secretions is critical. Failure to clear secretions predisposes patients to the development of pneumonia, the leading cause of mortality in the acutely injured patient with SCI. Several mechanisms may be employed to assist patients with producing an effective cough. Manually assisted cough (i.e., "quad coughing") is performed by providing an upward thrust on the abdomen while the patient attempts to exhale. Before performing a cough, secretions may be mobilized by percussion or use of devices similar to the "pneumovest," which loosen secretions by gentle vibration to the chest wall. Routine suctioning can also be used to extract secretions. The use of an insufflation/exuflation device is beneficial in combating atelectasis, as well as managing secretions. It is also very well tolerated by patients.

Another effect of paralysis on respiratory function relates to the positioning of the diaphragm in the abdominal cavity. The diaphragm, like other muscles, is at a mechanical disadvantage near the end range of contraction. In the neurologically intact person, the optimal position of the diaphragm is partially maintained by the tone of the abdominal musculature. In patients with SCI who have midthoracic level injuries and higher, the diaphragm tends to remain partially collapsed, placing it at a mechanical disadvantage. This explains why the use of an abdominal binder, which enhances abdominal tone, aids respiration, and also why patients with SCI, in contrast to neurologically intact people, have improved respiratory function in the supine position.

Cardiovascular System

The impact of SCI on the cardiovascular system is apparent from the time of initial injury throughout the life span of the patient with SCI. Acutely, the patient may experience bradycardia, orthostastic hypotension, difficulty with thermoregulation and autonomic dysreflexia. In the chronic phase of SCI, patients are at increased risk of developing coronary artery disease as compared with non-SCI, age-matched controls. In fact, coronary artery disease is the leading cause of death in the chronic phase of SCI.

Bradycardia

Spinal cord-injured patients are at increased risk of developing bradyarrhythmias. The incidence of bradycardia is especially high during the first 2 weeks following injury. As with non-SCI patients, tracheal suctioning can increase vagal tone resulting in bradycardia. Treatment generally consists of atropine in patients who are symptomatic or have a persistent rate of less than 44 bpm, although placement of a transvenous pacemaker may be required in more severe cases.

Orthostatic Hypotension

The loss of sympathetic outflow to the vascular smooth muscles impairs the body's ability to autoregulate blood pressure. Normally, blood vessels in the lower extremities constrict with changes in position to maintain perfusion pressures. This response is impaired in immobilized patients. Therefore, blood will pool in the extremities, decreasing cerebral perfusion and causing orthostatic hypotension. By conventional definition, orthostatic hypotension occurs when there is a decrease in systolic blood pressure (SBP) by 20 mmHg, or a decrease in diastolic blood pressure (DBP) of 15 mmHg or more. Many spinal cord-injured patients have baseline SBP of 90 mmHg or less, making symptoms a more reliable parameter to follow in diagnosis and treatment. Patients with SCI often experience symptomatic hypotension with position changes, especially when moving from supine to more upright positions. Patients should be cautioned to avoid rapid changes in position. Simple adjustments, such as raising the head for several minutes before transferring out of bed, can be effective in decreasing episodes of orthostatic hypotension. Additionally, the use of compression stockings and abdominal binders may help to prevent pooling of blood in the extremities. Maintaining adequate fluid intake is important, and one should not be started on fluid restriction for an intermittent bladder catheterization program until the orthostatic symptoms have improved.

When the use of behavioral interventions and compressive garments fail to control the symptoms of orthostasis, pharmacological agents can be added to the treatment regimen. Sodium chloride tablets (1 g four times a day), catecholamines, such as midodrine (2.5–10 mg three times a day), or a salt-retaining mineralcorticoid, such as fludrocortisone (0.05–0.1 mg daily), may be useful adjuncts. The medication should be given approximately 1 hour before activity known to cause hypotensive episodes. Patients should be monitored closely for hypertension when taking these medications.

Autonomic Dysreflexia

At the other end of the blood pressure spectrum from orthostasis is autonomic dysreflexia (AD), which may result in a dangerous elevation in blood pressure. AD is defined as an acute sympathetic discharge triggered by a noxious stimulus below the level of the SCI. It occurs in patients with lesions above the sympathetic splanchnic outflow tract (usually T6 and above, but may be seen in levels as low as T10). The noxious stimulus produces afferent impulses that are transmitted to the dorsal column and spinothalamic tract, where they stimulate sympathetic neurons. In neurologically intact persons, descending supraspinal inhibitory impulses would modulate this sympathetic discharge. However, these inhibitory impulses are blocked in patients with SCI (Fig. 3). The result is unopposed sympathetic tone below the level of the injury, causing peripheral and splanchnic vasoconstriction and elevated blood pressure. The parasympathetic system, via the vagus nerve, functions normally in patients with SCI; therefore, vagal tone attempts to compensate for the increase in blood pressure by decreasing the heart rate. Additionally, the inhibitory spinal pathways increase parasympathetic tone above the level of injury. Thus, parasympathetic tone predominates above the level of the lesion, whereas sympathetic tone is prominent below the level of the lesion.

Hypertension is the hallmark of AD. Remembering that patients with SCI often have baseline blood pressures lower than their non-SCI counterparts, hypertension in this patient population is defined as SBP more than 20 to 40 mmHg above baseline, or DBP more than 15 mmHg above baseline. Patients will often complain of a pounding headache. They may also exhibit flushing, sweating, and piloerection above the level of injury, as well as anxiety and blurred vision. Upon examination, the patient may have bradycardia (secondary to vagal stimulation of the carotid sinus), although tachycardia and cardiac arrhythmias are also seen. Table 7 lists common signs and symptoms of dysreflexia.

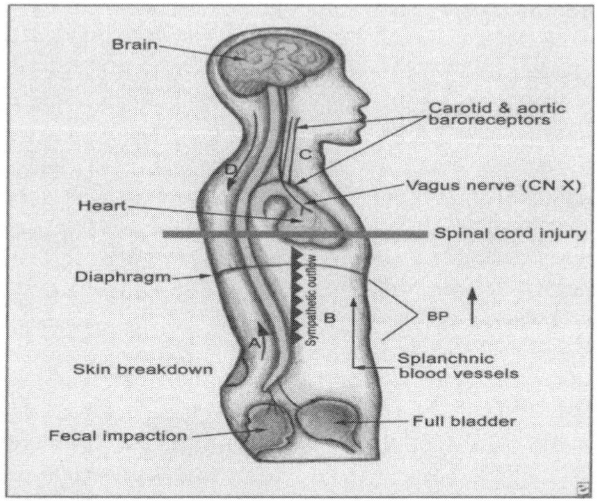

Fig. 3. Autonomic nervous system.

Table 7
Signs and Symptoms of Autonomic Dysreflexia

Parasympathetic response

- Pounding headache
- Nasal congestion
- Pupillary constriction
- Profuse perspiration above the level of the lesion
- Flushing
- Bradycardia

Sympathetic response

- Hypertension
- Piloerection

The most common cause of dysreflexia is either urinary infection or retention. Other causes include fecal impaction, pressure ulcers, restrictive clothing, invasive procedures (which include catheterizations), and infections. Any noxious stimulus may trigger AD, including an ingrown toenail. The focus of treatment is to correct the underlying cause. Table 8 outlines the approach to treating AD.

Table 8
Management of Autonomic Dysreflexia

1. Sit patient up, remove any restrictive clothing, check blood pressure.
2. If patient has an indwelling catheter, check for occlusions.
3. If patient does not have catheter, catheterize using xylocaine to anesthetize the urethra before insertion of catheter; obtain urine specimen for urinalysis and culture.
4. Repeat blood pressure; if more than 150/90, consider anti-hypertensive before performing rectal examination.
5. Apply xylocaine to rectum, wait 5 minutes, examine rectal vault, removing any impaction; monitor blood pressure frequently because exam may worsen hypertension.
6. Repeat blood pressure; if more than 150/90, treat with short-acting anti-hypertensive medication.
7. Assess for other noxious stimuli, including pressure ulcers.
8. Repeat blood pressure; if still elevated, consider transfer to emergency room for treatment of hypertensive crisis.

Medication options include antihypertensives, such as 0.5 to 1 inch of nitropaste, applied to a clearly visible area (being careful not to forget to remove the nitropaste once the AD is controlled), 10 mg of nifedipine (chewed and swallowed), 25 mg of hydralazine, and 0.1 mg of clonidine. Oral medications may result in rebound hypotension once the cause of the dysreflexia is identified and treated. One benefit of nitropaste is that it can be removed quickly once the AD has been treated. If a pressure ulcer is the suspected trigger, the patient should be positioned so that pressure is not applied over the area of the wound. In refractory cases, intravenous antihypertensives may be required.

Gastrointestinal System

SCI patients experience disorders of both the upper and lower gastrointestinal (GI) tracts. The upper GI abnormalities are generally easily treated, if recognized; however, the management of lower GI pathology, including neurogenic bowel, is often more challenging.

Upper GI Tract

The incidence of peptic ulcer disease is 22% during the acute injury period. The unopposed vagal tone present acutely after SCI leads to increased gastric acid production. Additional risk factors for peptic stress ulceration include administration of steroids, nonsteroidal anti-inflammatory exposure, and malnutrition. Prophylaxis with either an H-2 blocker, sucralfate, or a proton pump inhibitor is indicated during the first 6 to 8 weeks following injury. Patients should also begin oral intake as soon as medically possible. Patients with a history of peptic ulcer disease or those with ongoing risk factors should continue treatment beyond the acute injury phase.

With injuries at or above the T1 level, patients with SCI are also prone to delayed gastric emptying, which manifests as nausea, vomiting after meals, epigastric distension, and decreased appetite. The diagnosis is made by gastric emptying scan or an upper GI series with small bowel follow through. Both tests will reveal a delayed gastric emptying time. Potentially reversible causes, such as electrolyte abnormalities and constipation, should be corrected. Acute decompression with nasogastric tube may be indicated in extreme cases. Pharmacotherapy with prokinetic agents, such as metoclopromide, erythromycin, and domperidol, can be beneficial.

Patients with SCI may also develop gastroesophageal reflux disease (GERD). This occurs secondary to decreased pressure in the lower esophageal sphincter, which allows gastric contents to reflux into the lower esophagus. Patients with GERD complain of heartburn, regurgitation of partially digested food, dysphagia, recurrent hiccoughs, or an unpleasant acidic taste in the mouth. The condition can be exacerbated by medications that cause decreased lower esophageal pressures, including those with anticholinergic properties. Treatment begins with behavioral modifications. Patients should avoid recumbent positions following meals. It is recommended that no meals be consumed late in the evening. Eliminating or decreasing intake of known food triggers—fatty meals, acidic or highly spiced foods, and caffeine, for example—may decrease symptoms. If symptoms persist despite behavioral changes, pharmacological treatments are advised. The use of a proton pump inhibitor is generally adequate to control GERD symptoms. The addition of an H-2 blocker, particularly for added nighttime suppression, may be helpful in refractory cases.

During the acute injury period, patients with SCI are also at increased risk of developing gallstones (especially those with injuries above T6), as well as other abdominal pathologies, such as pancreatitis and appendicitis, which may be difficult to detect clinically in patients with impaired sensation. The patient may report nausea or have unexplained emesis after meals. The physician must have a high index of suspicion and perform the appropriate blood and radiologic tests to evaluate for biliary disease or other abdominal pathologies. This includes a complete blood count, electrolytes, liver function tests, amylase, and lipase as needed. In addition, an ultrasound or computed tomography scan of the abdomen should be considered if the diagnosis is unclear. Recurrent vomiting may also be a sign of superior mesenteric artery (SMA) syndrome, which occurs when the duodenum is compressed between the abdominal aorta and the SMA. Patients with SCI are at increased risk of developing SMA syndrome, which may be exacerbated by supine position and/or loss of retroperitoneal fat. An upper GI series is helpful in making the diagnosis. Treatment includes sitting the patient upright or positioning the patient on the left side.

Management of Neurogenic Bowel

Effective management of bowel function is critically important to both the physical and psychological well-being of the patient with SCI. Stool incontinence can be devastating to patients, leading to social isolation, loss of income secondary to work absenteeism, and depression. Therefore, the ultimate goal of the bowel program should be regular, predictable bowel movements without episodes of incontinence. Achieving this goal often requires a trial-and-error period about which patients should be advised from the onset. The bowel program must be practical for the patient and/or caregiver, or it will be of little or no benefit.

The design of the bowel program depends on the underlying cause of the neurological impairment. Patients with upper motor neuron (UMN) injuries have lesions above the conus medullaris with normal-to-increased resting rectal tone. The hallmark of UMN lesions is constipation. Whereas patients with SCI have decreased lower GI motility, there are reflexes that remain intact in patients with UMN injuries. The gastrocolic, colo-colonic and rectocolic reflexes are all helpful in evacuating stool. To utilize the gastrocolic reflex (contraction of the colon occurring with gastric distension), patients should be instructed to perform their bowel program 20 to 30 minutes after eating, when feasible. For patients with UMN injuries, the "3-2-1" bowel program may be initiated once the patient can tolerate feeding that consists of a stool softener (100 mg of docusate sodium) three times per day, a stimulant (two Senokot® tablets) given 8 hours before initiation of the bowel program, and a suppository. An integral part of the bowel program is digital stimulation, which is performed by inserting a finger into the rectum and sweeping in a clockwise direction to initiate the rectocolic reflex—contraction of the colon occurring with stimulation of the rectal mucosa. This will often trigger evacuation of stool in the lower rectal vault. Once the vault is empty, a suppository is inserted to stimulate contraction of the lower colon and evacuation of stool located higher in the descending colon. Repeat digital stimulation (three to five times) should be performed to check for stool that may remain in the rectal vault. Ideally, the bowel program should be performed at the same time of day to facilitate "retraining" of the bowel. Bowel programs are generally performed every 1 to 3 days.

For those patients who remain constipated, laxatives, such as lactulose, polyethylene glycol, bisacodyl tablets, milk of magnesium, or cascara, may replace or be used in combination with components of the 3-2-1 program. Ultimately, the goal is to eliminate medications as the time from injury increases.

In lower motor neuron (LMN) lesions, continence is often lost as a result of weakness of the pelvic floor muscles with a flaccid external anal sphincter. Because spinal mediated reflexes are absent, digital stimulation and contact irritant suppositories are largely ineffective, necessitating manual disimpaction. The stool is kept firm by use of bulking agents to aid manual disimpaction. Performing disimpaction more than once per day may be required to maintain continence. Assistive techniques, such as the Valsalva maneuver, abdominal massage in a clockwise direction, increase in physical activity, standing, and completing the bowel program in a commode chair rather than in bed, can also greatly facilitate the process.

Genitourinary System

Before the 1970s, renal disease was the leading cause of mortality in chronically injured spinal cord patients. Since the advent of intermittent catheterization programs, the prevalence of renal disease has decreased dramatically. The goals of the bladder management program are similar to that of the bowel program. These include safe, effective elimination of urine while maintaining continence.

The urinary system consists of the upper urinary tract, which includes the kidneys and ureters, as well as the lower urinary tract, which includes the bladder and urethra. The kidneys function to secrete, concentrate, and excrete urine. The ureters act as conduits transmitting urine to the bladder by passive and active forces, which are activated by pacemaker cells located at the proximal portion of the ureter. In the absence of intrinsic renal disease, the upper urinary tract continues to function normally. Pathology of the lower tract can result in upper tract deterioration and frank renal disease.

Input to the lower urinary tract is predominantly via the sympathetic and parasympathetic nervous systems. There is supraspinal input from the pons and frontal lobe, which is primarily inhibitory. In spinal cord-injured patients, this inhibition is blocked. There are spinal reflexes, which remain intact, except in patients with LMN lesions. A simplistic view of the autonomic influence over bladder function is that sympathetic input facilitates storage of urine, whereas parasympathetic input propels urine out of the bladder. Activation of the sympathetic system produces relaxation of the

smooth muscle lining the bladder (via β-2 receptors originating from T11–L2) and contraction of the bladder neck, trigone, and urethral sphincter (via α-1 receptors), facilitating storage of urine at low pressures. Parasympathetic input, via the S2–S4 nerve roots, causes excitation of cholinergic muscarinic receptors resulting in contraction of the bladder wall and expulsion of urine. It should be noted that the parasympathetic system simultaneously inhibits sympathetic outflow to prevent contraction of the urethra during attempted voiding. In patients with dyssynergia, there is co-contraction of the bladder and detrusor resulting in the generation of high bladder pressures, often with little urine output. Increased pressure may be transmitted proximally to the kidneys, placing patients at risk of developing hydronephrosis and renal disease.

Evaluation of bladder function includes the use of portable ultrasound to measure bladder volume, and is a fast and easy way to evaluate bladder storage and emptying capacity. A bladder ultrasound cannot, however, measure pressure, which is the key parameter to assessing the patient's risk of developing hydronephrosis. A routine kidney, ureter, and bladder X-ray (KUB) will show calcifications that may be present in the bladder, kidneys, or ureters. To adequately evaluate the pressures in the bladder during filling and voiding, a formal urodynamic study is required.

Bladder Management

Many patients present acutely in spinal shock. These patients' bladders are areflexic, meaning the bladder will retain urine. Therefore, it is advisable to place an indwelling catheter to remove the urine. Alternatively, patients can be started on an intermittent catheterization program, but during the initial stage after injury, an indwelling catheter helps regulate fluid intake and output, and is the management of choice.

Once patients are medically stable, a discussion regarding long-term management options should commence. The goals of the bladder program include maintaining low bladder pressures and continence while minimizing infections and the risk of upper tract deterioration. As with the prescription of the bowel program, patient preference must be considered. Ideally, the clinician will present all available management strategies, including the pros and cons of each, and the ultimate decision will be made by the patient.

Treatment is determined by the underlying pathology. For patients who are unable to effectively store urine (UMN lesions), several options exist. These include reflex or spontaneous voids (with the use of an external catheter—most often used in men as a condom catheter because there is no

Table 9
Bladder Management Options

	Pros	*Cons*
Reflex voiding	• Non-invasive	• May generate high pressures • May have high post-void residual volumes • Need UDS to evaluate pressures generated with voids
Intermittent catheterization	• Allows for catheter-free periods • Improved self-image	• Requires repeated catheterizations • Difficult for patients with poor hand function • Non-compliance with schedule may increase UTIs and generate high volumes and pressures
Indwelling urethral catheter	• Relatively easy for patients and caregivers to maintain • Suitable for patients with poor hand function • Less frequent catheter changes	• Increased UTIs • Increased risk of bladder cancer with long-term (>10 years) use • Risk of urethral erosion • Decreased bladder capacity • Interferes with sexual intercourse
Indwelling suprapubic catheter	• Relatively easy for patients and caregivers to maintain • Suitable for patients with poor hand function • Less frequent catheter changes • Does not interfere with sexual intercourse	• Increased UTIs • Increased risk of bladder cancer with long-term (>10 years) use • Decreased bladder capacity

UDS, urodynamic study; UTI, urinary tract infection.

adequate external collecting system for females), indwelling catheter (suprapubic or urethral), intermittent catheterization, or surgical interventions (Table 9). Careful monitoring of postvoid residuals in those patients who are able to void is needed to ensure adequate emptying because urinary stasis increases occurrence of urinary tract infections. Anticholinergic medications decrease bladder contractions, facilitating storage of urine. α-Agonists increase urethral sphincter pressures—also increasing the bladder's capacity to store urine. Surgical options include sphincter augmentation, bladder augmentation, and placement of a fascial sling, which increases bladder outlet resistance.

For patients who have an impaired ability to empty the bladder, there are myriad treatment options. Crede (direct pressure applied over the lower abdomen) and/or valsalva maneuvers may provide enough pressure to cause expulsion of urine from the bladder. This technique is indicated for patients with LMN injuries (i.e., cauda equina lesions). Patients should be cautioned that they may inadvertently increase bladder pressures to dangerously high levels, thereby increasing the risk of hydronephrosis. For this reason, these maneuvers are not advised for patients with known dyssynergia. Indwelling catheters provide reliable evacuation of urine.

For patients who have adequate hand function, an intermittent catheterization program provides a near-physiological voiding pattern. For patients who have urinary leakage between catheterizations, anticholinergic medications can be administered. Patients must understand that failure to comply with the catheterization schedule may lead to high bladder volumes and pressures, and ultimately may progress to upper tract deterioration. The benefits of an intermittent catheterization program over an indwelling catheter include improved self-image, decreased incidence of bladder stones, and development of bladder cancer.

Chronic indwelling catheters, including urethral and suprapubic catheters, are generally quite easy for patients and their caregivers to manage. Negatives consequences associated with indwelling catheters include increased incidence of bladder stones and cancer for long-term (>10 years) users. Additionally, the presence of the catheter may hinder attempts at intimacy.

Patients with neurogenic bladder require routine screening for development of stones, fibrosis, hydronephrosis, renal disease, and bladder cancer. Annually, a KUB and urinalysis culture and sensitivity will screen for bladder or renal stones, proteinuria, which may suggest underlying renal disease, and infection. The presence of bacturia in patients that have indwelling catheters is quite common. Generally, asymptomatic bacturia is not treated. Exceptions include patients who are scheduled to undergo invasive procedures, such as cystoscopy or urodynamic studies. Renal sonograms are generally obtained every 1 to 2 years or if there is clinical evidence suggestive of nephrolithiasis. Patients with indwelling catheters should have cystoscopy evaluations every 3 to 5 years to screen for bladder cancer. Those at higher risk, i.e., smokers and those with a history of abnormal cystoscopy findings, may require more frequent examinations. Of course, patients with persistent hematuria or constitutional symptoms consistent with an underlying malignancy should be screened immediately. urodynamic studies are indicated whenever there is a change in the patients voiding pattern.

Sexuality and Fertility

Soon after SCI, patients often inquire about the ability to resume ambulation. Patients are less likely to initiate a discussion about sexual function; however, many are concerned about this important part of human intimacy. It is important for health care professionals to initiate discussions about sexuality before discharge from the hospital or rehabilitation center. Patients should understand that intimacy is not confined to sexual intercourse. There is less research examining sexuality in women following SCI relative to men. Women with SCI often experience decreased libido. Altered self-image, as well as impaired sensation, may contribute to decreased sexual satisfaction. However, there are studies indicating women of all injury levels remain capable of experiencing orgasm. Couples should be encouraged to explore new erogenous zones above the level of the injury (e.g., breasts, neck, ears), which may provide pleasure and foster intimacy.

For men with erectile dysfunction, there are several treatment options available. More recently, the phosphodiesterase class of medications, including sildenafil and tadalifil, has been used with success in the SCI population. Hypotension is a potential adverse side effect within this class, as well as headache and flushing, and patients should be educated to recognize the difference between these side effects and those of autonomic dysreflexia in persons with injuries above T6. In addition, these patients should be made aware of the contraindication to using any nitrates when using these products. Generally, these medications are indicated in patients with either reflexogenic or psychogenic erections. Intracorporeal injections with prostaglandin E1, α-blockers, or vasodilators are another treatment option. Patients should be informed about the possibility of priapism with these medications. Additional treatments include penile implants and vacuum and ring devices. Penile implants are effective but have a relatively high failure rate, and may cause infections or penile erosion. The vacuum and ring device is somewhat cumbersome but effective in maintaining erections. These devices are contraindicated in patients with sickle cell disease.

Male fertility is variably affected by SCI. Achieving ejaculation does not insure successful reproduction. Retrograde ejaculation is reported to occur in 37 to 100% of men with SCIs. Less than 10% of couples will have successful spontaneous pregnancies. Therefore, patients who experience infertility should consider an evaluation by a reproductive medicine specialist soon after the decision to attempt pregnancy is made. Semen analysis in men with SCI reveals decreased sperm count, as well as decreased sperm motility. Couples have had relatively good outcomes with in vitro fertilization, gamete intrafallopian transfer, intracytoplasmic sperm injection, and intrauterine insemination procedures. However, the cost can be prohibitive, and these services may not be covered by insurance plans.

In contrast to their male counterparts, fertility in the female patient with SCI is generally unaffected by the injury. Initially, female patients may experience amenorrhea lasting up to 6 months. With the resumption of regular menses, fertility returns to the pre-injury baseline. Pregnancy presents a unique set of potential problems for women with SCI. Women may develop pressure ulcers, recurrent urinary tract infections, increased spasticity, or decreased pulmonary function during pregnancy. There is a slightly increased incidence of preterm labor in women with SCI. AD may develop in susceptible women during labor. Preeclampsia can be difficult to distinguish from AD; however, once the diagnosis of AD has been made, epidural anesthesia is the treatment of choice. The epidural should continue at least 12 hours after delivery or until the dysreflexia resolves.

Endocrine/Metabolic Disorders

Metabolic abnormalities occur throughout the lifespan of patients with SCI. Acutely, patients may experience hypercalcemia, significant bone loss, or abnormal bone deposition. Immobilization hypercalcemia can appear as early as 2 weeks after an SCI. Increased risk factors include male gender, age less than 21 years, complete neurological injuries, high cervical levels of SCI, dehydration, and a prolonged period of immobilization. Presenting symptoms can be vague and include abdominal discomfort, nausea, constipation, diffuse musculoskeletal pain, and change in mental status. Treatment does not differ from that of non-SCI patients. First-line treatment consists of hydration with intravenous fluids. Diuretics, such as furosemide, are also helpful in decreasing serum calcium. Calcium-sparing diuretics, such as hydrochlorothiazide, are contraindicated. More recently, bisphosphonates (i.e., intravenous pamidronate given as a single bolus over 8 hours) have proven effective in treating hypercalcemia.

Heterotopic ossification (HO), deposition of bone within muscular fascial planes, becomes clinically significant in up to 20% of patients with SCI. HO appears to be more common in men, those with cervical or thoracic level injuries, and those with motor complete injuries. The hip is the most common site of HO formation in patients with SCI, followed by the knee and shoulder. Presenting symptoms may include acute swelling of the extremity, loss of passive range of motion (ROM), increased spasticity or low-grade fever. The differential of HO includes acute DVT, cellulites, acute fracture, and a septic joint. The initial diagnosis can be made by triple-phase bone scan. Abnormalities on plain X-rays are subtle early in the course of HO, and it may take up to 3 weeks to see some changes. Serum markers, such as alkaline phosphatase, are nonspecific. An elevation of serum creatine phosphokinase (CPK) may be a more reliable predictor of HO. Treatment with bisphosphonates has been shown to decrease the rate of new bone formation in patients with HO. However, it has no effect on bone that has already been deposited. Pharmacological treatment includes oral administration of etidronate at 20 mg/kg/day for 6 months if the CPK level is elevated at the time of diagnosis, or 20 mg/kg/day for 3 months, followed by 10 mg/kg/day for an additional 3 months if the CPK level is normal. With this regimen, they reported faster resolution of edema with less rebound formation after the medication was discontinued. Passive and active assistive ROM to the affected limb is necessary to prevent further loss of ROM at the joint.

Patients with SCI develop osteoporosis as early as 6 weeks following injury. Following injury, there is a marked increase in osteoclastic activity leading to net bone resorption. Rapid bone loss continues for up to 14 to 16 months following SCI, placing patients at increased risk of developing pathological fractures. Falls during transfers are the most common cause of osteoporotic fractures. In patients with severe osteoporosis, fractures may occur in the absence of trauma. Symptoms of acute fracture in the patient with SCI include fever, acute pain, swelling, or increased spasticity. Treatment of acute fractures usually consists of immobilization with a cast or splint, and usually dos not necessitate surgery. However, open or displaced fractures may require surgical fixation. Research into possible treatments to prevent bone loss following SCI including the use of bisphosphonates is ongoing. Although there seems to be some benefit for patients with incomplete injuries, evidence that this helps increase bone mineral density in a patient with a neurologically complete spinal cord injury is inconclusive.

In the chronic stage of SCI, patients may develop insulin resistance leading to an increased risk of developing type II diabetes mellitus. The precise etiology is not fully understood. Symptoms of hyperglycemia include polydipsia and polyuria. In the SCI-patient population, polyuria may include increased intermittent catheterizations volumes, new-onset urinary incontinence, or autonomic dysreflexia. Urinary tract infection should be ruled out as the etiology of the increased urination. One other confounding factor in the patient with SCI includes the relatively high incidence of anticholinergic medication usage, which itself may cause polydipsia. A simple urinalysis is helpful to clarify infection from glucosuria. The measurement of hemoglobin A1C is helpful in making the diagnosis of diabetes mellitus.

Table 10
Goals of Spasticity Treatment

1. Decrease pain.
2. Prevent or decrease medical complications (i.e., pressure ulcers or contractures).
3. Facilitate activities of daily living.
4. Ease rehabilitation.
5. Save caregiver's time.
6. Improve sleep.
7. Facilitate functional mobility.
8. Decrease frequency or intensity of spasms.

Spasticity

Spasticity is a common sequela of SCI affecting approximately 67% of all patients. It is defined as velocity-dependent resistance to passive stretch. The pathophysiology of spasticity, which is associated with UMN injuries, is not fully understood. One hypothesis is that a lack of supraspinal inhibition results in repeated muscle contraction. Known exacerbating factors of spasticity include infection, stress, change of weather, prolonged supine position, and noxious stimuli below the level of the SCI lesion, such as a pressure ulcer. The mere presence of spasticity does not warrant treatment, but rather treatment is appropriate when spasticity interferes with function, splint use, sleep, or is painful for the patient. Treatment may consist of focal or systemic interventions. The treating physician should establish clear goals with patients and caregivers before initiating treatment (Table 10).

There are a myriad of treatment options available to manage spasticity. Therefore, it is important to design a treatment plan that will achieve carefully selected goals. Therapeutic modalities for treatment include ROM to affected limbs and avoiding the supine position for extended periods of time. For patients with primarily focal spasticity, injection therapies may be more appropriate than systemic oral medications. Focal treatments include neuromuscular blocking agents, such as botulinum toxin, which acts to block transmission of acetylcholine at the neuromuscular junction, or chemical denervation with alcohol or phenol, which act by denaturing proteins. Table 11 outlines the pharmacological options available for systemic management of spasticity.

Table 11
Anti-Spasticity Medications

Medication	*Mechanism of action*	*Dosage*	*Precautions/ side effects*
Lioresal (Baclofen)	Centrally acting GABA-B agonist	Start 5 mg TID-QID; max dose 80 mg/day	• Abrupt cessation may cause seizures • Sedation
Diazepam (Valium)	Centrally acting GABA-A agonist	Start 2 mg BID-TID, titrate for effect, dose limited by side effects	• Sedation • Patients may build tolerance • Abrupt cessation may cause withdrawal syndrome
Tizanidine (Zanaflex)	Centrally acting α-2 agonist	Start 2 mg TID-QID, max dose 36 mg/day	• May cause hypotension
Clonidine	Centrally acting α-2 agonist	Start TTS-1 to skin weekly, max dose TTS 0.4 mg/day	• Hypotension
Dantrolene	Act peripherally to inhibits release of Ca^{2+} from sarcoplasmic reticulum	Start 25 mg QD, max dose 400 mg/day in divided doses	• Hepatotoxicity, monitor liver function tests • Can cause muscle weakness
Intrathecal Baclofen	Centrally acting GABA-B agonist	Start 50–100 µg/day, max dose limited by side effects	• Abrupt cessation may cause seizures • Requires surgical implantation • Requires monthly pump refills

TID, three times a day; QID, four times a day; BID, twice a day; GABA, γ-aminobutyric acid; QD, daily.

Neuropathic Pain

Studies examining pain in patients with SCI report an incidence of 66 to 94%. One study found 30 to 40% of patients reported experiencing severe disabling pain, with 23 to 37% of patients with SCI willing to trade the possibility of bowel, bladder, or sexual function recovery for pain relief.

The pathophysiology of neuropathic pain is not clearly understood. The gate control theory, proposed by Melzack and Wall, states nonpainful sensory input inhibits nociceptive activity. Therefore, patients with a lack of nonpainful sensory input, such as those who are insensate secondary to SCI, will have increased nociception. Painful input is carried within the spinothalamic tract in the anterior portion of the spinal cord via α, β, δ, and C fibers to the thalamus and finally to the somatosensory areas of the cerebral cortex. Neurotransmitters, such as somatostatin, substance P, cholesystikinin, glutamate, aspartate, norepinephrine, and serotonin, are thought to play a key role in pain transmission and perception. An alternative hypothesis is that there is a loss of spinal inhibition resulting in recruitment of adjacent neurons with amplification of pain. There is also evidence that a decreased level of γ-aminobutyric acid activity leads to allodynia and hyperalgesia. Overall, there is no clear etiology, but it is likely that the cause of neuropathic pain is multifactorial.

There is no consistent pain classification used in SCI, but the Bryce/Ragnarsson Scale incorporates all types of pain separated by location and character of the pain. Nociceptive pain is usually secondary to overuse of the upper extremities because individuals with SCI rely on their upper extremity (especially the shoulders and hands) for all functional activities, such as transfers, wheelchair propulsion, and activities of daily living. Neuropathic pain is also extremely common and can be debilitating for the patient, affecting all domains of a patient's life.

Potential treatments for neuropathic pain include antidepressants, anticonvulsants, and occasionally opioids. Tricyclic antidepressants are somewhat useful in treating neuropathic pain. The anticholinergic side effects of this class of medications, including urinary retention and sedation, may be of benefit in patients with SCI who have hyperreflexic bladder and/or poor sleep, but unfortunately, constipation may occur or worsen with anticholinergic use. Anticonvulsants, such as gabapentin and topiramate, have been successfully used to treat pain in patients with SCI. Opioid medications may be useful in the short-term in treating severe pain; however, patients should understand that constipation is a major side effect of this class of medication and careful monitoring of the bowel program is required. Adjunctive therapies including the use of transcutaneous electrical nerve stimulation units, ROM, desensitization exercises, biofeedback, and psychological counseling may be useful in all cases and should be attempted.

Psychological Issues

SCI is a life-altering event for patients and their families. It is therefore not surprising that patients with SCI have an increased incidence of depres-

Table 12
Mnemonic for Depressive Symptoms

SIG E CAPS:

S LEEP: insomnia or hypersomnia
I NTEREST: loss of interest or pleasure in activities, poor hygiene
G UILT: excessive guilt, worthlessness, hopelessness and helplessness

E NERGY: fatigue, loss of energy

C ONCENTRATION: diminished ability to concentrate or indecisiveness
A PPETITE: decreased or increased; more than 5% weight loss or gain
P SYCHOMOTOR: retardation or agitation
S UICIDALITY: suicidal ideation or plan, access to lethal means, prior attempt, comorbid alcohol or drug abuse

Adapted from Kaplan HI, Saddock BJ. Comprehensive Textbook of Psychiatry, 5th ed. Baltimore: Williams and Wilkin, 1989.

sion as compared with the general population. One study found an incidence of 25% in men and 47% in women with SCI. The suicide rate for individuals with SCI is five times the age–sex-specific suicide rate in the United States. Suicide rates are highest 1 to 5 years post-injury. Certainly there is a period of normal grieving that occurs following SCI, but depression should not be accepted as an expected part of recovery. In fact, most patients with SCI do not experience clinical depression. It is imperative that all members of the rehabilitation team be aware of signs of evolving depression in this patient population. The mnemonic SIG E CAPS (*see* Table 12) is helpful in assessing patients for depression.

An additional mnemonic, SAD PERSONS (*see* Table 13), is used to assess the risk for suicide. Substance abuse, which is increased in the SCI population, is a major risk factor for suicide. The highest risk for suicide continues through 5 years following injury, and it is imperative that physicians and other health care personnel continue to monitor patients for depression well after the acute phase of injury.

Pharmacological interventions are often times appropriate for patients with depression. Medications should be considered for individuals who present biological, somatic, and/or mood-related symptoms of sufficient severity to disrupt the person's life and activities of daily living. Additionally, psychological support should be initiated. For patients with active suicidal ideation, acute hospitalization should be strongly considered. Involvement of family or other social support systems are also helpful.

Table 13
Mnemonic for Suicide Risk

SAD PERSONS:

S EX: most common among white males
A GE: increasingly prevalent among adolescents; elderly at high risk
D EPRESSION

P REVIOUS ATTEMPTS: increases risk 50 to 100 times
E THANOL ABUSE: 25 to 35% of suicides occur among people with alcohol dependency
R ATIONAL THINKING: disorganized ideation, psychosis
S OCIAL SUPPORTS: dearth of family or friends for comfort and support, living alone
O RGANIZED PLAN: method, time, setting, availability of means
N O SPOUSE: lack of an intimate system heightens risk
S ICKNESS: 35 to 40% of suicides have significant, chronic physical illness or disability

Adapted from Consortium for spinal cord medicine clinical practice guidelines. Depression following spinal cord injury: a clinical practice guideline for PCP. Washington DC: Paralyzed Veterans of America, 1998.

Rehabilitation

"Rehabilitation" includes meeting SCI-specific medical (as previously outlined) and rehabilitative needs (Table 14) and is extremely important to help the individual who suffered the injury meet their potential in terms of physical, social, emotional, recreational, vocational, and functional recovery. The rehabilitation process for newly injured patients should begin immediately. Although patients may initially be too ill to engage in rigorous therapy, bedside activities including ROM can be helpful in preventing the development of joint contractures and pressure ulcers. Patients may also begin to work on mobility within the bed, as well as transferring from the bed to a chair or bedside commode. The most basic of functional tasks—feeding, grooming, dressing, transferring to and from the bed or wheelchair, and wheelchair propulsion—are often addressed during the initial hospitalization. Early mobilization of patients not only helps to prevent medical morbidity (contractures, pressure ulcers, cardiovascular deconditioning, etc.) but may also benefit the patient's psychological outlook on their newly acquired disability. One of the primary goals of rehabilitation during the early recovery period is to convey to patients that life with an SCI can still be fulfilling.

One benefit of the inpatient rehabilitation setting is the presence of the interdisciplinary health care team. A typical "team" may consist of a physi-

Table 14
Sample Problem List

Medical Problem list	*Interventions*
Respiratory	Monitor vital capacity; perform incentive spirometry, assisted cough, deep breathing techniques, chest PT, and respiratory treatments.
Gastrointestinal	Stress ulcer prophylaxis.
Nutrition	Perform calorie count; monitor weekly weights.
Neurogenic bowel	Initiate bowel program and adjust as needed; patient and family training.
Neurogenic bladder	Proper intake and output; discuss bladder options; family training.
DVT prophylaxis	Check admission doppler study; adequate pharmacological prophylaxis; monitor LE circumference.
Skin	Proper mattress; turn Q 2° initially; heel protectors; frequent weight shifts; proper cushion; teach patient to use mirror to check skin.
Orthostasis	Change positions slowly; ace wrap or LE stockings and abdominal binder; use tilt table; pharmacological intervention, if needed.
HO	Monitor hip and knee ROM; X-rays and bone scan if suspect.
Spasticity	Stretching/ROM; modalities; medications; injections; intrathecal Baclofen.
Autonomic dysreflexia	Monitor closely.
Hypercalcemia	Monitor for symptoms; fluids, medications.

Rehabilitation issues:

- Mobility
- Adjustment to disability
- Communication
- SCI education
- Sexuality
- Recreation
- Discharge planning
- ADL
- Cognitive
- Swallowing
- Vocational
- Driving
- Family training
- Equipment evaluation

Adapted from Kirshblum SC, Ho C, Druin E, Nead C, Drastal S. Rehabilitation after spinal cord injury. In Kirshblum SC, Campagnolo D, DeLisa JE, eds. Spinal Cord Medicine. Philadelphia: Lippincott, Williams and Wilkins. 2002, pp. 275–298.

PT, physical therapy; DVT, deep venous thrombus; Q, every; HO, heterotopic ossification; ROM, range of motion; LE, lower extremity; ADL, activities of daily living.

atrist who specializes in SCI medicine, a physical therapist, an occupational therapist, a rehabilitation nurse, a psychologist, a speech pathologist, a vocational counselor, a recreational therapist, a social worker, and a nutritionist, as well as the patient and his or her family. Each team member plays a vital role in the rehabilitation process providing care, as well as patient and family education. As the length of stay shortens in acute rehabilitation, coordination of the entire team has become more important to allow for a timely and safe discharge. The focus of the inpatient rehabilitation period is to improve patient function to facilitate a safe discharge back to the community.

Projected functional outcomes are based on the initial neurological level of injury and whether the injury is classified as neurologically complete or incomplete. Projected goals for persons with a complete injury are outlined in Table 15 and should be individualized based on a person's age, medical comorbidities, and family support.

The projected long-term goals are a starting point for the rehabilitation prescription to eventually achieve. The treatment team should be guided by these long-term functional goals, but the rehabilitation program should be individualized to meet each person's strengths, weaknesses, and individual circumstances (Table 16). Short-term goals are progressive steps that should be attained to achieve the long-term goals. The patient should understand the goals projected to become an active participant in their program.

For the high cervical levels (C1–C4), the important aspects of rehabilitation include the training of how to instruct others with their care, use of environmental control units, independence in power mobility, as well as psychological, vocational, and peer support. For each level of injury, additional goals are mastered and the proper equipment is tried and prescribed as needed. Because there is a large variety of wheelchairs and specialized equipment now available, including voice activated computer systems, implanted electrical stimulation controls for the upper extremities, bladder function, standing, and ambulation, the patient is best served being in a larger and specialized SCI unit in order to be exposed to all options available.

The basic tasks of transferring to and from the bed or wheelchair, repositioning in bed, and propelling a wheelchair should be accomplished before moving to higher level skills, such as standing and/or walking. C7 is the level at which most patients can achieve a degree of independence in terms of performing the majority of their mobility skills and activities of daily living independently. Patients should be advised that gait training may not begin until after they have been discharged from the inpatient rehabilitation setting. Basic dressing and grooming skills are also stressed. The

Table 15
Projected Functional Outcomes at 1 Year Post-Injury by Level

	C1–C4	*C5*	*C6*	*C7*	*C8–T1*
Feeding	Dep	Ind. with adaptive equipment after set-up	Ind. with or w/o adaptive equipment	Ind	Ind
Grooming	Dep	Min assist with equipment after set up	Some assist to Ind. with adaptive equipment	Ind. with adaptive equipment	Ind
UE dressing	Dep	Requires assistance	Ind	Ind	Ind
LE dressing	Dep	Dep	Requires assistance	Some assist to Ind. with adaptive equipment	Usually Ind
Bathing	Dep	Dep	Some assist to Ind with equipment	Some assist to Ind. with equipment	Ind with equipment
Bed mobility	Dep	Assists	Assists	Ind to some assist	Ind
Weight shifts	Ind. in power Dep in manual wc	Assists unless in power wc	Ind	Ind	Ind
Transfers	Dep	Maximum assist	Some assist to Ind. on level surfaces	Ind. with or without board for level surfaces	Ind
WC propulsion	Ind. with power Dep in manual	Ind. In power; Ind. to some assist in manual with adaptations on level surfaces	Ind.—manual with coated rims on level surfaces	Ind.—except curbs and uneven terrain	Ind
Driving	Unable	Ind with adaptations	Ind. Adaptations	Car with hand control or adapted van	Car with hand controls or adapted van

Table 15 *(Continued)*

Potential outcomes for complete paraplegics

	T2–T9	*T10–L2*	*L3–S5*
ADL (grooming, feeding, dressing, bathing)	Ind	Ind	Ind
Bowel/Bladder	Ind	Ind	Ind
Transfers	Ind	Ind	Ind
Ambulation	Standing in frame, tilt table, or standing wheelchair. Exercise only	Household ambulation with orthoses. Can try ambulation outdoors	Community ambulation is possible
Braces	Bilateral KAFO forearm crutches or walker	KAFOs with forearm crutches	Possibly KAFO or AFOs, with canes/crutches

Adapted from Kirshblum SC, Ho C, Druin E, Nead C, Drastal S. Rehabilitation after spinal cord injury. In Kirshblum SC, Campagnolo D, DeLisa JE, eds. Spinal Cord Medicine. Philadelphia: Lippincott, Williams and Wilkins. 2002, pp. 275–298.

Ind, independent; Dep, dependent; UE, upper extremity; LE, lower extremity; w/c, wheelchair; ADL, activities of daily living; KAFO, knee–ankle–foot orthosis.

Table 16
Sample Physical and Occupational Therapy Prescription

Diagnosis:	C7 ASIA A Tetraplegia
Goals:	*see* outlined goals
Precautions:	Skin, respiratory, sensory, orthostasis, safety, risk for autonomic dysreflexia and others as needed for the specific patient—i.e., bleeding if on Coumadin.

Physical therapy:

- PROM to bilateral LE, with stretching of hamstrings and hip extensors.
- Mat activities.
- Tilt table as tolerated. Start at 15°, progress 10° every 15 min within precautions up to 80°.
- Sitting balancing (static and dynamic).
- Transfer training from all surfaces including mat, bed, wheelchair and floor.
- Wheelchair propulsion training and management.
- Teach and encourage weight-shifting.
- Standing table as tolerated.
- Deep breathing exercises.
- FES for appropriate candidates.
- Family training.
- Community skills.
- Teach home exercise program.

Occupational therapy:

- Passive, active-assisted, active ROM/exercises to bilateral UEs.
- Allow for some finger tightness to enhance grasp.
- Bilateral UE strengthening.
- Motor coordination skills.
- ADL program with adaptive equipment as needed (dressing, grooming, feeding).
- Functional transfer training (bathroom, tub, car, etc.).
- Splinting and adaptive equipment evaluation.
- Desktop skills.
- Shower program.
- Kitchen and home-making skills.
- Wheelchair training (parts and management).
- Home evaluation.
- Family training.
- Teach home exercise program.

Adapted from Kirshblum SC, Ho C, Druin E, Nead C, Drastal S. Rehabilitation after spinal cord injury. In Kirshblum SC, Campagnolo D, DeLisa JE, eds. Spinal Cord Medicine. Philadelphia: Lippincott, Williams and Wilkins. 2002, pp. 275–298.

ASIA, American Spinal Cord Injury Association; PROM, passive range of motion; LE, lower extremity; FES, functional electrical stimulation; UE, upper extremity.

education of patients and their caregivers commences soon after SCI. In addition to verbal instruction, written information can serve as a helpful resource before and after discharge. Psychological and vocational counseling are also extremely important during this early period.

During the postacute period, several interventions can be considered. For patients with specific functional goals for each level of cervical injury, tendon transfer surgery may improve upper extremity function. The goals of the surgery should be very specific, and patients must understand that there is the potential for a decrease in upper extremity function following tendon transfer. After a period of relative immobility during the immediate postoperative period, intense therapy is required to maximize the benefits of the surgery.

Predicting Outcomes

The ability to predict the extent of neurological recovery after a traumatic SCI is extremely important. In recent years, our knowledge of the course of neurological recovery has increased to where we can predict, within 1 week of injury, the recovery of strength in the arms and legs in the early years post-injury. The most accurate method used to prognosticate such recovery is a standardized physical examination performed early after the injury, utilizing the International Standards for Neurological Classification of Spinal Cord Injury.

Persons with a motor-complete injury will usually regain one motor level by 1 year after their injury. Recovery of strength is greater and earlier in those individuals with some initial motor strength immediately caudal to the level of injury. The greater the initial strength of the muscle, the faster the muscle will recover to strength of 3/5 or greater. Persons with an initially complete cervical level of injury will not be able to regain the motor strength required for ambulation. Persons with an initially incomplete injury have a better prognosis for future ambulation if there is motor sparing, as opposed to sensory sparing only. For individuals with an initially sensory-incomplete lesion, sparing of pin sensation is a better predictor of functional ambulation at 1 year relative to those with light touch alone spared. Approximately 70% of individuals diagnosed with an incomplete cervical injury may regain the ability to ambulate at 1 year, with approximately 46% regaining the ability for community ambulation.

Recovery from injuries below the cervical spine, resulting in paraplegia, has not been studied to the degree of tetraplegia, but some of the generalizations regarding prediction of recovery are the same. In thoracic level and high lumbar level injuries (neurological level of injury above L2) one can usually only test for sensory modality change to document an improvement in neurological level of injury because there are no corresponding key muscle groups between T1 and L2. The prognosis for regaining functional ambulation in persons with complete paraplegia is 5%; however, the lower the level of injury, the greater the potential capability. Individuals with incomplete paraplegia have the best prognosis for ambulation. Of individuals with initial incomplete paraplegia, 80% regain hip flexors and knee extensors at 1 year. The mechanism of recovery often includes recovery of the spinal roots and spinal cord and therefore differs from the mechanism of recovery of leg function in tetraplegic subjects. The majority of motor recovery occurs within the first 6 months post-injury, with the greatest rate of change within the first 3 months. Motor strength improvement continues during the second year at a slower pace and smaller degree. The etiology of the traumatic SCI only plays a role in determining whether the injury is more likely to be neurologically complete or not.

For the purposes of prognostication, magnetic resonance imaging (MRI) is the most superior of all radiological tests. A number of studies have related MRI findings to the neurological status and recovery after SCI and found that the degree and type of MRI change correlates with the severity and prognosis of the injury. A hemorrhage on an acute MRI correlates with the poorest prognosis, followed by contusion and edema. A normal study (no MRI abnormality) correlates with the best prognosis. If a hemorrhage is initially seen on MRI, this usually suggests a complete injury. If a hemorrhage is present in patients who present with an incomplete injury, those patients usually have less chance of recovery relative to patients with other MRI findings. If no hemorrhage is seen on the initial MRI, those patients will most likely have an incomplete lesion and a significantly better prognosis for motor recovery in the upper and lower extremities, as well as improvement in their AIS classification. The degree and extent of cord edema on MRI has an inversely proportional affect as a prognostic indicator for initial impairment level and future recovery. If the edema involves multiple levels, there is a poorer prognosis and a greater chance of having a complete lesion. In general, MRI can be used to augment the physical examination in prognosticating recovery of patients with cervical SCI. However, by itself, MRI is not as accurate a predictor as the physical examination.

Community Reintegration

Recalling that the average age of injury for patients with SCI is just 37.7 years, it is important for all members of the rehabilitation team to begin addressing vocational and recreational issues early in the course of rehabilitation. Data from the National Spinal Cord Injury Statistical Center suggests more than 63% of patients with SCI are employed or in school at the time of their injury. Post-injury employment rates were 31.8% for those with paraplegia and 26.4% for those with tetraplegia. People with higher pre-injury education levels were more likely to be employed after their injury.

Time away from work is also essential for full integration into the community. Increasingly, recreation activities are being modified for people with disabilities. The Internet provides access to information on activities available in individual communities.

Research in SCI

The future of SCI rehabilitation is full of promise. Research directions will focus on facilitating nerve regeneration within the central nervous system, as well as limiting secondary injury to the cord. While the search for a cure continues, patients should be encouraged to maintain full and active lives. Although we all want a cure, what we have is hope and rehabilitation.

Key References and Suggested Additional Reading

American Spinal Injury Association/International Medical Society of Paraplegia International Standards for Neurological and Functional Classification of Spinal Cord Injury Patients, Revised 2000. Reprinted 2002. Chicago, IL.

Bach JR. Alternative methods of ventilatory support for the patient with ventilatory failure due to spinal cord injury. J Am Paraplegia Soc 1991; 14:158–174. Review.

Baker ER, Cardenas DD. Pregnancy in spinal cord injured women. Arch Phys Med Rehabil 1996; 77:501–507. Review.

Banovac K, Sherman AL, Estores IM, Banovac F. Prevention and treatment of heterotopic ossification after spinal cord injury. J Spinal Cord Med 2004; 27:376–382.

Bauman WA, Adkins RH, Waters RL. Cardiovascular risk factors: Prevalence in 300 subjects with SCI. J Spinal Cord Med 1996; 19:56A.

Bauman WA, Spungen AM. Disorders of carbohydrate and lipid metabolism in veterans with paraplegia or quadriplegia: a model of premature aging. Metabolism 1994; 43:749–756.

Bennett CJ, Seager SW, Vasher EA, et al. Sexual dysfunction and electroejaculation in men with spinal cord injury: review. J Urol 1988; 139:453–456.

Berkowitz M, O'Leary PK, Kruse DL, et al. Spinal Cord Injury: Analysis of Medical and Social Costs. New York: Demographics, 1998.

Bracken M, Holford T. Effects of timing of methylprednisolone or naloxone administration on recovery of segmental and long-tract neurological function in NASCIS 2. J Neurosurg 1993; 80:954–955.

Bracken MB, Shepard MJ, Holford TR, et al. Administration of methylprednisolone for 24 or 48 hours or tirilazad mesylate for 48 hours in the treatment of acute spinal cord injury. JAMA 1997; 277:1597–1604.

Bryce TN, Ragnarsson KT. Pain after spinal cord injury. Phys Med Rehabil Clin N Am. 2000; 11:157–168.

Colachis SC III. Autonomic hyperreflexia with spinal cord injury. J Am Paraplegia Soc 1992;15:171–186.

Consortium for Spinal Cord Medicine. Acute management of autonomic dysreflexia: adults with spinal cord injury presenting to health care facilities. Washington, DC: Paralyzed Veterans of America, 2001.

Consortium for Spinal Cord Medicine. Clinical Practice Guidelines. Depression following spinal cord injury: a clinical practice guideline for PCP. Washington DC: Paralyzed Veterans of America, 1998.

Consortium for Spinal Cord Medicine. Clinical Practice Guidelines. Prevention of thromboembolism in spinal cord injury. Washington, DC: Paralyzed Veterans of America, 2001.

Crozier KS, Graziani V, Ditunno JF Jr, Herbison GJ. Spinal cord lesion level. Arch Phys Med Rehabil 1991; 72:119–121.

Cushman LA, Dijkers M. Depressed mood during rehabilitation of persons with spinal injury. J Rehabil 1991; 2:35–38.

DeVivo MJ, Black D, Stover S. Causes of death during the first 12 years after spinal cord injury. Arch Phys Med Rehabil 1993; 74:248–254.

DeVivo MJ, Black K, Stover S. Long term survival and causes of death. In Stover SL, DeLisa JA, Whiteneck GF, eds. Spinal Cord Injury Clinical Outcomes from the Model Systems. Gaithersburg, MD: Aspen, 1995, p. 297.

DeVivo, MJ, Black KJ, Richard S, Stover SL. Suicide following spinal cord injury. Paraplegia 1991; 29: 620–627.

Dinoff BL, Richards JS, Ness TJ. Use of topiramate for spinal cord injury-related pain. J Spinal Cord Med 2003; 26:401–403.

Ditunno J, Flanders A, Kirshblum SC, Graziani V, Tessler A. Predicting outcome in traumatic spinal cord injury. In Kirshblum SC, Campagnolo D, DeLisa JE, eds. Spinal Cord Medicine. Philadelphia: Lippincott, Williams and Wilkins. 2002, pp. 108–122.

Estenne M, DeTroyer A. Mechanism of the postural dependence of vital capacity in tetraplegic subjects. Am Rev Respir Dis 1987; 135:367–371.

Frank RG, Umlauf RL, Wonderlich SA, Askanazi GJ, Buchelew SP, Elliott TR. Differences in coping styles among persons with spinal cord injury: a cluster-analytic approach. J Consult Clin Psychol 1987; 55:727–731.

Frankel HL, Mathias CJ, Spalding JMK. Mechanism of reflex cardiac arrest in tetraplegic patients. Lancet 1975; 2:1183–1185

Fuhrer M, Garber SDR. Pressure ulcers in community-resident persons with spinal cord injury: Prevalence and risk factors. Arch Phys Med Rehabil 1993; 74:1172–1177.

Gans WH Zaslau S Wheeler S Galea G Vapnek JM. Efficacy and safety of oral sildenafil in men with erectile dysfunction and spinal cord injury. J Spinal Cord Med 2001; 24:35–40.

Garland DE, Stewart CA, Adler RH, et al. Osteoporosis after spinal cord injury. J Orthop Res 1992; 10:371–378.

Garstang SV, Kirsblum SC, Wood KE. Patient preference for in-exsufflation for secretion management in spinal cord injury. J Spinal Cord Med 2000; 23: 8–85.

Gerridzen RG, Thijssen AM, Dehoux E. Risk factors for upper urinary tract deterioration in chronic spinal cord-injured patients. J Urol 1992; 147:416–418.

Gore RM, Mintzer RA, Calenoff L. Gastrointestinal complications of spinal cord injury. Spine 1981; 6:538–544.

Hurlbert RJ. The role of steroids in acute spinal cord injury: an evidenced-based analysis. Spine 2001;26(24 Suppl):S39–S46.

Jackson AB, Dijkers M, DeVivo MJ, Poczatek RB. Demographic profile of new traumatic spinal cord injuries: change and stability over 30 years. Arch Phys Med Rehabil 2004; 85:1740–1748.

Jackson AB, Groomes TE. Incidence of respiratory complications following spinal cord injury. Arch Phys Med Rehabil 1994; 75:27–275.

Johnstone BR, Jordan CJ, Buntine JA. A review of surgical rehabilitation of the upper limb in quadriplegia. Paraplegia 1988; 26:317–339.

Kirshblum SC, Donovan WH. Neurologic assessment and classification of traumatic spinal cord injury. In: Kirshblum SC, Campagnolo D, DeLisa JE, eds. Spinal Cord Medicine. Philadelphia: Lippincott, Williams & Wilkins, 2002:82–95.

Kirshblum SC, Ho C, Druin E, Nead C, Drastal S. Rehabilitation after Spinal Cord Injury. In: Kirshblum SC, Campagnolo D, DeLisa JE, eds. Spinal Cord Medicine. Philadelphia: Lippincott, Williams and Wilkins. 2002; 275–298.

Kirshblum SC, O'Connor K. Levels of injury and outcome in traumatic spinal cord injury. Phys Med Rehabil Clin N Am 2000; 11:1–27.

Kosiak M. Etiology of decubitus ulcers. Arch Phys Med Rehabil 1961; 42: 19–29.

Linsenmeyer TA. Evaluation and treatment of erectile dysfunction following spinal cord injury:a review. J Am Paraplegia Soc 1991; 14:43–51.

Locke JR, Hill DE, Walzer Y. Incidence of squamous cell carcinoma I patients with long-term catheter drainage. J Urol 1985; 133:1034–1035.

Long C, Lawton EB. Functional significance of spinal cord lesion level. Arch Phys Med Rehabil 1955; 36:249–255.

Maloney FP. Pulmonary function in quadriplegia: effects of a corset. Arch Phys Med Rehabil 1979; 60:261–265.

Massagli TL, Cardenas DD. Immobilization hypercalcemia treatment with pamidronate disodium after spinal cord injury. Arch Phys Med Rehabil 1999; 80:998–1000.

Mathias CJ. Bradycardia and cardiac arrest during tracheal suction mechanisms in tetraplegic patients. Eur J Intens Care Med 1976; 2:147–156.

Maury M. About orthostatic hypotension in tetraplegic individuals: reflections and experience. Spinal Cord 1998; 36:87–90.

Maynard FM, Daurnas RS, Waring WP. Epidemiology of spasticity following traumatic spinal cord injury. Arch Phys Med Rehabil 1990; 71:566–569.

Maynard FM, Glen GR, Fountain S, Wilmot C, Hamilton R. Neurological prognosis after traumatic quadriplegia. J Neurosurg 1979; 50:611–616.

McKinley WO, Jackson AB, Cardenas DD, et al. Long-term medical complications after traumatic spinal cord injury: a regional model systems analysis. Arch Phys Med Rehabil 1999; 80:1402–1410.

Merli, G, Crabbe S. Doyle L, et al. Mechanical plus pharmacological prophylaxis for deep vein thrombosis in acute spinal cord injury. Paraplegia 1992; 30:558–562.

Merli GJ, Crabbe S,Paluzzi RG, et al. Etiology, incidence, and prevention of deep vein thrombosis in acute spinal cord injury. Arch Phys Med Rehabil 1993; 74:1199–1205.

Merli G, Herbison G, Ditunno J, et al: Deep vein thrombosis in acute spinal cord-injured patients. Arch Phys Med Rehabil 1988; 69:661–664.

Mukand J, Karlin L, Barrs K, et al. Midodrine for the management of orthostatic hypotension in patients with spinal cord injury: a case report. Arch Phys Med Rehabil 2001; 82:694–696.

National Pressure Ulcer Advisory Panel (NPUAP). Pressure ulcers prevalence, costs, and risk assessment; consensus development conference statement. Decubitus 1989; 2:24–28.

National Spinal Cord Injury Statistical Center: Spinal Cord Injury: Facts and Figures at a Glance 2005. Birmingham: University of Alabama at Birmingham, 2005.

Nepomuceno C, Fine PR, Richards JS, et al. Pain in patients with spinal cord injury. Arch Phys Med Rehabil. 1979; 60:605–609.

Nesathurai S. Steroids and spinal cord injury: Revisiting the NASCIS2 and NASCIS3 trials. J Trauma Injury Infect Crit Care 1998; 45:1088–1093.

Popolo GD Marzi VL Mondaini N Lombardi G. Time/duration effectiveness of sildenafil versus tadalafil in the treatment of erectile dysfunction in male spinal cord-injured patients. Spinal Cord 2004; 42:643–648.

Long C, Lawton EB. Functional significance of spinal cord lesion level. Arch Phys Med Rehabil 1955; 36:249–255.

Maloney FP. Pulmonary function in quadriplegia: effects of a corset. Arch Phys Med Rehabil 1979; 60:261–265.

Massagli TL, Cardenas DD. Immobilization hypercalcemia treatment with pamidronate disodium after spinal cord injury. Arch Phys Med Rehabil 1999; 80:998–1000.

Mathias CJ. Bradycardia and cardiac arrest during tracheal suction mechanisms in tetraplegic patients. Eur J Intens Care Med 1976; 2:147–156.

Maury M. About orthostatic hypotension in tetraplegic individuals: reflections and experience. Spinal Cord 1998; 36:87–90.

Maynard FM, Daurnas RS, Waring WP. Epidemiology of spasticity following traumatic spinal cord injury. Arch Phys Med Rehabil 1990; 71:566–569.

Maynard FM, Glen GR, Fountain S, Wilmot C, Hamilton R. Neurological prognosis after traumatic quadriplegia. J Neurosurg 1979; 50:611–616.

McKinley WO, Jackson AB, Cardenas DD, et al. Long-term medical complications after traumatic spinal cord injury: a regional model systems analysis. Arch Phys Med Rehabil 1999; 80:1402–1410.

Merli, G, Crabbe S. Doyle L, et al. Mechanical plus pharmacological prophylaxis for deep vein thrombosis in acute spinal cord injury. Paraplegia 1992; 30:558–562.

Merli GJ, Crabbe S,Paluzzi RG, et al. Etiology, incidence, and prevention of deep vein thrombosis in acute spinal cord injury. Arch Phys Med Rehabil 1993; 74:1199–1205.

Merli G, Herbison G, Ditunno J, et al: Deep vein thrombosis in acute spinal cord-injured patients. Arch Phys Med Rehabil 1988; 69:661–664.

Mukand J, Karlin L, Barrs K, et al. Midodrine for the management of orthostatic hypotension in patients with spinal cord injury: a case report. Arch Phys Med Rehabil 2001; 82:694–696.

National Pressure Ulcer Advisory Panel (NPUAP). Pressure ulcers prevalence, costs, and risk assessment; consensus development conference statement. Decubitus 1989; 2:24–28.

National Spinal Cord Injury Statistical Center: Spinal Cord Injury: Facts and Figures at a Glance 2005. Birmingham: University of Alabama at Birmingham, 2005.

Nepomuceno C, Fine PR, Richards JS, et al. Pain in patients with spinal cord injury. Arch Phys Med Rehabil. 1979; 60:605–609.

Nesathurai S. Steroids and spinal cord injury: Revisiting the NASCIS2 and NASCIS3 trials. J Trauma Injury Infect Crit Care 1998; 45:1088–1093.

Popolo GD Marzi VL Mondaini N Lombardi G. Time/duration effectiveness of sildenafil versus tadalafil in the treatment of erectile dysfunction in male spinal cord-injured patients. Spinal Cord 2004; 42:643–648.

Frankel HL, Mathias CJ, Spalding JMK. Mechanism of reflex cardiac arrest in tetraplegic patients. Lancet 1975; 2:1183–1185

Fuhrer M, Garber SDR. Pressure ulcers in community-resident persons with spinal cord injury: Prevalence and risk factors. Arch Phys Med Rehabil 1993; 74:1172–1177.

Gans WH Zaslau S Wheeler S Galea G Vapnek JM. Efficacy and safety of oral sildenafil in men with erectile dysfunction and spinal cord injury. J Spinal Cord Med 2001; 24:35–40.

Garland DE, Stewart CA, Adler RH, et al. Osteoporosis after spinal cord injury. J Orthop Res 1992; 10:371–378.

Garstang SV, Kirsblum SC, Wood KE. Patient preference for in-exsufflation for secretion management in spinal cord injury. J Spinal Cord Med 2000; 23: 8–85.

Gerridzen RG, Thijssen AM, Dehoux E. Risk factors for upper urinary tract deterioration in chronic spinal cord-injured patients. J Urol 1992; 147:416–418.

Gore RM, Mintzer RA, Calenoff L. Gastrointestinal complications of spinal cord injury. Spine 1981; 6:538–544.

Hurlbert RJ. The role of steroids in acute spinal cord injury: an evidenced-based analysis. Spine 2001;26(24 Suppl):S39–S46.

Jackson AB, Dijkers M, DeVivo MJ, Poczatek RB. Demographic profile of new traumatic spinal cord injuries: change and stability over 30 years. Arch Phys Med Rehabil 2004; 85:1740–1748.

Jackson AB, Groomes TE. Incidence of respiratory complications following spinal cord injury. Arch Phys Med Rehabil 1994; 75:27–275.

Johnstone BR, Jordan CJ, Buntine JA. A review of surgical rehabilitation of the upper limb in quadriplegia. Paraplegia 1988; 26:317–339.

Kirshblum SC, Donovan WH. Neurologic assessment and classification of traumatic spinal cord injury. In: Kirshblum SC, Campagnolo D, DeLisa JE, eds. Spinal Cord Medicine. Philadelphia: Lippincott, Williams & Wilkins, 2002:82–95.

Kirshblum SC, Ho C, Druin E, Nead C, Drastal S. Rehabilitation after Spinal Cord Injury. In: Kirshblum SC, Campagnolo D, DeLisa JE, eds. Spinal Cord Medicine. Philadelphia: Lippincott, Williams and Wilkins. 2002; 275–298.

Kirshblum SC, O'Connor K. Levels of injury and outcome in traumatic spinal cord injury. Phys Med Rehabil Clin N Am 2000; 11:1–27.

Kosiak M. Etiology of decubitus ulcers. Arch Phys Med Rehabil 1961; 42: 19–29.

Linsenmeyer TA. Evaluation and treatment of erectile dysfunction following spinal cord injury:a review. J Am Paraplegia Soc 1991; 14:43–51.

Locke JR, Hill DE, Walzer Y. Incidence of squamous cell carcinoma I patients with long-term catheter drainage. J Urol 1985; 133:1034–1035.

Roth EJ, Fenton LL, Gaebler-Spira DJ, Frost FS, Yarkony GM. Superior mesenteric artery syndrome in acute traumatic quadriplegia: case reports and literature review. Arch Phys Med Rehabil 1991; 72:417–420.

Roth EJ, Nussbaum SB, Berkowitz M, et al. Pulmonary function testing in spinal cord injury: correlation with vital capacity. Paraplegia 1995; 33:454–457.

Segal JL, Milne N, Brunnemann SR, Lyons KP. Metoclopramide-induced normalization of impaired gastric emptying in spinal cord injury. Am J Gastroenterol 1987; 82:1143–1148

Singh RS, Craig MC, Katholi CR, Jackson AB, Mountz JM. Predictive value of creatine phosphokinase and alkaline phophatase in identification of heterotopic ossification in patients after spinal cord injury. Arch Phys Med Rehabil 2003; 84:1584–1588.

Sipski ML. The impact of spinal cord injury on female sexuality, menstruation and pregnancy: a review of the literature. J Am Paraplegia Soc 1991; 14:122–126.

Sipski ML, Alexander CJ, Rosen RC. Orgasm in women with spinal cord injuries: a laboratory-based assessment. Arch Phys Med Rehabil 1995; 76: 1097–1102.

Spinal Cord Injury Thromboprophylaxis Group. Prevention of venous thromboembolism in the acute treatment phase after SCI: A randomized multicenter trial comparing low-dose heparin plus intermittent compression with enoxaparin. J Trauma 2003; 54:1116–1126.

Spinal Cord Injury Thromboprophylaxis Investigators. Prevention of venous thromboembolism in the rehabilitation phase after spinal cord injury: prophylaxis with low-dose heparin or enoxaparin. J Trauma 2003; 54:1111–1115.

Stiens SA, Bergman SB, Goetz LL: Neurogenic bowel dysfunction after spinal cord injury: Clinical evaluation and rehabilitative management. Arch Phys Med Rehabil 1997; 78(Suppl 3):S86–S102.

Tai Q, Kirshblum S, Chen B, Millis S, Johnston M, DeLisa JA. Gabapentin in the treatment of neuropathic pain after spinal cord injury: a prospective, randomized, double-blind, crossover trial. J Spinal Cord Med 2002; 25:100–105.

To TP, Lim TC, Hill ST, et.al. Gabapentin for neuropathic pain following spinal cord injury. Spinal Cord 2002; 40:282–285.

Waters RL, Adkins RH, Yakura JS, Sie I. Motor and sensory recovery following incomplete tetraplegia. Arch Phys Med Rehabil 1994; 75:306–311.

Wicks AB, Menter RR. Long-term outlook in quadriplegic patients with initial ventilator dependency. Chest 1986; 90:406–410.

Wittenberg RH, Peschke U, Botel U. Heterotopic ossification after spinal cord injury. Epidemiology and risk factors. J Bone Joint Surg Br 1992; 74:215–218.

Yarkony GM. Enhancement of sexual function and fertility in spinal cord-injured males. Am J Phys Med Rehabil 1990; 69:81–87.
Yeziersky RP. Pain following spinal cord injury: the clinical problem and experimental studies. Pain 1996; 68:185–194.
Yekutrel M, Brooks ME, Ohry A, et al. The prevalence of hypertension, ischemic heart disease and diabetes in traumatic spinal cord-injured patients and amputees. Paraplegia 1989; 27:58–62.
Young RR. The physiology of spasticity and its response to therapy. Ann NY Acad Sci 1988; 531:146–149.

Yarkony GM. Enhancement of sexual function and fertility in spinal cord-injured males. Am J Phys Med Rehabil 1990; 69:81–87.

Yeziersky RP. Pain following spinal cord injury: the clinical problem and experimental studies. Pain 1996; 68:185–194.

Yekutrel M, Brooks ME, Ohry A, et al. The prevalence of hypertension, ischemic heart disease and diabetes in traumatic spinal cord-injured patients and amputees. Paraplegia 1989; 27:58–62.

Young RR. The physiology of spasticity and its response to therapy. Ann NY Acad Sci 1988; 531:146–149.

Roth EJ, Fenton LL, Gaebler-Spira DJ, Frost FS, Yarkony GM. Superior mesenteric artery syndrome in acute traumatic quadriplegia: case reports and literature review. Arch Phys Med Rehabil 1991; 72:417–420.

Roth EJ, Nussbaum SB, Berkowitz M, et al. Pulmonary function testing in spinal cord injury: correlation with vital capacity. Paraplegia 1995; 33:454–457.

Segal JL, Milne N, Brunnemann SR, Lyons KP. Metoclopramide-induced normalization of impaired gastric emptying in spinal cord injury. Am J Gastroenterol 1987; 82:1143–1148

Singh RS, Craig MC, Katholi CR, Jackson AB, Mountz JM. Predictive value of creatine phosphokinase and alkaline phophatase in identification of heterotopic ossification in patients after spinal cord injury. Arch Phys Med Rehabil 2003; 84:1584–1588.

Sipski ML. The impact of spinal cord injury on female sexuality, menstruation and pregnancy: a review of the literature. J Am Paraplegia Soc 1991; 14:122–126.

Sipski ML, Alexander CJ, Rosen RC. Orgasm in women with spinal cord injuries: a laboratory-based assessment. Arch Phys Med Rehabil 1995; 76: 1097–1102.

Spinal Cord Injury Thromboprophylaxis Group. Prevention of venous thromboembolism in the acute treatment phase after SCI: A randomized multicenter trial comparing low-dose heparin plus intermittent compression with enoxaparin. J Trauma 2003; 54:1116–1126.

Spinal Cord Injury Thromboprophylaxis Investigators. Prevention of venous thromboembolism in the rehabilitation phase after spinal cord injury: prophylaxis with low-dose heparin or enoxaparin. J Trauma 2003; 54:1111–1115.

Stiens SA, Bergman SB, Goetz LL: Neurogenic bowel dysfunction after spinal cord injury: Clinical evaluation and rehabilitative management. Arch Phys Med Rehabil 1997; 78(Suppl 3):S86–S102.

Tai Q, Kirshblum S, Chen B, Millis S, Johnston M, DeLisa JA. Gabapentin in the treatment of neuropathic pain after spinal cord injury: a prospective, randomized, double-blind, crossover trial. J Spinal Cord Med 2002; 25:100–105.

To TP, Lim TC, Hill ST, et.al. Gabapentin for neuropathic pain following spinal cord injury. Spinal Cord 2002; 40:282–285.

Waters RL, Adkins RH, Yakura JS, Sie I. Motor and sensory recovery following incomplete tetraplegia. Arch Phys Med Rehabil 1994; 75:306–311.

Wicks AB, Menter RR. Long-term outlook in quadriplegic patients with initial ventilator dependency. Chest 1986; 90:406–410.

Wittenberg RH, Peschke U, Botel U. Heterotopic ossification after spinal cord injury. Epidemiology and risk factors. J Bone Joint Surg Br 1992; 74:215–218.

4 Prosthetics and Orthotics

Heikki Uustal

Lower Extremity Amputation and Prosthetics

Incidence

More than 100,000 major lower limb amputations occur annually in the United States, and most are the result of dysvascular disease. There are more than 500,000 amputee survivors currently in the United States. There are at least 10 times more lower extremity amputations than there are upper extremity amputations. The primary cause of lower limb amputation in the age group older than 50 years is diabetes and vascular disease. The primary cause of lower limb amputation in the age group younger than 50 years is trauma. The primary cause of upper limb amputation is also trauma. The distribution and relative energy costs for lower limb amputation are outlined in Table 1.

Ideal Length

Transtibial amputations are ideally done at the junction of the proximal to middle third of the tibia, but can be as short as 1 cm distal to the tibial tubercle (Fig. 1). Transfemoral amputations are generally performed to maintain as much length as possible. Amputation above the lesser trochanter of the femur will be fitted essentially as hip disarticulation.

From: *Essential Physical Medicine and Rehabilitation*
Edited by: G. Cooper © Humana Press Inc., Totowa, NJ

Table 1
Distribution of Lower Limb Amputations and Energy Costs

Level of amputation	*Distribution*	*Increased energy cost*
Symes	3	15%
Transtibial	59	25–40%
Knee disarticulation	1	40–60%
Transfemoral	35	60–70%
Hip disarticulation	2	100% or greater

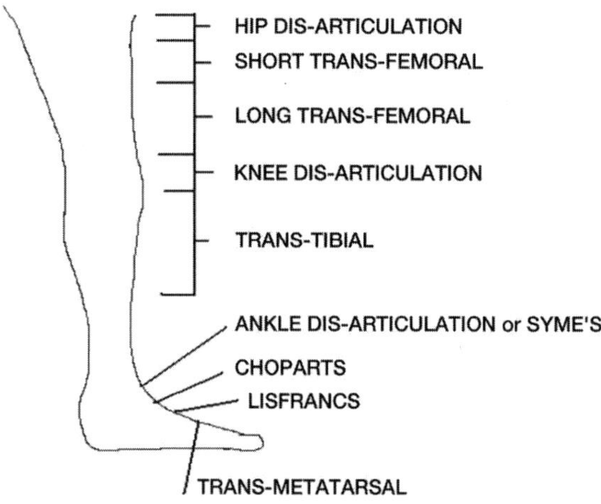

Fig. 1. Diagram of levels of lower limb amputation.

Rehabilitation Program

- Day 0: Amputation.
- Days 1–4: Acute hospital postoperative stay.
- Days 5–21: Preprosthetic program as outpatient or at subacute rehabilitation facility.
- Days 21–28: Suture removal and casting for preliminary prosthesis.
- Months 2 and 3: Prosthetic training with preliminary prosthesis.
- Months 3–6: Fitting of permanent prosthesis (replacement every 4–5 years).

Medicare Functional Levels (Restrictions for Prosthetic Components)

- Level 0: Nonambulatory.
- Level 1: Household ambulator or transfers only.
- Level 2: Limited community ambulator.
- Level 3: Unlimited community ambulator.
- Level 4: High-energy activities and recreational sports.

Current Prosthetic Design by Level of Amputation

Partial Foot Amputation

Partial foot amputation requires a custom insert in a proper orthopedic shoe with appropriate toe filler. Acceptable levels of amputations include toe amputation, ray resection, and transmetatarsal amputation. Less desirable levels include Lisfranc and Choparts level of amputation because of plantigrade migration of calcaneous from loss of dorsiflexor insertions.

Modified Syme's

This is a level of amputation most commonly found in traumatic injury and not for dysvascular disease. It preserves the full length of the tibia and the end-bearing articular cartilage of the tibia, but removes the medial and lateral malleolus to obtain a flat weight-bearing surface. The purpose of a Syme's amputation is partial end-bearing and a long lever length for good control of the prosthesis. This relies on good soft-tissue coverage, including the heel pad from the plantar surface of the foot, inserted directly onto the articular cartilage of the tibia. The prosthetic design would generally include a split foam liner inside a laminated socket. This would include partial end-bearing and partial bearing at the patellar tendon. It is commonly laminated directly to the specialized Syme's-type prosthetic foot with no movable ankle joint but a low-profile energy-storing keel. The functional outcome at this level is very high, with running and jumping being easily accomplished.

Transtibial Amputation

The most common socket design for transtibial amputation is a patellar tendon-bearing total-contact socket with a soft interface material. The outer rigid portion of the socket is often of a laminated material but can also be a high-temperature thermal plastic. The soft interface materials are commonly a closed-cell foam material, such as Pelite or Bock-Lite. The foam

Table 2
Prosthetic Feet
(Examples of Commercial Products Currently Available)

Response	*No ankle motion*	*Simulated motion*	*Single-axis*	*Multi-axis*
No energy	SACH Foot	SAFE Foot	Single-axis Foot	Greisinger Foot
Energy	Seattle Foot	Luxon DP Foot		College Park

SACH, solid ankle cushion heel; SAFE, solid ankle flexible endoskelton; DP, dynamic pylon.

materials are most commonly used for the preliminary prosthesis. However, a silicone or urethane gel material is most commonly used for the permanent prosthesis. The suspension mechanism can be one of four types:

1. Supracondylar wedge.
2. Suction with a gel liner, pin, and shuttle lock.
3. Elastic suspension sleeve.
4. Supracondylar cuff or strap.

The overall construction of the prosthesis may be of an *endoskeletal* design, where the pipe or pylon transmits the body weight from the residual limb to the foot and is then covered with a soft foam cosmetic cover. The pylon connects the socket to the prosthetic foot and often incorporates the alignment mechanisms, shock absorbers, or torque absorbers. The endoskeletal design allows for ease of adjustability. The other type is an *exoskeletal* design, with a hard outer shell that transmits the weight from the socket continuously down to the prosthetic foot. The exoskeletal design gives better durability and, therefore, is most commonly used in children, construction workers, or for waterproof legs.

Prosthetic feet can be divided into several different categories (*see* Table 2):

1. The prosthetic foot can have no motion, single axis, multi-axis, or simulated motion.
2. The foot can have energy response (bounce) or no energy response.

Functional outcome at the transtibial level can be very high if there is good soft-tissue coverage of the residual limb and good fitting of the socket. Walking with no assistive device, and running or jumping can be accomplished if there is unilateral amputation. A prosthetic device should not be used to operate a pedal on a motor vehicle and, therefore, a right lower limb amputation would require a left-side accelerator pedal to resume driving.

Knee Disarticulation Amputation

The socket design for knee disarticulation includes partial end-bearing and partial bearing on the distal two-thirds of the thigh. This would include a rigid outer frame and flexible inner socket. The suspension mechanisms at this level are generally a self-suspending design using a gel liner with a locking strap or a split liner with a removable medial window similar to the Syme's amputation level. The biggest advantages at the knee disarticulation level are the full length of the femur, which allows good control of the prosthesis, and that the socket design does not need to incorporate ischial bearing and, therefore, stays out of the groin and is much more comfortable to the patient. Unfortunately, the knee disarticulation socket tends to be somewhat bulky in design and not all prosthetic knees are compatible with this design.

Transfemoral Amputation

The current transfemoral amputation socket includes a narrow medial-lateral (ML) dimension with ischial containment and total contact. Again, this would incorporate a flexible inner liner and a rigid outer frame, in addition to another soft interface material. The preliminary prosthesis would most likely include prosthetic socks as the interface material, and the permanent prosthesis would most likely include full suction of skin directly to the socket or a gel interface to provide suction into the socket. The weight-bearing is focused primarily at the ischial tuberosity and gluteal muscles, but there is significant weight-bearing across the entire muscle mass of the thigh. The preliminary prosthesis suspension mechanism includes a semi-suction design with prosthetic socks and the addition of an elastic waist belt. The permanent prosthesis is a full-suction design and no waist belt is generally required.

Prosthetic knees can be divided into roughly seven categories:

1. *Manual locking knees* are used primarily for marked weakness at hip extensors or multiple disabilities, including stroke or other neuromuscular disease (level 1 ambulators).
2. *Stance control knees* have a weight-activated locking mechanism, providing only fixed cadence ambulation for level 1 or level 2 ambulators.
3. *Pneumatic knees* provide adjustable swing control with variable cadence and are generally used for level 2 or level 3 ambulators.
4. *Hydraulic knees* provide adjustable swing and stance control with variable cadence for level 3 and level 4 ambulators.
5. *Polycentric knees* provide biomechanical stability from full extension to roughly 25° of flexion with fixed cadence and are generally reserved for knee disarticulation or long transfemoral amputation.

6. *Hybrid polycentric knees* incorporate pneumatic or hydraulic control mechanisms for stance stability and variable cadence, again for longer residual limbs (level 3 and 4 ambulators).
7. *Microprocessor-controlled hydraulic knees* include computer-controlled swing and stance, in addition to stumble control mechanisms to prevent falls, and are generally reserved for level 3 and level 4 ambulators.

The functional outcome at transfemoral amputation generally depends on proximal muscle strength, the residual limb length, and the overall status of the patient. With a long residual limb and normal muscle strength, a transfemoral amputee should be able to ambulate without any assistive device, but running and higher-level activities may be very demanding. Amputation of more than 50% of femur length will often require an assistive device for ambulation.

Hip Disarticulation

The socket design for hip disarticulation includes a custom-molded bucket that incorporates much of the pelvic structures. This would include a rigid outer frame around the involved side with weight-bearing primarily through the gluteal muscle and ischial tuberosity, and a semirigid or elastic component that wraps around the waist and pelvis on the contralateral side. A specialized hip joint is used, which stays in extension throughout the gait cycle and flexes only for sitting activities. Typically, very light-weight components are used for hip disarticulation amputation because of the lack of leverage for control of the prosthesis. A common selection of components would include a light-weight stance control knee and a single-axis or multi-axis foot. The functional outcome at hip disarticulation level is quite variable. Approximately 50% of patients at the hip disarticulation level do not use a prosthesis and ambulate with two forearm crutches, hopping on the remaining leg. The patients that do ambulate with a prosthesis will nearly always need at least one assistive device for stability. Some patients at this level would choose wheelchair mobility because of the high energy cost at this level of amputation.

Lower Extremity Orthotics

Introduction

Most lower limb orthoses are named by a universal terminology where the name describes the joints that are involved, as well as any special features. Most lower limb orthoses are custom made, but there are some that are custom fit or off-the-shelf. Most lower limb orthoses also incorporate some type of footwear and, therefore, we will discuss orthopedic shoes in the next section.

Orthopedic Shoes

Common features of an orthopedic shoe include the following:

1. Extra depth with removable innersole to accommodate an orthosis.
2. Blucher opening to allow easier access into the shoe.
3. Rounded and higher toe box.
4. Availability of very wide widths.
5. Strong heel counter to support rearfoot.

Options available for shoes include the following:

1. Crepe or leather sole.
2. High top.
3. Surgical opening.
4. Velcro closure.
5. High toe box.
6. Bunion last or contour.
7. Modifications at the heel, such as wedging, flaring, or lifts.
8. Outside buttress to support the arch.

Common indications for orthopedic shoes would include diabetic foot, dysvascular foot, orthopedic deformities, such as bunion or hammertoes, or to accommodate an orthosis.

Foot Orthosis

Generally, foot orthoses are divided into two categories: accommodative and corrective. The accommodative foot orthotic is generally soft to medium, multidensity materials that help redistribute pressure on the foot. These are often custom-made, but can be off-the-shelf if the foot has normal architecture. Common materials used are Thermocork, Plastazote, and leather. Indications would include diabetic and dysvascular foot with callous formation or ulceration. The corrective foot orthotic is often a semirigid material that helps control or change the positioning of rearfoot, midfoot, or forefoot. They should be custom-made and are fabricated from a firm Plastazote, cork, plastic, or even carbon fiber material. The indications for corrective foot orthotics include calcaneal varus or valgus, correctable pes planus, excessive pronation or supination, or chronic plantar fasciitis. Additional options for foot orthoses include a metatarsal pad to unload the metatarsal heads nos. 2, 3, and 4, or a metatarsal bar to unload 1–5.

University of California Biomechanics Laboratory Orthosis

This is a custom thermoplastic orthosis that controls the calcaneous and crosses the subtalar joint but generally stays at the level of the standard orthopedic shoe. It provides rigid rearfoot and midfoot control, and the indication is for early Charcot joint or posterior tibialis tendon dysfunction. The major drawback is the concern of tissue tolerance to such rigid control.

Supramalleolar Orthosis

This is a short, hinged ankle–foot orthosis (AFO) made of plastic or carbon to control ML instability of the ankle, short-term or long-term. It is generally tolerated better by children than adults, but can be used short-term for a variety of ligamentous or tendon sprain and strain injuries across the ankle.

Ankle–Foot Orthosis

This is a very common lower limb orthotic device that can be divided into categories of plastic or metal. The plastic design is used most often and is custom fabricated from a cast or molding of the patient's limb. Some off-the-shelf designs may be suitable for short-term use, but custom designs are better for long-term use. The general features of a plastic AFO would include the trimlines (degree of rigidity), degrees of dorsiflexion, and foot plate design.

1. *PLS design* is the most flexible design for flaccid footdrop, and is typically set in 5–7° of dorsiflexion with very low-profile three-quarters-length footplate.
2. *Just behind the malleolus* is a less flexible design with somewhat more ML control commonly set in 3–4° of dorsiflexion. This trimline is most commonly used after stroke or other disease with moderate or low tone.
3. *Midmalleolar trimline* is most commonly used in patients with increased tone, and provides excellent ML stability with little or no flexibility in the anterioposterior plane. This can also incorporate tone reducing features in the footplate or 3-point inversion control. Because of its rigid nature, this design is set at 0–3° of dorsiflexion.
4. *Anterior trimline* provides very rigid control with no motion in anterio-posterior or ML direction. This design is used for the most spastic patient and is usually set in a neutral position with a full footplate incorporating the toes to prevent curling of the toes over the edge.

Plastic AFOs can also incorporate several special features:

1. *Hinged joints*, which will allow some dorsiflexion and limited plantar flexion, but are less adjustable than metal AFO joints.
2. *Footplate designs* can incorporate three-quarter length, which stops just before the metatarsal heads for easier access into shoes, or a full length footplate with padding, which is generally used for the most spastic or most vulnerable foot.
3. *Inversion control features* include a high medial wall on the footplate and a large lateral phalange at the fibula to prevent inversion positioning of the foot in the brace.

Metal AFOs are still used for several indications, including the insensate foot, the foot with fluctuating edema, or when the need for adjustability or progressive changes in the device are indicated. The metal AFO has two metal uprights connected proximally by a rigid calf band and extends down to the ankle joint into a stirrup, which then attaches to the shoe. The ankle joint can be of two types:

1. *Single-channel ankle joints* can provide dorsiflexion assistance and a plantar flexion stop, and are the most commonly used.
2. *Dual-channel ankle joints* can provide control both in the dorsiflexion and plantar flexion directions, and can lock the ankle joint in any selected position. Using a set screw in the ankle joint makes adjustments easy. Hybrid designs can also incorporate metal uprights to a plastic footplate, which would then allow changing the shoe on a daily basis. A very wide shoe must be used to accommodate the ankle joint and the plastic footplate.

Patellar Tendon-Bearing Orthosis

This device provides proximal loading of the leg to unload the foot and ankle because of disease or injury. Generally, 50% unloading is expected with this device, and more can be accomplished with the use of assistive devices in both arms. Generally, there are two types of patellar tendon-bearing (PTB) orthoses used:

1. A *bi-valve plastic clamshell* is incorporated in the upper third of the tibia similar to a PTB socket in prosthesis. Metal uprights then extend down to an ankle joint and to an orthopedic shoe. This relies on consistent limb volume, and there can be concerns about tissue tolerance owing to the plastic shell at the knee.
2. A *calf corset design* PTB orthosis includes a laced corset, which incorporates the upper two-thirds of the tibia, and can accommodate volume changes easily. This device, however, is more user-dependent in terms of putting on the device correctly. It still incorporates metal uprights to a dual-channel ankle joint and then to a stirrup and the orthopedic shoe. Both types of PTB orthoses can be used for Charcot joint to help unload and limit mobility across the foot and ankle. They can also be used for dysvascular patients with chronic ulcerations on the feet.

Knee–AFO

A knee–AFO (KAFO) is commonly used to control the knee and the ankle, and can incorporate a combination of plastic and metal components. The thigh component can include a plastic thigh shell with Velcro strap closure or metal uprights with thigh bands. The thigh components of both types are connected to a knee joint. There are six common types of knee joints:

1. *Drop lock* will lock at full extension or unlocks to allow full flexion.
2. *Bail lock* is a spring-loaded joint that locks automatically as the leg reaches full extension, and can be unlocked by reaching back and pulling a metal loop in the back or gently bumping against the chair. This is com-

monly used in paraplegia when two KAFOs are necessary for "hands-free operation."
3. *Ratchet lock* has an incremental locking mechanism every 7–10° to gradually stretch the knee following contracture or spasticity.
4. *Offset knee joint* has a posterior offset axis to allow inherent stability from 0 to 30°.
5. *Trick knee* has a locking mechanism, but still allows up to 25° of flexion, even in its locked position, to mimic normal gait patterns.
6. *Stance-locking knee* is an electromechanical locking mechanism that locks the knee in extension at heel strike and releases at toe-off for normal swing phase.

KAFO designs can be all metal, plastic, carbon fiber, or a hybrid of any of these materials. KAFOs are commonly used for instability of the knee and ankle, such as stroke with hemiparesis, but also for other diseases, such as Guillain-Barré, polio, lumbar spinal injury, or severe peripheral neuropathy.

Hip–KAFO

A hip–KAFO (HKAFO) is a device that stabilizes the hip joint in addition to the knee and ankle joint. All of the features of the KAFO described under the previous subheading will be used, in addition to a hip joint and waist belt. Hip joints can allow free motion, limited motion, or can be locked. They are most often used for paraplegia for limited ambulation with bilateral crutches. Specialized designs include the reciprocal gait orthosis.

Hip joints can also be used in a hip abduction orthosis, which is used commonly after hip dislocation or in higher risk patients after total hip replacement. This device keeps the hip at 30° of abduction and blocks hip flexion at 70–90° to prevent dislocation.

Upper Extremity Prosthetics

Introduction

There are approximately 5000–10,000 major upper limb amputations per year, and they are most commonly caused by trauma. The most common group is males aged 15–50 years. In the younger age group of 1–15 years old, congenital deficiency and cancers can also lead to upper limb amputation. The distribution of amputation is generally two-thirds below the level of the elbow and one-third above. The levels of upper limb amputation are indicated in Fig. 2.

Digit Amputation

Functional issues should dictate prosthetic restoration versus reconstructive surgery at this level. Prosthetic restoration of single or multiple digits

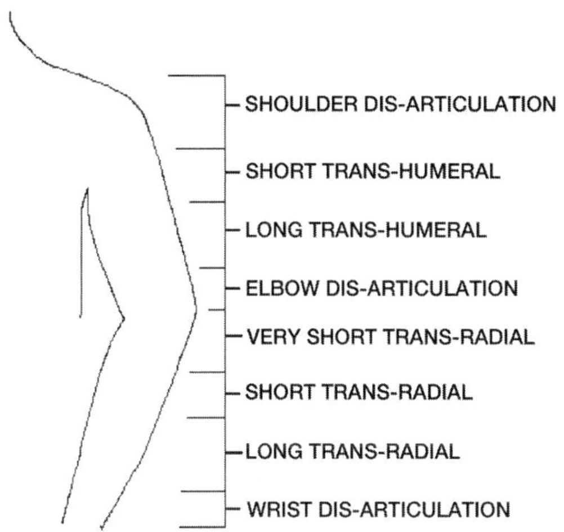

Fig. 2. Diagram for levels of upper limb amputation.

may conflict with function of the remaining digits and may cover sensate areas of the hand or digits. Each digit has a specialized function, and its importance to the individual patient may be determined by their functional activities. The thumb is the most important digit because it opposes all other fingers to give fine motor control and gross grasp. The index and middle fingers work together to give pinch and the best fine motor dexterity. The fourth and fifth fingers work together to provide gross grasp and a strong power grip. This may be most critical to laborers or those who rely on manipulating larger objects. Hand or finger reconstruction should always be considered, including toe transplantation to replace a thumb or other major digit. Many patients will choose to use a cosmetic prosthetic device for certain social activities, but no prosthetic device may be necessary for most of their functional tasks if there is at least the thumb and one finger remaining.

Mitt Amputation

With mitt amputation, there is loss of all fingers and thumb with preservation of the metacarpals. This is a very awkward and difficult level of amputation because there is no good prosthetic restoration available. Reconstructive surgery options are also limited and, therefore, further amputation at the level of the wrist may provide a more appropriate functional outcome.

Partial Hand Amputation

This refers to any combination of loss of digits and metacarpals, and can be particularly devastating if there is loss of the thumb. The function is difficult to restore through the use of prosthesis, and reconstructive surgery should be strongly considered. Custom silicone restoration prostheses may give a nice cosmetic outcome, but provide little or no functional improvement. In fact, most silicone restoration prostheses will have a glove-type suspension, which will cover sensate areas and limit active range of motion (ROM) of remaining segments. Prosthetic options at this level may include a Handi-Hook device strapped to the palm of the hand and controlled through a single cable to the opposite axilla. Sometimes, a unique prosthetic device may be fashioned for a specific task or activity.

Wrist Disarticulation Amputation

This level of amputation has distinct advantages with maximum pronation and supination preserved and good leverage for lifting, pushing, and pulling activities with or without a prosthesis. However, the disadvantages include a bulky distal end and limitations on some wrist and hand components because of lack of space. There are two prosthetic options:

1. A *body-powered prosthesis* is most commonly used at wrist disarticulation with a hook or hand terminal device. This will include a thin wrist unit to change or reposition terminal devices, which also helps to minimize length discrepancy between the amputated limb and the intact limb. A rigid socket with soft interface incorporates approximately two-thirds of the distal forearm and yet allows some remaining pronation and supination mobility of the prosthetic device. The suspension is a *figure-9 harness* with a control cable from the terminal device to an axilla loop proximally around the contralateral limb. The terminal device is opened by biscapular abduction or forward humeral flexion. The terminal device options include *voluntary opening hooks*, *voluntary closing hooks*, and *functional hands*. Use of the terminal device for functional grasp and manipulation of an object is very good at the wrist disarticulation level, but declines steadily with more proximal levels of amputation.
2. A *myoelectric prosthesis* may also be fabricated at the wrist disarticulation level and would include a suction socket with surface electrodes over the forearm flexors and extensors. Muscle activity is detected by the surface electrodes to control the motorized hand or hook terminal device. Some disadvantages of the myoelectric device include an overall bulkier and heavier prosthetic device and the necessity to recharge batteries on a regular basis.

Transradial Amputation

This level is divided into three distinct lengths as outlined in Fig. 2. The *long transradial amputation* preserves 55–90% of radius and ulna, and represents the ideal length because it preserves most of the pronation and supination ROM, allows good leverage for lifting, pushing, and pulling activities, and allows adequate room for most electric- or body-powered wrist units and terminal devices. For most individuals, a suction socket with a myoelectric terminal device is a good option with good functional outcome and cosmesis. No harnessing is required. However, other individuals involved in more heavy-duty or outdoor activities may still prefer a cable-powered prosthesis with hook or hand terminal device and figure-9 harness. The *short transradial amputation* preserves 30–55% of radius and ulna length and still provides moderate stability for lifting, pulling, and pushing activities with a prosthesis. However, no pronation or supination is preserved at this level. Prosthetic options include both myoelectric control and cable control as outlined in the Subheading entitled "Wrist Disarticulation Amputation." However, the myoelectric design may require suspension over the humeral condyles for additional support and rotational control. The cable prosthesis will now require a double wall socket with flexible elbow hinges to a triceps cuff and *figure-8 harness* with an additional suspension strap anteriorly.

With *very short transradial amputation* there is less than 30% of the radius and ulna remaining, but there must be preservation of biceps muscle insertion to maintain active elbow flexion. This is a difficult level to fit because of the limited length of the residual limb and the limited leverage for lifting, pushing, and pulling activities. The socket design must be supracondylar and may limit elbow flexion and extension. Myoelectric prosthetic control may still work at this level using a suction socket, but supplemental suspension may be necessary from an additional elastic sleeve or harness. A cable-powered prosthesis at this level may require a rigid elbow joint or step-up joint to improve elbow flexion ROM, in addition to the triceps cuff and figure-8 harness.

Elbow Disarticulation Amputation

The advantages of this level of amputation include better leverage for lifting, pushing, or pulling than transhumeral amputation. Also, the humeral condyles can be used to control internal and external rotation of the prosthesis. However, disadvantages include a bulky distal end, which makes for a bulky socket design with little or no room for elbow joints. Myoelectric prosthetic designs may be limited at this level because of the lack of space needed for electrically controlled elbow joints. Therefore, a *hybrid system* using cable power at the elbow to figure-8 harness should be used along with an electronic hand or wrist rotator using the biceps and triceps muscle for myoelectric control. A cable-powered prosthesis would include a rigid socket with thin soft interface, socket trimlines below the acromion, a figure-8 harness, external locking elbow joint, and dual-control cable system. The posterior control cable will operate the terminal device and position the elbow. A second anterior cable will be used for locking and unlocking the elbow mechanism. At this level of amputation, external elbow joints must be used owing to lack of space. Proper positioning of the attachment points of the posterior control cable are critical, both on the socket and on the forearm shell. The initial pull on the posterior control cable using biscapular abduction will initiate elbow flexion. Once the elbow is properly positioned, the elbow must be locked with a "down, back, and out" maneuver of the shoulder, then further biscapular abduction or forward humeral flexion will open the terminal device. Once the object is grasped in the terminal device, it is difficult to reposition the elbow; therefore, initial elbow positioning is critical.

Transhumeral Amputation

Functional use of any prosthesis declines rapidly at this level. Similar to transradial amputation, there are three distinct levels of amputation at the humerus. *Long transhumeral amputation* preserves 50–90% of humeral length and is ideal for this level of amputation, with the greatest leverage for lifting, pushing, and pulling activities but allowing adequate room for appropriate electric elbow units. Prosthetic options at this level would include a full cable-powered prosthesis, myoelectric prosthesis, hybrid prosthesis, and cosmetic prosthesis. A full cable-powered prosthesis would include a rigid socket with soft interface, figure-8 harness, dual-control cables, internal locking elbow unit, rigid forearm shell, wrist unit, and terminal device. Control of the cable-powered device is the same as elbow disarticulation. Elbow flexion is first initiated by biscapular abduction to pull on the posterior control cable. Once the elbow is positioned, it could be locked with the "down, back, and out" maneuver at the shoulder. Further excursion of the posterior control cable will now open the terminal device. Because of the difficulty with repostioning the elbow once the terminal device is activated, a hybrid prosthesis with cable-powered elbow and electric controlled hand is often recommended to allow independent functioning of the elbow and the hand devices. A fully myoelectric prosthesis can be used at this level using biceps and triceps muscle sites to control elbow flexion/extension and hand open/close. This is accomplished by signaling the prosthesis to switch from elbow to hand function with co-contraction of the biceps and triceps muscles. The disadvantages of myoelectric control at this level include increasing cost and increasing weight of the prosthetic device. *Short transhumeral amputation* preserves 30–50% of humerus, but the ability to push, pull, or lift with the prosthesis is significantly limited. The socket design will commonly include the acromion to provide extra stability and weight-bearing of the prosthesis. This will eliminate much of the active ROM of the shoulder, hence reducing excursion for a cable-powered system and limited ability to reach with the prosthesis. Prosthetic designs otherwise are similar to those described for the long transhumeral amputation. *Very short transhumeral amputation* preserves only 30% or less of humeral length. This is also commonly called "humeral neck amputation" and is functionally grouped together with shoulder disarticulation because there is no effective way to capture the movement of the humerus. It is still important to leave the short segment of humerus in place because it provides better contour of the shoulder, better cushioning of the shoulder, and the potential of residual muscles attached to the humerus, which may be used for myoelectric control.

Shoulder Disarticulation Amputation

This level is functionally very difficult to fit with a prosthesis because control of the prosthesis comes exclusively from proximal, trunk-based muscles for myoelectric control or scapulo-thoracic movement for cable control. The socket design will cover the entire shoulder like a cap to distribute the weight of the prosthesis. A shoulder joint with passive positioning can be used or the shoulder can be fixed in one position in the prosthesis. Generally, a myoelectric control prosthesis at shoulder disarticulation level will be difficult to control and difficult to weight-manage. Some patients will choose a hybrid design with a fixed passive shoulder joint, cable-powered elbow joint, and myoelectrically controlled hand to minimize the weight and complexity. This prosthetic device will be, at best, a helper for the remaining limb. Some patients will choose a light-weight cosmetic prosthesis or no prosthesis at all.

Forequarter Amputation

At this level of amputation, there is loss of the entire upper limb and scapula. There is no effective control mechanism for cable power and there are very few residual muscles for myoelectric control. Most patients will choose a cosmetic prosthesis or no prosthesis at all at this level.

Specialty Terminal Devices

There are a variety of specialized terminal devices for specific tasks. Many of them are available for cable-powered or myoelectric control systems.

1. *Robotic terminal devices*, such as the Greifer or Steeper, provide parallel jaws for better grip of both small and large objects.
2. *Waterproof terminal devices* including a myoelectric hook for active outdoor and sports use.
3. *Activity-specific terminal devices* can be designed for golf, skiing, photography, swimming, or even certain types of sports gloves and mitts. There is also a series of mechanic's tools and kitchen utensils that are plugged directly into the wrist unit of the prosthesis.

Upper Extremity Orthotics

Introduction

Upper limb orthoses can be described by the joints or segments that they cross and any special design features incorporated. These should also be described as a static, dynamic, or hybrid system. A static orthosis remains fixed in one position with no movement across the joint. A dynamic orthosis increases or decreases movement across the joint. In contrast to lower limb orthoses, many upper limb orthoses can be fabricated from a kit or purchased off the shelf from a catalog or medical supplier.

Finger Orthosis

There are three common types of finger orthoses used:

1. For fracture, ligamentous injury, or inflammatory disease a *static gutter splint* or *circumferential splint* is used to eliminate motion across interphalangeal (IP) joints.
2. For contracture across an IP joint, a *dynamic finger orthosis* with spring wire or rubber bands is used.
3. For progressive deformity from disease, such as rheumatoid arthritis, a specialized finger orthosis called a *ring orthosis* can be used. This is used to control swan neck deformity and Boutonniere's deformity.

Hand–Finger Orthosis

These are commonly used to control the digits or metacarpophalangeal (MCP) joints from a device positioned across the palmar or dorsal surface of the hand.

1. For rheumatoid arthritis at the base of the thumb or deQuervain's tendonitis, the thumb can be controlled with a static hand–finger orthosis stabilizing the thumb commonly called a *thumb spica*.

2. Median nerve injury at the distal forearm or wrist will cause loss of motor function of the thumb. A *short opponens orthosis* is fabricated from plastic to position the thumb opposite the fingers while maintaining first web space.
3. Ulnar nerve injury causes "intrinsic minus" hand positioning with hyperextension of the MCPs. This can be treated with a *hand–finger orthosis with MCP block* in slight flexion. This allows better functioning of the long finger flexors and extensors.
4. Flexion–extension contracture across the MCP joints can be treated with a dynamic hand–finger orthosis commonly called a *knuckle bender* using spring wire or rubber bands.

Wrist–Hand–Finger Orthoses

These devices range from very simple, off-the-shelf products to complex, custom-made devices.

1. The simplest and most common device to cross the wrist is the *cock-up splint* for carpal tunnel syndrome. This device positions the wrist in its neutral or slightly extended position to minimize pressure within the carpal tunnel.
2. Stroke patients with little or no function in the affected hand can be positioned properly with a *static wrist–hand–finger orthosis*, maintaining the wrist in neutral, MCPs in slight flexion, and IP joints in extension. The thumb must always be maintained in its position of opposition to the fingers.
3. Low radial nerve injury causes wrist drop and inability to extend the fingers. A *dynamic wrist–hand–finger orthosis* with extension positioning of the wrist and fingers using outriggers and rubber bands should be used. The patient can still flex the fingers and wrist for grasp and functional activities. However, when the patient relaxes, the rubber bands extend the fingers to open the hand.
4. With C6-level quadriplegia, active wrist extension is preserved but finger flexion and grasp is lost. A *tenodesis or flexor hinge orthosis* is commonly used to restore grasp or prehension. This is a dynamic wrist–hand–finger orthosis that uses active wrist extension to drive the second and third fingers against the thumb for grasp. There are several designs available both by kit and custom fabrication.

Elbow Orthosis

Flexion or extension contractures at the elbow are common after immobilization of the upper limb from fractures, burns, surgery, or other injury. A *dynamic elbow orthosis* with adjustable tension in flexion or extension is commonly used to stretch the contractures. Elbow orthoses with adjustable ROM joints are also available postoperatively to slowly restore active movement at the joint as healing occurs.

Shoulder Orthoses

Generally, there are two types of devices applied across the shoulder joint:

1. In acute injury or surgery, the shoulder can be fixed in nearly any position using an *airplane* or *gunslinger* type of device. This provides unloading of the weight of the limb to prevent subluxation of the gleno-humeral joint, and can allow limited or no movement for healing of soft or bony tissues.
2. Following stroke or brachial plexus injury, the gleno-humeral joint may be at risk for subluxation and chronic pain. A *non-elastic humeral cuff* or *sling* can be applied to maintain gleno-humeral positioning.

Definitions

Prosthesis: A device that replaces an absent body part.

Prosthetics: The field of design and fabrication of the devices to replace a body part.

Prosthetist: A certified practitioner who designs and fabricates a prosthesis.

Orthosis: A device that supports an existing body part.

Orthotics: The field of design and fabrication of any type of brace device.

Orthotist: The certified practitioner who designs and fabricates an orthosis.

Key References and Suggested Additional Reading

Braddom RL, ed. Physical Medicine and Rehabilitation. Philadelphia: W.B. Saunders, 2000:263–352.

Cuccurullo SJ ed. Physical Medicine and Rehabilitation Board Review. New York: Demos Medical Publishing, 2004:409–487.

Delisa JA, ed. Physical Medicine and Rehabilitation: Principles and Practice. Philadelphia: Lippincott, Williams, and Wilkins, 2005:1325–1391.

Meier RH, Atkins DJ, eds. Functional Restoration of Adults and Children With Upper Extremity Amputation. New York: Demos Medical Publishing, 2004: 159–287.

Seymour R, ed. Prosthetics and Orthotics: Lower Limb and Spine. Lippincott, Williams, and Wilkins, 2002.

5 Cardiac Rehabilitation

Mathew N. Bartels

Epidemiology of Heart Disease

Cardiac disease is a leading cause of morbidity and mortality in the adult population in the United States. The rates of morbidity and mortality from cardiac disease have been steadily declining owing to more aggressive management and public heath awareness. Still, the death rate of coronary artery disease (CAD) was 228.1 per 100,000 population in 1970, and 94.9 per 100,000 in 1994. CAD is also one of the main causes of disability in the United States, with an estimated 7.9 million Americans age 15 years and older with disabilities from cardiovascular conditions in 1991–1992, representing approximately 19% of disabilities from all conditions. Cardiac disease also accounts for a large portion of the total health care expenditures. In 1992, there were 3.9 million hospital admissions, including 2.1 million hospital admissions for myocardial infarction (MI), 800,000 admissions for congestive heart failure (CHF), and 550,000 admissions for arrhythmias. Procedures are also a large part of the hospitalizations, with more than 1 million cardiac catheterizations and 300,000 coronary artery bypass grafts (CABG) performed.

Additionally, new technologies and advances in care of end-stage CHF, transplant, and implantable devices have led to ever increasing numbers of patients with cardiac disease who can benefit from rehabilitation services. The survival from acute events and the widespread use of surgical procedures also has led to an ever increasing number of individuals with dual disability as well, with CAD, CHF, stroke, spinal cord injury, peripheral vascular disease, or other traditional rehabilitation diagnoses as comorbidi-

From: *Essential Physical Medicine and Rehabilitation*
Edited by: G. Cooper © Humana Press Inc., Totowa, NJ

ties. A good understanding of the basic principles in management of cardiac rehabilitation will help to care for these patients in the rehabilitation setting.

Types of Heart Disease

There are generally four types of cardiac disease that will commonly be encountered by the practicing physiatrist.

1. Because of protocols and improvement in acute management, cardiac rehabilitation of the post-MI patient is now usually handled in an acute 3- to 5-day hospital stay, followed by outpatient rehabilitation.
2. Post-surgical patients, including those who have had CABG, valve replacement, cardiac defect repairs, and devices implanted (automatic internal cardiac defibrillators, etc.), usually will have a smooth and uncomplicated course. Advances in surgery have also made CABG less invasive for many (minimally invasive CABG, off-pump CABG, and robotic surgery are just a few new techniques), but have also expanded the populations to whom these interventions are being offered. This can increase the risk of complications postoperatively in more debilitated patients, and the presence of comorbidities and the possibility of a long, debilitating postoperative course is increased, leading to the need for more intensive rehabilitation interventions.
3. Unlike in the past, the patient with severe CHF or severe arrhythmias is now being referred for cardiac rehabilitation. With appropriate precautions and monitoring, rehabilitation can be very successful in these populations.
4. Finally, the population of transplant patients has their own unique physiology and issues, which make the services of rehabilitation especially helpful in that population.

All of these different populations will be discussed separately in later portions of this chapter.

Overview of Cardiac Rehabilitation

Unfortunately, although rehabilitation services are often available for patients who are eligible for cardiac rehabilitation, only 10–15% of the 1 million survivors of acute MI go on to take part in a cardiac rehabilitation program. The basic goals of cardiac rehabilitation are to restore and improve cardiac function, reduce disability, identify and improve cardiac risk factors, and increase cardiac conditioning. A cardiac rehabilitation program achieves these goals through a program of education, behavior modification, secondary prevention, and exercise. A program of rehabilitation may allow an older debilitated individual to resume activities of normal life without significant cardiac symptomatology. Each of the different types of

Table 1
Coronary Artery Disease Risk Factors

Reversible risks	*Irreversible risks*
• Sedentary lifestyle • Cigarette smoking • Hypertension • Low HDL cholesterol (<0.9 mmol/L [35 mg/dL]) • Hypercholesterolemia (>5.20 mmol/L [200 mg/dL]) • High lipoprotein A • Abdominal obesity • Hypertriglyceridemia (>2.8 mmol/L [250 mg/dL]) • Hyperinsulinemia • Diabetes mellitus	• Age • Male gender • Family history of premature CAD (before age 55 in a parent or sibling) • Past history of CAD • Past history of occlusive peripheral vascular disease • Past history of cerebrovascular disease

CAD, coronary artery disease; HDL, high-density lipoprotein.

cardiac disease lend themselves to a different form of rehabilitation, and the benefits of cardiac conditioning and improved survival are well-documented by numerous studies.

Classic Post-MI Cardiac Rehabilitation Program

Risk-Factor Modification

An essential part of any cardiac rehabilitation program is achievement of a healthier lifestyle through a program of cardiac risk-factor modification. Cardiac risk factors (Table 1) are divided into two major groups: reversible and irreversible risk factors. Irreversible risk factors include male gender, past history of vascular disease, age, and family history. The patient and family have to be educated on the presence of risks, and where appropriate, family counseling can be added. Early and aggressive attention to reversible risk factors is essential in individuals with significant irreversible risks. Reversible risk factors for cardiac disease include obesity, sedentary lifestyle, hyperlipidemia, cigarette smoking, and conditions such as diabetes mellitus and hypertension. Modification of these risk factors is a part of a cardiac rehabilitation program, and should be part of a "heart healthy" lifestyle for all individuals. These same principles also need be applied to the disabled population because they often are at further increased risk through weight loss, immobility, and deconditioning.

Diabetes

Close control of blood sugars has been shown to decrease the risk of cardiac disease through the slowing of the development of atherosclerosis and secondary conditions, such as nephrogenic hypertension. Exercise training can also help to improve diabetic control. The exact benefits of exercise training in combination with good glucose control are still being elucidated.

Hypertension

Control of hypertension has been shown to be beneficial in individuals with normal cardiograms. Reduction of dietary salt and increased exercise to improve conditioning in combination with pharmacological management can significantly improve blood pressure. The major agents for the control of hypertension are divided into β-blockers, α-blockers, diuretics, calcium channel blockers, and angiotensin-converting enzyme inhibitors. Because of the combination of antihypertensive effects and lower myocardial cardiac oxygen consumption through decreased inotropy and heart rate, β-blockers are the most effective agents. Diuretics and angiotensin-converting enzyme inhibitors have also been shown in large trials to have beneficial effects on decreasing cardiac mortality. The cardiac effects of calcium channel blockers are not clear, but some early data may indicate an actual increase in MI with certain agents, and it is recommended that rehabilitation physicians seek the advice of the treating cardiologist or internist for assistance in the optimal management of each individual patient.

Hypercholesterolemia

Lowering cholesterol levels and increasing high-density lipoprotein is associated with decreased risk of cardiac disease. Patients can decrease their lipids by adhering to a low-cholesterol, low-fat diet along with weight reduction, even without the addition of exercise. The American Heart Association recommends that the total amount of calories from fat in the diet should not exceed 30%. Control of cholesterol can be achieved through a three-step program, as outlined in the National Cholesterol Education Program guidelines. Phase 1 is an adoption of nutritional guidelines, lifestyle changes, and general improvement in health habits. Phase II adds fiber supplements and possibly nicotinic acid. Phase III includes lipid-lowering drugs. Lipid-lowering programs have been shown to retard the progression of CAD. With the addition of physical activity, high-density lipoprotein cholesterol concentration can rise 5–16%, but the data on the lowering of low-density lipoprotein cholesterol is still controversial.

Obesity

The multiple metabolic syndrome of obesity, diabetes, hypertension, and hyperlipidemia is associated with increased morbidity and mortality, and the obesity is at the center of the syndrome. Weight loss can decrease blood pressure, improve lipid profile, and improve diabetic control, as well as improve the ability to perform exercise. Attention to proper weight needs to be part of any cardiac rehabilitation program.

Cigarette Smoking

Cigarette smoking is one of the greatest single modifiable risk factors for cardiac disease. Smoking cessation is associated with a 30% decrease in 10-year mortality in individuals with angiographically demonstrated CAD or MI. Smoking accelerates atherosclerosis, contributes to hypertension, and is associated with a sedentary lifestyle. Smokers tend to be less compliant in cardiac rehabilitation programs, and exercise is not associated with decreased cigarette use. However, cardiac rehabilitation coupled with counseling for smoking cessation can lead to a decrease in smoking. Although smoking cessation programs are not a primary rehabilitation function, awareness of available resources and appropriate referrals for patients should be available for all smokers with cardiac or other disease.

Cardiac Anatomy

A good understanding of cardiac anatomy helps in providing cardiac rehabilitation. Of particular importance is a familiarity with the normal distribution of the major arteries of the heart with ischemic distributions and valvular anatomy. Some important functional and anatomical issues are briefly covered here.

The cardiac conduction system facilitates the appropriate sequencing of the contraction of the atria and ventricles at the physiologically appropriate rate. Conduction blocks can occur as a result of MIs, aging, and other conditions. Abnormalities of cardiac conductions, such as congenital defects and accessory tracts, can lead to arrhythmias, both atrial and ventricular, which can lead to life-threatening arrhythmias.

Normally, there are left and right coronary arteries arising from the base of the aorta in the left and right aortic sinuses. The left main coronary artery divides into the left anterior descending and the circumflex arteries, whereas the right coronary artery continues on as a single vessel. Approximately 60% of individuals have right-dominant circulation. Approximately 10–15% of individuals have the posterior descending arise from the left circumflex, in left-dominant circulation. About 30% of individuals have the

Table 2
The Distributions of Infarcts by Anatomy

	Area of infarct	*Associated syndrome*
Left anterior descending	• Anterior wall and septum	• Papillary muscle necrosis • Left heart failure • Left ventricular aneurysm • Anterior wall thrombus • Conduction block • Sudden death
Left circumflex	• Apex and lateral wall	• Apical thrombus • Left heart failure
Left main coronary artery	• Anterior and lateral wall apex	• Massive congestive heart failure • Left ventricular aneurysm • Anterior wall thrombus • Conduction block • Sudden death
Right coronary artery	• Inferior wall and right ventrical	• Sinus node arrest • Bradycardia • Right ventricular failure • Peripheral edema

posterior descending arise from the left circumflex and right coronary arteries in what is described as balanced circulation. Table 2 lists the anatomy and the distributions of infarcts with a description of associated cardiac syndromes.

Cardiac Physiology

The heart is among the most metabolically active organs in the body. Oxygen extraction is nearly maximal at all levels of activity and is nearly 65% (compared with 36% for brain and 26% for the rest of the body). The heart prefers to metabolize aerobically, but is able to perform both anaerobic and aerobic metabolism. Cardiac metabolism uses 40% carbohydrates, with fatty acids making up most of the rest. Coronary blood flow is limited to diastole, especially in the endocardium. In order to meet the demands of exercise, the coronary arteries must dilate, using nitric oxide-mediated pathways. The goal of medical, rehabilitation, and surgical therapies is to restore normal blood flow to the myocardium.

The ability of the heart to generate an increase in cardiac output (CO) is related to the increase in venous return, which increases the length of the myocardial fibers in diastole prior to the initiation of cardiac contraction. With stretch, the overlap of the actin and myosin fibers is maximized and the strength of contraction is maximized. With overstretching, the overlap of myosin and actin begins to decrease, and the strength of contraction declines. This relationship is seen in the Frank–Starling relationship. This is part of the contractile changes in patients with cardiomyopathy, who are so overstretched that they can only increase CO by decreasing myofibril length. Atrial contraction is also important because atrial filling of the ventricles can add 15–20% to the total CO, especially with increased heart rate and in conditions with decreased ventricular compliance. Loss of this atrial "kick" is important in heart failure combined with atrial dysfunction, such as atrial fibrillation.

Basic Cardiac Vocabulary

Aerobic Capacity

Aerobic capacity (VO_2Max) is the work capacity of an individual, and is expressed in milliliters oxygen per kilogram per minute. Oxygen consumption (VO_2) has a linear relationship with workload, increasing up to a plateau which occurs at the VO_2Max. VO_2 reaches steady state after approximately 3–6 minutes of exercise. A decrease in efficiency is represented by an increase in the slope of the line between VO_2 and workload. The work done at submaximal effort is expressed as a percentage defined by VO_2 divided by VO_2Max. The use of percent VO_2Max allows for normalization of data across individuals and for comparison of activities. VO_2Max has been demonstrated to decrease with age in longitudinal studies, such as the Baltimore Longitudinal Study of Aging.

Heart Rate

Heart rate (HR) has a linear increase in relation to VO_2 or other measures of work. Maximum HR is determined by age and can be roughly estimated by subtracting the age of the individual in years from 220. Even with exercise, the maximum HR continues to decline with age. The slope of the line between HR and VO_2 is an indication of physical conditioning.

Stroke Volume

Stroke volume (SV) is the quantity of blood pumped with each heartbeat. The majority of SV increase occurs in early exercise, with the major determinant of SV being diastolic filling time. SV changes very little in supine exercise, being near maximum at rest, whereas in erect position, it increases in a curvilinear fashion until it reaches maximum at approximately 40% of VO_2Max. SV also decreases with advancing age and in cardiac conditions, which results in decreased compliance, such as left ventricular hypertrophy.

Cardiac Output

CO is the product of the HR and SV. CO increases linearly with work, and in early exercise, is mostly dependent on increased SV, whereas in late exercise, it is mostly determined by increased HR. In general, the relationship between CO and VO_2 is linear with a break in the slope at the anaerobic threshold. The maximum CO is the primary determinant of VO_2Max. CO declines with age without any change in linearity or slope. The CO seen in submaximal work is parallel but lower in upright work compared with supine work. VO_2Max and maximal CO are less in supine than erect positions.

Myocardial Oxygen Consumption

Myocardial oxygen consumption (MVO_2) is the actual oxygen consumption of the heart. MVO_2 rises in a linear fashion with workload, being limited by the anginal threshold. Although MVO_2 can be determined directly with cardiac catheterization, the usual practice is estimate the MVO_2 by using the rate pressure product (RPP). The RPP is the product of the HR and the systolic blood pressure (SBP) divided by 100. In general, activities with the upper extremities and exercises with isometric components to them have a higher MVO_2 for a given VO_2. Activities performed while supine demonstrate a higher MVO_2 at low intensity and a lower MVO_2 at high intensity when compared with activities performed in the erect position. Finally, the MVO_2 increases for any activity when performed in the cold, after smoking, or after eating.

Aerobic Training

Aerobic training is the term to describe exercises that increase cardiopulmonary capacity. The basic principles of aerobic training are dependent on intensity, duration, frequency, and specificity of the exercise.

- *Intensity* of exercise is defined by either the intensity of the exercise performed or the physiological response of the individual. Exercise programs can be directed at a target HR or RPP, a rating of perceived exertion, or at a fixed level of exercise intensity on a treadmill or cycle ergometer. Often, target HR is used for simplicity in writing exercise prescriptions. Often intensity of exercise can be set at 80–85% of the maximum HR determined on a baseline exercise tolerance test (ETT). It is generally accepted that exercises that evoke 60% or more of the maximal HR will have at least some training effect.

- *Duration* of exercise is usually 20–30 minutes, excluding a 5- to 10-minute warm-up and a similar cooling down period after exercising. In general, exercise at lower intensity requires a longer duration to achieve a training effect than exercises at higher intensity.
- *Frequency* of training is defined as the number of exercise periods in a given time, usually expressed in sessions per week. Training programs should be done three times a week at a minimum, and a low exercise program may require five times a week to achieve a training effect.
- *Specificity* of exercise refers to the types of activities that are performed. If a goal is to increase ambulation, walking exercise is preferred because it will give the best benefit. This principle dictates that the types of activities and muscle groups targeted in exercise should be based on the needs of the individual in vocational and recreational activities. This is also referred to as the law of specificity of conditioning, and is commonly referred to in cardiac conditioning programs.

Effects of Exercise Training

- *Aerobic capacity*: The VO_2Max will increase with training. Resting VO_2 is not changed, and VO_2 at a given workload does not change. The changes are specific to the muscle groups that are trained.
- *Cardiac output*: Resting CO is not changed with training. The maximum CO increases with aerobic training. The relationship between VO_2 and CO does not change during training.
- *Heart rate*: The resting HR decreases after aerobic training, and is lower at any given workload. The maximum HR is not changed.
- *Stroke volume*: The SV is increased at rest and at all levels of exercise after aerobic training. It is the increase in SV that permits a decrease in HR at a given workload.
- *Myocardial oxygen capacity*: The maximum MVO_2 does not change, because it is determined by the anginal threshold. However, at any given workload, the MVO_2 is decreased with training. This allows individuals to increase their exercise capacity and improve function. Training will allow performance of activities at MVO_2 below the anginal threshold that were above the anginal threshold before training. Pharmacological interventions can affect the resting and submaximal MVO_2, but only a revascularization procedure, such as angioplasty or coronary bypass sur-

Table 3
Sample Metabolic Equivalent (MET) Levels

Energy costs of activities of daily living	*METs*	*Energy costs of avocational activities*	*METs*
Sitting at rest 1		Backpacking (45 pounds)	6–11
Dressing	2–3	Baseball (competitive)	5–6
Eating	1–2	Baseball (noncompetitive)	4–5
Hygene (sitting)	1–2	Basketball (competitive)	7–12
Hygene (standing)	2–3	Basketball (noncompetitive)	3–9
Sexual intercourse	3–5	Card playing	1–2
Showering	4–5	Cycling, 5 mph	2–3
Tub bathing	2–3	Cycling, 8 mph	4–5
Walking, 1 mph	1–2	Cycling, 10 mph	5–6
Walking, 2 mph	2–3	Cycling, 12 mph	7–8
Walking, 3 mph	3–3.5	Cycling, 13 mph	8–9
Walking, 3.5 mph	3.5–4	Karate	8–12
Walking, 4 mph	5–6	Running 12 minutes/mile	8–9
Climbing up stairs	4–7	Running 11 minutes/mile	9–10
Bed-making	2–6	Running 9 minutes/mile	10–11
Carrying 18 pounds upstairs	7–8	Skiing crosscountry, 3 mph	6–7
Carrying suitcase	6–7	Skiing crosscountry, 5 mph	9–10
Housework (general)	3–4	Skiing downhill	5–9
Mowing lawn (push power mower)	3–5	Skiing water	5–7
Ironing	2–4	Swimming (backstroke)	7–8
Snow shoveling	6–7	Swimming (breaststroke)	8–9
		Swimming (crawl)	9–10
		Television	1–2
		Tennis (singles)	4–9

Continued

gery, can actually affect the maximum MVO_2. A way to look at this is using metabolic equivalents (METs) to assess energy demand for various activities. The MVO_2 at a given MET level will decline, allowing a patient to perform more activities with less risk. A sample of METs is shown in Table 3.

- *Peripheral resistance*: The peripheral resistance (PR) decreases in response to exercise training. The PR is decreased at rest and at all levels of exercise. The decreased PR leads to a lower RPP and a lower MVO_2 at a given workload and at rest.

In summary, training causes benefits in cardiac patients in two major areas: (1) reduced cardiac risk and (2) improved cardiac conditioning.

Table 3 *(Continued)*
Sample Metabolic Equivalent (MET) Levels

Energy costs of vocational activities	*METs*
Assembly line work	3–5
Carpentry (light)	4–5
Carry 20–44 pounds	4–5
Carry 45–64 pounds	5–6
Carry 65–85 pounds	7–8
Chopping wood	7–8
Desk work	1.5–2
Digging ditches	7–8
Handyman	5–6
Janitorial (light)	2–3
Lift 100 pounds	7–10
Painting	4–5
Sawing hardwood	6–8
Sawing softwood	5–6
Sawing (power)	3–4
Shoveling 10 pounds, 10 per minute	6–7
Shoveling 14 pounds, 10 per minute	7–9
Shoveling 16 pounds, 10 per minute	9–12
Tools (heavy)	5–6
Typing	1.5–2
Wood splitting	6–7

Adapted from Dafoe, WA. Table of Energy Requirements for Activities of Daily Living, Household Tasks, Recreational Activities, and Vocational Activities. In: Pashkow FJ, Dafoe WA, eds. Clinical Cardiac Rehabilitation: A Cardiologist's Guide. Baltimore, MD: Wiiliams and Wilkins; 1993: 359–376.

Cardiac rehabilitation after acute MI reduces the risk of mortality by 20–25% in a 3-year follow-up. This benefit has been seen in multiple groups, including in the elderly, women, and postbypass patients.

Abnormal Physiology

Cardiac disease alters normal cardiac physiology. Myocardial infarction decreases the ejection fraction (EF) of the heart, ischemic heart disease will lower the MVO_2 and VO_2Max that can be achieved. Valvular heart disease will decrease the maximum CO, either through stenosis or through valvular insufficiency. The end result of the valve disease is a decreased MVO_2 and VO_2Max and increased VO_2 at any level of submaximal exercise. CHF leads to lower VO_2Max, lower SV, higher resting HRs, and decreased CO. Arrhythmias will decrease CO by lowering SV and altering HRs. In severe disease, cardiac transplantation can correct many of the abnormalities from CHF, but a persistently high HR in a deinnervated heart and a limited ability to increase SV can limit exercise response. The rehabilitation considerations in working with patients who have each of these diseases is discussed in detail later in the Heading entitled "Cardiac Rehabilitation Programs in Special Conditions." The effects of these conditions on physiological responses to exercise are compared with normal individuals in Table 4.

Cardiac Rehabilitation Programs

Cardiac rehabilitation programs consist of primary prevention and secondary prevention with cardiac rehabilitation after manifestation of cardiac disease.

Primary prevention programs focus on the reduction of cardiac risk factors. Education alone can have a profound effect on the rate of cardiac disease. Increased physical activity decreases obesity, lowers SBP, and modifies lipid profiles. Primary prevention should begin in childhood in order to establish healthy behavior patterns for life. Ideally, educational interventions should be started in schools with parental support.

Secondary risk-factor modification programs include all of the features of primary prevention programs. Secondary prevention decreases second cardiac events and lowers mortality post-MI. Multiple studies demonstrate the benefits of lowering cholesterol, including the Oslo Study, the Western Electric Study, the Multiple Risk Factor Intervention Trial, Helsinki Heart Study, the National Heart, Lung, and Blood Institute Type II Study, and others. Cessation of cigarette smoking is essential because the risk of heart disease can return to that of nonsmokers after 2 years of not smoking. Secondary programs can also improve hypertension and diabetes management.

Cardiac Rehabilitation of the Post-MI Patient

The rehabilitation of the post-MI patient follows the principles of the classic model of cardiac rehabilitation as first described by Wenger et al. Cardiac rehabilitation is traditionally divided into four stages or phases. Phase I is the acute phase, immediately following the MI up to discharge. Phase I rehabilitation is characterized by early mobilization. Phase II is the convalescent phase, which is done at home and continues the program

Table 4
Abnormal Physiology in Response to Exercise (as Compared With Normal Individuals)

	Aerobic capacity (VO_2Max)	*Cardiac output*	*Heart rate*	*Stroke volume*	*Myocardial oxygen capacity (MVO_2)*	*Peripheral resistance*
Ischemic heart disease	Lower	Unchanged or lower	Lower, unchanged, or higher	Unchanged or lower	Lower	Lower, unchanged, or higher
Myocardial infarction	Lower	Lower	Lower, unchanged, or higher	Unchanged or lower	Lower	Unchanged or higher
Congestive heart failure	Lower	Lower	Unchanged or higher	Lower	Lower	Higher
Valvular heart disease	Lower	Lower	Unchanged or higher	Lower, unchanged, or higher	Unchanged or lower	Unchanged or higher
Arrhythmias	Unchanged or lower	Unchanged or lower	Lower, unchanged, or higher	Unchanged or lower	Unchanged or lower	Unchanged
Cardiac Transplant	Lower	Lower	Higher at rest, lower at maximum effort	Lower	Lower	Unchanged or higher

Table 5
Wenger Protocol

Step	*Activity*
1	Passive range of motion (ROM); ankle pumps; introduction to the program; self-feeding.
2	As above; also dangle at side of bed.
3	Active-assisted ROM; sitting upright in a chair, light recreation, and use of bedside commode.
4	Increased sitting time; light activities with minimal resistance; patient education.
5	Light activities with moderate resistance; unlimited sitting; seated activities of daily living (ADL).
6	Increased resistance; walking to bathroom; standing ADL; up to 1-hour group meetings.
7	Walking up to 100 feet; standing warm-up exercises.
8	Increased walking; walk down stairs (not up); continued education.
9	Increased exercise program, review energy conservation, and pacing techniques.
10	Increase exercises with light weights and ambulation; begin education on home exercise program.
11	Increased duration of activities.
12	Walk down two flights of stairs; continue to increase resistance in exercises.
13	Continue activities, education, and home exercise program teaching.
14	Walk up and down two flights of stairs; complete instruction in home exercise program and in energy conservation and pacing techniques.

Adapted from Bartels MN. Cardiac rehabilitation. In: Physical Medicine and Rehabilitation: The Complete Approach. Grabois M, ed. Chicago: Blackwell Science, 2000.

started in phase I until the myocardial scar has matured. Phase III is the training phase; this usually starts after 4–6 weeks, and is the classic exercise program of conditioning and education. Phase IV is the maintenance phase, and is devoted to keeping the aerobic conditioning gains made in phase III. Risk-factor modifications are taught and reemphasized throughout all phases.

Acute Phase (Phase I)

The innovation in Dr. Wenger's model of cardiac rehabilitation was early mobilization. The classic Wenger cardiac rehabilitation program is outlined in Table 5. The goal of the original program was to get individuals from bed rest to climbing 2 flights of stairs in 14 days. Under current practices, clinicians have modified the classic program of cardiac rehabilitation to allow stays of 3–5 days after MI. The 14 steps of the classic program are now condensed. Patients are encouraged to be sitting out of bed and in a chair by days 1–2 (steps 1–5), with short distance ambulation and bathroom privileges by days 2–3 (steps 6–9). By days 4–5, the patient learns the home exercise program, climbs stairs, and increases duration of ambulation (steps 10–13). Prior to discharge, the patient has a low-level ETT for risk stratification and completes learning the home program (step 14). Education is started at this time. Cardiac monitoring should be performed under the supervision of a trained physical or occupational therapist or nurse during phase I. The post-MI HR rise should be kept to within 20 bpm of baseline, and the SBP rise within 20 mmHg of baseline. Any decrease of SBP of 10 mmHg or more should stop exercise. The intensity target for the phase I program is activities up to 4 METs, which is within the range of most daily activities.

Convalescent Phase (Phase II)

The convalescent phase is designed to allow the scar over the infarction to mature. The target HR is determined during a low-level ETT, which is performed before discharge and at the end of phase I. This exercise test is performed to a level of 70% maximum HR or a MET level of 5. A Borg rating of perceived exertion scale of 7 (modified scale) or 15 (old scale) can also be used to determine the maximum tolerated exercise. The Borg scale and Modified Borg scale are shown in Table 6. The low-level ETT also has a role for cardiac risk stratification. The classic program consisted of six monitored phase II sessions of 1 hour each with a home exercise program over 6 weeks in the uncomplicated patient. Patients at high risk with the need for monitoring are included in Table 7. A full-level ETT can be performed at the end of the 6-week healing period in preparation for phase III rehabilitation.

Training Phase (Phase III)

The training phase of the cardiac rehabilitation program is started after the symptom-limited full-level ETT. This HR maximum is the one that is used to determine the maximum exertion to be performed by the patient during aerobic training. In patients who are low risk, a program designed to achieve 85% of the maximum HR is safe. Gradation of the program to lower target HRs needs to be tailored to the individual patient based on the results of the ETT and the reason for cessation of exercise. For patients with life threatening arrhythmias or chest pain, a lower target HR should be chosen. Even a target HR of 65–75% of the maximum can be safe and effective in a regular program, and target rates as low as 60% can still yield

Table 6
Borg Scale

Borg scale	*Perceived exertion*	*Modified Borg scale*	*Perceived exertion*
		0.0	Nothing at all
		0.5	Very, very weak
		1.0	Very weak
		1.5	
		2.0	Weak (light)
6		2.5	
7	Very, very light	3.0	Moderate
8		3.5	
9	Very light	4.0	Somewhat strong
10		4.5	
11	Fairly light	5.0	Strong (heavy effort)
12		5.5	
13	Somewhat hard	6.0	
14		6.5	
15	Hard	7.0	Very strong
16		7.5	
17	Very hard	8.0	
18		8.5	
19	Very, very hard	9.0	Very, very strong
20		9.5	
		10.0	Maximal

a training benefit. For the patients at higher risk, monitoring at each increase in activity level is appropriate.

The classic duration of a cardiac training program is 3 sessions per week for 6–8 weeks. As limitations of availability, facilities, and financing imposed by managed care have arisen, creative new at-home programs for low-risk post-MI patients have been developed. These include community-based programs and home programs. In all of these programs, it is important that the patient be able to self-monitor during their exercise program. Guidelines for self-monitoring are covered in detail elsewhere (*see* Key References and Suggested Additional Reading). Each exercise session should begin with a stretching session, followed by a warm-up session, the training exercise, and ending with a cool-down period. It is important to remember that conditioning benefit is related to the specificity of training, and that the conditioning applies to the specific muscles exercised.

Table 7
Patients at High Risk During Cardiac Rehabilitation

Ischemic risk

- Postoperative angina
- LVEF <35%
- NYHA grade III or IV CHF
- Ventricular tachycardia of fibrillation in the postoperative period
- SBP drop of 10 points or more with exercise
- Excessive ventricular ectopy with exercise
- Incapable of self-monitoring
- Myocardial ischemia with exercise

Arrhythmic risk

- Acute infarction within 6 weeks
- Active ischemia by angina or exercise testing
- Significant left ventricular dysfunction (LVEF <30%)
- History of sustained ventricular tachycardia
- History of sustained life-threatening supraventricular arrhythmia
- History of sudden death, not yet stabilized on medical therapy
- Initial therapy of patients with automatic implantable cardioverter defibrillator
- Initial therapy of a patient with a rate adaptive cardiac pacemaker

LVEF, left ventricular ejection fraction; NYHA, New York Heart Association; CHF, congestive heart failure; SBP, systolic blood pressure.

Maintenance Phase (Phase IV)

Although often the least discussed, the maintenance phase of a cardiac conditioning program is the most important part of the program. If the patient stops exercising, the benefits gained from phase III can be lost in a few weeks. The patient should be taught the importance of an ongoing exercise program from the beginning of the cardiac rehabilitation program, and the concept reemphasized throughout. The actual exercises need to be integrated into the patient's lifestyle and interests to assure compliance. The secondary prevention measures also need to be integrated into the patient's lifestyle. The ongoing exercises should be performed at the target HR for at least 30 minutes, three times a week, if at a moderate level. If at a low level, exercises need to be performed five times a week. During the maintenance phase, electrocardiogram monitoring is not necessary.

Cardiac Rehabilitation Programs in Special Conditions

With recent advances in medical technology, there are many conditions that are being referred to cardiac rehabilitation programs. Heart failure, valvular heart disease, life-threatening arrhythmias, pre- and posttransplant patients, and patients who have just received left ventricular assist devices, just to name a few, are all now entering rehabilitation programs. Each of these groups is described in this section.

Angina Pectoris

For patients with a stable angina, cardiac rehabilitation can be utilized to improve efficiency of performance below the anginal threshold. It is important to remember that the actual MVO_2 (and thus the maximum HR) at which angina occurs will not change with conditioning. A full-level ETT should be done in order to determine the maximum HR and rule out the potential of life-threatening events. The program of rehabilitation can begin at phase III (training). The primary goal of rehabilitation in this group of patients is aimed at increasing work capacity and education in primary/secondary prevention strategies. Increased conditioning and efficiency of exercise may significantly decrease disability caused by their recurrent chest pain.

Cardiac Rehabilitation After Revascularization Procedures

Post-CABG

Rehabilitation after CABG has a number of benefits. The patients start in a phase III program as soon as healing is completed. Because of the lower level of invasiveness with new techniques, such as minimally invasive CABG, off- pump CABG, robotic surgery, and other techniques, a larger number of patients with severe pre-existing cardiac disease can now tolerate surgery. Unlike the past, patients with low EFs and CHF are also considered candidates for revascularization. There is a role for a symptom-limited cardiac stress test if continued ischemia is considered a risk. Testing can be safely performed at 3–4 weeks after surgery. The exercise test should determine maximal functional capacity, maximal HR, exercise blood pressure response, exercise-induced arrhythmias, and anginal threshold. A complete education program to help modify risk factors and supervised and unsupervised home programs can help with the management of risk of recurrent heart disease.

Cardiac rehabilitation after CABG has two stages: the immediate postoperative period and the later maintenance stage. The in-hospital period usually only lasts 5–7 days. This phase has three parts: (1) intensive mobilization starting postoperative day 1, (2) progressive ambulation and daily exercises, and (3) discharge planning and exercise prescription for the maintenance stage.

Early mobilization should only be delayed for an unstable postoperative course or severe CHF. Early mobilization has several benefits, including decreasing effects of immobility and preventing cardiac deconditioning. Days 2–5 include progressive ambulation and daily exercise. Initial ambulation aims for assistance with distances of 150–200 feet, followed by independent ambulation by the third day. In the last few days prior to discharge, the patient is given a program of self-monitored exercise that allows for a gradual return to previous levels of activity.

The at-home program for a CABG patient is usually conducted as an outpatient procedure. Inpatient rehabilitation may be needed for high-risk patients or those who have had postoperative complications or significant comorbidities. Patients should be stratified according to risk into either low-, moderate-, or high-intensity programs. A low-intensity program is in the area of 2–4 METs, with a target HR of 65–75% of maximum HR. A moderate-intensity program is from 3 to 6.5 METs, with target HR 70–80% of maximum HR. A high-intensity program is from 5 to 8.5 METs with a target HR of 75–85% of maximum HR. In the presence of β-blockade, the target HR is 20 bpm above the resting HR or at a target HR determined through an ETT aiming at a target MET level. Assignment of level of exercise is determined by the objective criteria and patient observation in the postoperative period. A level of exercise that equals a rating of perceived exertion (RPE) of 13 on the Borg scale is a level of training where the patient can be safely prescribed in the outpatient setting. The inpatient program for high-risk patients has to be tailored to the specific needs of the patient in cooperation with the patient's cardiologist.

Postpercutaneous Transluminal Coronary Angioplasty

The rehabilitation of patients after percutaneous transluminal coronary angioplasty (PTCA) is essentially the same as after CABG. Patients with PTCA tend to be younger and have disease limited to only one or two vessels. The exercise program is similar to that of the post-CABG patient with the benefit of no significant postoperative recovery. There can be a role for diagnostic exercise testing before the PTCA, followed by a functional exercise test immediately after PTCA to set parameters for exercise presciption. Although ideal, this approach may not be practical in all settings or with all patients. Risk-factor modification in outpatient programs with both supervised and unsupervised home programs are possible. As after CABG, high-risk patients require closer monitoring and closer physician supervision. For low-risk post-PTCA patients, the usual risk stratification is done.

Cardiac Rehabilitation After Cardiac Transplant Surgery

As cardiac transplantation has improved, the numbers of patients with cardiac transplantation have increased. Five- and 10-year survival has improved, and the focus of rehabiliation programs is to recover from preoperative invalidism and general muscle weakness. Cardiac physiology after transplant is somewhat different with loss of vagal inhibition to the sinoatrial node, causing an elevated resting HR (often near 100 bpm). There is a reduced SV, but the heart has normal compliance, and CO still increases via the Frank–Starling mechanism. Because there is also no direct sympathetic innervation to the heart, circulating catecholamines induce chronotropic and inotropic responses to increase CO. This leads to a situation of resting tachycardia with a blunted HR response to exercise. Peak HRs are 20–25% lower than in matched controls, and HR recovery after exercise is delayed. Resting hypertension is often seen owing to the effects of antirejection medications. If there is any rejection or ischemic injury at the time of transplant, there may be an element of diastolic dysfunction caused by myocardial stiffness.

Deconditioning can be seen pre- and posttransplant. Transplant recipients have a 10–50% loss of lean body mass from the lack of activity and high-dose steroids in the perioperative period. This leads to a decrease in maximum work output and maximum oxygen uptake. At submaximal exercise levels, perceived exertion, minute ventilation, and the ventilatory equivalent for oxygen are all higher, whereas oxygen uptake is the same. At rest, HR and SBP are higher, and with maximum effort work capacity, CO, peak HR, peak SBP, and peak oxygen uptake are all lower. Resting and exertional diastolic blood pressure are higher after cardiac transplantation than in normal controls.

Exercise testing can be done but dyspnea, faintness, and electrocardiogram changes need to be followed vigilantly as the donor-denervated heart cannot demonstrate ischemia through anginal pain. In long-standing transplants, accelerated atheroschlerosis may develop and lead to cardiac ischemia.

Cardiac rehabilitation after heart transplant must address conditioning, as well as cardiac function. In the initial postoperative period, aggressive mobilization is done, similar to post-CABG patients. At the time of discharge, after patients have learned self-monitoring, patients are encouraged to increase ambulation to 1 mile. The home program consists of progressive ambulation, with the pace designed to be at a level of 60–70% of peak effort for 30–60 minutes three to five times a week. The RPE, using the Borg scale, should be maintained at 13 to 14, with the level of activity increasing incrementally to stay at this level. Education about the complicated medical regimen and possible vocational rehabilitation also need to be considered. The benefit of rehabilitation posttransplant includes increased work output, improved exercise tolerance, and improved quality of life.

Valvular Heart Disease

In valvular heart disease, the major problem is often deconditioning along with CHF. In patients receiving surgical correction of the valvular disease, a post-CABG-type program is used. In uncorrected valvular heart disease with heart failure, the program resembles the program for CHF. Training can increase physical work capacity by 60%, decrease RPE, and decrease the RPP by 15% in uncorrected valve disease. Postoperative anticoagulation needs to be accounted for, and in those patients, low-impact exercises are used to avoid hemarthroses and bruising. Otherwise, the training program is similar to that followed for the post-CABG patient.

Cardiomyopathy

One of the fastest growing subsets of the cardiac rehabilitation population is in CHF among individuals with an EF of 30% or less. The major issue is that this population is at higher risk of sudden death and has a high degree of depression because of their chronic cardiac disability. Limited exercise capacity is common in heart failure and is one of the earliest findings.

Patients with heart failure demonstrate inconsistent responses to exercise, and the hemodynamic alterations do not always correlate with overall exercise capacity. In CHF, exercise can cause a drop in EF, a decrease in stroke volume, exertional hypotension, and syncope. In severe CHF, there can be a failure to generate a dynamic exercise response at all. Low endurance and fatigue are also common in CHF, and prolonged fatigue can be seen for hours to days after heavy exertion. Additional factors, such as atrial fibrillation, fluid overload, and medication noncompliance, may further decrease exercise tolerance. Despite these limitations, exercise duration and efficiency can increase by as much as 18–34%, and peak oxygen uptake can increase by 18–25%. Patients will have lower HRs at rest and during submaximal exercise, raised anaerobic thresholds, and increased maximal work loads. This improvement in efficiency of exercise can mean the difference between independent living and dependency for a patient with CHF.

In CHF, unstable angina, decompensated CHF, and unstable arrhythmias are contraindications to cardiac rehabilitation. Screening functional exercise testing is indicated to allow patients to have safe programs, and estimation of EF can be helpful. Prolonged warm-ups and cool downs are needed because these patients often have abnormal hemodynamic responses to exercise. Dynamic exercise is preferred with a target HR 10 bpm below any significant end point. Isometric exercise should be avoided where possible, and limited to 2-minute intervals when performed. Cardiac exercise is best supervised initially until the patient is able to self-monitor to prevent complications. Patients with severe left ventricular dysfunction (EF < 30%) will need telemetry during warm-up, exercise and cool down. In time, this can be stopped once safe exercise levels have been established.

Cardiac Arrhythmias

The risk of death from cardiac arrhythmia during rehabilitation exercises is very low, with one arrest per 112,000 patient hours of exercise reported between 1980 and 1984. Thus, only high-risk patients need continuous monitoring. For patients with life-threatening arrhythmias, the automatic internal cardiac defibrillators is commonly used. Modifications for cardiac rehabilitation program in these patients are limited to not exceeding the target rate that the device is set at. The support and reassurance that can be given to these patients during the exercise program is also important because anxiety about recurrent arrhythmia is a frequent concern.

Key References and Suggested Additional Reading

American Association for Cardiovascular and Pulmonary Rehabilitation. Guidelines for Cardiac Rehabilitation and Secondary Prevention Programs, 4th ed. Champaign, IL: Human Kinetics, 2004.

American College of Chest Physicians. Cardiac rehabilitation services. Ann Intern Med 1988; 109:671–673.

American College of Sports Medicine. ACSM's Guidelines for Exercise Testing and Prescription, 6th ed. Philadelphia: Lippincott, Williams and Wilkins, 2000.

April EW. Anatomy. Philadelphia: John Wiley and Sons, 1984, pp. 143–161.

Bartels MN. Cardiopulmonary assessment. In: Grabois M, ed, Physical Medicine and Rehabilitation: The Complete Approach. Chicago: Blackwell Science, 2000:351–372.

Bartels MN. Cardiac rehabilitation. In: Grabois M, ed, Physical Medicine and Rehabilitation: The Complete Approach. Chicago: Blackwell Science, 2000.

Berne RB, Levy MN. Cardiovascular Physiology. St Louis: CV Mosby, 1986:1435–1456.

Billingham ME. Graft coronary disease: the lesions and the patients. Transplant Proc 1989; 21:3665–3666.

Borg G. Psychopathological bases of perceived exertion. Med Sci Sports Exerc 1982; 14:377–381.

Braunwald E, Sonnenblick EH, Ross J. Normal and abnormal circulatory function. In: Braunwald E, ed. Heart Disease. Philadelphia: W. B. Saunders, 1992, pp. 351–392.

Bresike JF, Levy RI, Kelsey SF, et al. Effects of therapy with cholstyramine on progression of coronary arteriosclerosis: results of the NHLBI Type II Coronary intervention study. Circulation 1984; 69:313–324.

Brown G, Albers JJ, Fisher LD, et al. Regression of coronary artery disease as a result of intensive lipid lowering therapy in men with high levels of apolipoprotein B. N Engl J Med 1990; 323:1289–1298.

Cannistra LB, Balady GJ, O'Malley CJ, et al. Comparison of the clinical profile and outcome of women and men in cardiac rehabilitation. Am J of Cardiol 1992; 69:1274–1279.

Cannom DS, Rider AK, Stinson EB, et al. Electrophysiologic studies in the denervated transplanted human heart. Amer. J. Cardiol 1975; 36:859.

Chandrasheckhar Y, Anand IS. Exercise as a coronary protective factor. Am Heart J 1991; 122:1723–1739.

Christopherson LK. Cardiac transplantation: a psychological perspective. Circulation 1987; 75:57–62.

Dafoe, WA. Table of energy requirements for activities of daily living, household tasks, recreational activities, and vocational activities. In: Pashkow FJ, Dafoe WA, eds. Clinical Cardiac Rehabilitation: A Cardiologist's Guide. Baltimore, MD: Lippincott, Williams and Wilkins; 1993: 359–376.

DeBusk RF, Haskell WL, Miller NH. Medically directed at-home rehabilitation soon after clinically uncomplicated acute myocardial infarction: a new model for patient care. Am J Cardiol 1985; 55:251–257.

De Marneffe M, Jacobs P, Haardt R, Englert M. Variations of normal sinus node function in relation to age: role of autonomic influence. Eur Heart J 1986; 7:662.

Dubach P, Froelicher VF. Cardiac rehabilitation for heart failure patients. Cardiology. 1989; 76:368–373.

Dubach P, Froelicher V, Klein J, et al. Use of the exercise test to predict prognosis after coronary artery bypass grafting. Am J Cardiol 1989; 63:530.

Fletcher BJ, Lloyd A, Fletcher GF. Outpatient rehabilitative training in patients with cardiovascular disease: emphasis on training method. Heart Lung 1988; 17:199–205.

Fletcher GF, Blair SN, Blumenthal J, et al. Statement on exercise. Benefits and recommendations for physical activity programs for all Americans. A statement for health professionals by the Committee on Exercise and Cardiac Rehabilitation of the Council on Clinical Cardiology. American Heart Association. Circulation 1992; 86:76–84.

Frick MH, Elo O, Haapa K, et al. Helsinki Heart Study: Primary prevention trial with Gemfibrizol in middle aged men with dyslipidemia. N Engl J Med 1987; 317:1237–345.

Froelicher VF. Exercise testing and training: clinical applications. J Am Coll Cardiol 1983; 1:114–125.

Gordon T, Kannel WB, McGee D. Death and coronary attacks in men after giving up cigarette smoking: a report from the Framingham study. Lancet 1974; 2:1375.

Graves EJ. 1992 Summary: National Hospital Discharge Survey. Advance data from vital and health statistics; no. 249. Hyattsville, MD: National Center for Health Statistics, 1994.

Guyton AC. Textbook of Medical Physiology, 7th ed. Philadelphia: W. B. Saunders, 1986.

Hausdorf G, Banner NR, Mitchell A, et al. Diastolic function after cardiac and heart lung transplantation. Br Heart J 1989; 62:123–132.

Heck CF, Shumway SJ, Kaye MP. The registry of the international society for heart transplantation: sixth official report 1989. J Heart Transplant 1989; 8: 271–276.

Humphry R, Bartels MN. Exercise, cardiovascular disease and chronic heart failure: a focused review. Arch Phy Med Rehabil 2001; 82(Suppl 1): S76–S81.

Ignarro LJ. Endothelium derived nitric oxide: actions and properties. FASEB J 1989; 3:31–36.

Juneau M, Geneau S, Marchand C, Brosseau R. Cardiac rehabilitation after coronary bypass surgery. (review). Cardiovasc Clin 1991; 21:25–42.

Juneau M, Rogers F, Desantos V, et al. Effectiveness of self monitored, home based, moderate intensity exercise training in sedentary midddle aged men and women. Am J Cardiol 1987; 60:66–70.

Kannel WB, Plehn JF, Cupples LA. Cardiac failure and sudden death in the Framingham Study. Am Heart J 1988; 115: 869–75.

Kavanaugh T. Exercise training in patients after heart transplantation. Herz 1991; 16:243–250.

Kavanaugh T, Yacoub MH, Campbell R, Mertens D. Marathon running after cardiac transplantation: a case history. J Cardiac Rehab 1986; 6:16–20.

Kavanaugh T, Yacoub M, Mertens DJ, Kennedy J, Campbell RB, Sawyer P. Cardiorespiratory responses to exercise training after orthotopic cardiac transplantation. Circulation 1988; 77:162–171.

Krone RJ. The role of risk stratification in the early management of myocardial infarction. Ann Intern Med 1992; 116:223–237.

Krone RJ, Gillespie JA, Weld FM, Miller JP, Moss AJ. Low level exercise testing after myocardial infarction: usefulness in enhancing clinical risk stratification. Circulation 1985; 71:80–89.

Lavie CJ, Miliani RV. Effects of cardiac rehabilitation programs on exercise capacity, coronary risk factors, behavioral characteristics, and quality of life in a large elderly cohort. Am J Cardiol 1995; 76:177–179.

Lavie CJ, Miliani RV, Boykin C. Marked benefits of cardiac rehabilitation and exercise training in an elderly cohort. J Am Coll Cardiol 1994; 23:439 (abstract).

Lavie CJ, Miliani RV, Littman AB. Benefits of cardiac rehabilitation and exercise training in secondary coronary conditioning in the elderly. J Am Coll Cardiol 1993; 22:678–683.

Lee AP, Ice R, Blessey R, et al. Long-term effects of physical training in coronary patients with impaired ventricular function. Circulation 1979; 60: 1519.

Leren P. The effect of plasma cholesterol lowering diet in male survivors of myocardial infarction. Acta Med Scand 1967; 466:1–92.

Loen AS, Certo C, Comoss P, et al. Scientific evidence of the value of cardiac rehabilitation services with emphasis on patients following myocardial infarction. J Cardiopulm Rehabil 1990; 10:79–87.

Martin JE, Dubbert PM, Cushman WC. Controlled trial of aerobic exercise in hypertension. Circulation 1990; 81:1560–1567.

McKirnan MD, Sullivan M, Jensen D, et al. Treadmill performance and cardiac function in selected patients with coronary heart disease. J Am Coll Cardiol 1984; 3:253–261.

Moldover JR, Bartels MN. Cardiac rehabilitation. In: Braddom RL, ed. Rehabilitation Medicine, 2nd ed. Philadelphia: W. B. Saunders, 2000.

Morris CK, Froelicher VF. Cardiovascular benefits of physical activity. Herz 1991; 16:222–236.

Newell JP, Kappagoda CT, Stoker JB, Deverall PB, Watson DA, Linden RJ. Physical training after heart valve replacement. Br Heart J 1980; 44:638–649.

O'Conner GT, Burling JE, Yusuf S, et al. An overview of randomized trials of rehabilitation with exercise after myocardial infarction. Circulation 1989; 80:234–244.

Oldridge N, Furlong W, Feeny D, et al. Economic evaluation of cardiac rehabilitation soon after acute myocardial infarction. Am J Cardiol 1993; 72: 154–161.

Oldridge NB, Guyatt GH, Fischer ME, Rimm AA. Cardiac rehabilitation after myocardial infarction: combined experience of randomized clinical trials. JAMA 1988; 260:945–950.

Packer M. Sudden unexpected death in patients with congestive heart failure: a second frontier. Circulation 1985; 72:681–685.

Pashkow F. Rehabilitation strategies for the complex cardiac patient. Cleve Clin J Med 1991; 58:70–75.

Pashkow FJ. Issues in contemporary cardiac rehabilitation: a historical perspective. J Am Coll Cardiol 1993; 21: 822–824.

Paskow FJ. Complicating conditions. In: Pashkow FJ, Pashkow P, Schafer M, eds. Successful Cardiac Rehabilitation: The Complete Guide for Building Cardiac Rehabilitation Programs. Loveland, CO: Heart Watchers Press, 1988, pp. 228–247.

Pashkow F, Schafer M, Pashkow P. HeartWatchers—low cost, community centered cardiac rehabilitation in Loveland, Colorado. J Cardiopulm Rehabil 1986; 6:469–473.

Perk J, Hedback B, Engvall J. Effects of cardiac rehabilitation after coronary bypass grafting on readmissions, return to work, and physical fitness: a case control study. Scand J Soc Med 1990; 18:45–51.

Pollock ML, Foster C, Anholm JD, et al. Diagnostic capabilities of exercise testing soon after myocardial revascularization surgery. Cardiology 1982; 69:358.

Pycha C, Gulledge AD, Hutzler J, Kadri N, Maloney JD. Psychological response to the implantable defibrillator. Psychosomatics. 1986; 27:841–845.

Rosenblum DS, Rosen ML, Pine ZM, Rosen S, Stein J. Health status and quality of life following cardiac transplantation. Arch Phys Med Rehabil 1993; 74:490–493.

Rushkin J, McHale PA, Harley A, et al, Pressure-flow studies in man: effects of atrial systole on left ventricular function. J Clin Invest 1970: 49:472.

Salomen JT. Stopping smoking and long term mortality after acute myocardial infarction. Br Heart J 1980; 43:463.

Shabetai R. Beneficial effects of exercise training in compensated heart failure. Circulation 1988; 78: 775–776.

Shekelle RB, Shyrock AM, Paul O, et al. Diet, serum cholesterol, and death from coronary heart disease: the Western Electric Study. N Engl J Med 1981; 304:65–70.

Sire S. Physical Training and occupational rehabilitation after aortic valve replacement. Eur Heart J 1987; 8:1215–1220.

Sivarajan E, Lerman J, Mansfield L. Progressive ambulation and treadmill testing of patients with acute myocardial infarction during hospitalization: a feasibility study. Arch Phys Med Rehabil 1977; 58:241–244.

Stamler J, Wentworth D, Neaton JD, for the MRFIT Research Group: Is the relationship between serum cholesterol and risk of premature death from coronary heart disease continuous and graded? Findings in 356,222 primary screenees of the Multiple Risk Factor Intervention Trial (MRFIT). JAMA 1986; 256:2823–2828.

Starling RC, Cody RJ. Cardiac transplant hypertension. Am J Cardiol 1990; 65:106–111.

Sullivan MJ, Higginbotham MB, Cobb FR. Exercise training in patients with severe left ventricular dysfunction. Circulation 1990; 81(Suppl II): II-5–II-13.

The Expert Panel: Report of the National Cholesterol Education Program Expert Panel on the Detection, Evaluation, and Treatment of High Blood Cholesterol in Adults. Arch Int Med 1988; 148:36–39.

Thompson PD. The benefits and risks of exercise training in chronic coronary artery disease. JAMA 1988; 259: 1537–1540.

Tran ZW, Weltman, A. Differential effects of exercise on serum lipid and lipoprotein levels seen with changes in body weight: A meta analysis. JAMA 1985; 254:919–924.

US Bureau of the Census, Statistical Abstract of the United States: 1993 (113th ed.) Washington, D.C., 1993.

US Bureau of the Census, Statistical Abstract of the United States: 1995 (115th ed.) Washington, D.C., 1995.

Vaitkevicius PV, Fleg JL, Engel JH, et al. Effects of age and aerobic capacity on arterial stiffness in healthy adults. Circulation 1993; 88: 1456–1462.

Van Camp S, Peterson R, Cardiovascular complications of outpatient cardiac rehabilitation programs. JAMA 1986; 256: 1160–1163.

Wainright RJ, Brennand-Roper DA, Maisey MN, et al. Exercise Thallium-201 myocardial scintigriphy in the follow-up of aortocoronary bypass graft surgery. Br Heart J 1980; 43:56.

Wenger NK, Rehabilitation of the coronary patient: status 1986. Prog Cardiovasc Dis 1986; 29:181.

Wenger N, Gilbert C, Skoropa M. Cardiac conditioning after myocardial infarction. An early intervention program. J Cardiac Rehabil 1971; 2:17–22.

Wenger N, Hellerstein H, Blackburn H, Castronova M. Uncomplicated myocardial infarction: current physician practice in patient management. JAMA 1973, 224:511–514.

Winkle RA, Mead RH, Ruder MA, et al. Long term outcome with the automatic implantable cardiac-defibrillator. J Am Coll Cardiol 1989; 13:1353–1361.

Wittels EH, Hay JW, Gotto AM. Medical Costs of coronary artery disease in the United States. Am J Cardiol 1990; 65:432–440.

Yusuf S, Aikenhead J, Theodoropoulos S, Shalla N, Wittes J, Yacoub M. Mechanism of cardiac output during dynamic exercise in cardiac transplant patients. J Am Coll Cardiol 1986; 7:225A (abstract).

Yusuf S, Theodoropoulos S, Mathias CJ, et al. Increased sensitivity to the denervated transplanted human heart to isoprenaline both before and after beta-adrenergic blockade. Circulation 1987; 75: 696–704.

6 Pulmonary Rehabilitation

Mathew N. Bartels

Background

In physical medicine and rehabilitation, pulmonary rehabilitation has traditionally meant the management of individuals with chronic respiratory insufficiency owing to neuromuscular or other central nervous system diseases. The management of ventilatory insufficiency in these populations is important, but focusing only on this population ignores the importance of the provision of rehabilitation services to people with primary lung disease, or the application of these principles to individuals with dual disabilities, such as stroke and concomitant emphysema. In view of this, this chapter covers both chronic ventilatory support in neuromuscular and other diseases, as well as the rehabilitation of individuals with severe lung disease.

Rehabilitation in Severe Lung Disease

Although there are a large number of lung diseases, several diagnoses are the primary beneficiaries of pulmonary rehabilitation. Among these are interstitial lung disease (ILD), emphysema and chronic obstructive lung disease (COPD), cystic fibrosis (CF), and pulmonary hypertension (PH). COPD is a major cause of death and illness in the United States, and the use of pulmonary exercise was started in this group of patients. To date, the data on the benefits of pulmonary rehabilitation are mostly in this group. A basic review of the epidemiology of COPD shows that it is the fourth highest cause of death in the United States, with the estimated national prevalence ranging from 14 to 20 million people. Chronic disability owing to COPD

From: *Essential Physical Medicine and Rehabilitation*
Edited by: G. Cooper © Humana Press Inc., Totowa, NJ

ranks second only to cardiac disease in payments from social security for chronic disability. Most COPD is caused by chronic exposure to cigarette smoke, and 15% of all smokers will progress to COPD. Most smokers who develop COPD have a history of smoking for 20 or more pack-years. The incidence of the other pulmonary conditions, including ILD, CF, and PH are a small fraction of the numbers of individuals with COPD. Smoking is also not a causative agent in these other conditions, but smoking and its associated bronchitis and COPD can be contributors to a more severe course in any lung condition. Because of the major role of smoking, counseling and smoking cessation should be considered an integral part of any pulmonary rehabilitation program. The rehabilitation standards from the COPD experience will be used as a description of the essentials of an effective pulmonary rehabilitation program, with the special needs of ILD, CF, and PH discussed separately.

It is important to remember that there are limited treatment options for individuals with severe pulmonary conditions and that pulmonary rehabilitation is one of the only treatments that can alleviate the impact of these diseases. The National Emphysema Treatment Trial of Lung Volume Reduction Surgery was a milestone in the acceptance of pulmonary rehabilitation. From the National Emphysema Treatment Trial, it was determined for the first time that rehabilitation was mandatory for the preparation for surgery and recovery after surgery. In view of this, the American College of Chest Physicians (ACCP) has now started to recommend pulmonary rehabilitation as a part of the plan of treatment for individuals who will undergo major chest procedures, and also for individuals with untreatable severe disease.

Pulmonary rehabilitation is a comprehensive approach to the management of the patient with lung disease that includes a multifaceted approach to treatment. The focus of the rehabilitation program is to alleviate the physiological effects of the disease process, as well as to help to decrease the psychosocial effects of the illness on the individual. The history of pulmonary rehabilitation dates back 50 years. The early mobilization programs ran counter to the standard wisdom in the past by exercising individuals with respiratory limitations.

In 1994, the National Institutes of Health held a workshop on pulmonary rehabilitation research that established the following definition of pulmonary rehabilitation:

> *Pulmonary rehabilitation is a multidisciplinary continuum of services directed to persons with pulmonary disease and their families, usually by an interdisciplinary team of specialists, with the goal of achieving and maintaining the individual's maximum level of independence and functioning in the community.*

The key aspects focus on the multidisciplinary approach, with a full range of services provided to the patient and their family. Working within these parameters is a natural setting for rehabilitation medical input. The current failings of research into pulmonary rehabilitation fall into three areas: (1) lack of clearly consistent data; (2) lack of well-controlled longitudinal studies; and (3) lack of research about other conditions, such as restrictive or pulmonary vascular conditions. Still, the clear clinical consensus is that pulmonary rehabilitation is a useful part of the comprehensive treatment of the patient with severe COPD. In 1997, the ACCP and the American Association of Cardiovascular and Pulmonary Rehabilitation released a joint ACCP/American Association of Cardiovascular and Pulmonary Rehabilitation statement of evidence-based guidelines regarding pulmonary rehabilitation. The benefits of rehabilitation were also restated in the *Journal of the American Medical Association* consensus statement on management of pulmonary diseases.

Benefits of Exercise and Participation in Pulmonary Rehabilitation

Exercise Capacity

Measuring the outcomes of pulmonary rehabilitation is often difficult because studies often use different outcome measures. The most common measures are the 6- or 12-minute walk and the symptom-limited maximum exercise test. Although on first glance these techniques may appear to have a resemblance to each other, they are in fact quite different. The 6- or 12-minute walk is a submaximal exercise test, measuring the greatest sustained effort that an individual can comfortably perform, and the walk test has to be performed meticulously in order to have validity and reproducibility. Because the test can measure efficiency of exercise, it will measure improvement in efficiency of an individual who undergoes exercise training.

The maximal exercise test evaluates the maximum capacity of the individual, and also can be used as a measure of efficiency in performing exercise. However, there is a safety risk because a small number of maximal exercise tests can lead to complications or death, and because of the difficulty of performing the test on supplemental oxygen (special equipment) and interpreting the results of the exercise test afterward. In experienced hands, these are not prohibitive, but not all programs will have easy access to the testing.

Each of these testing techniques has its benefits and problems when applied to the pulmonary population. There also have been somewhat unclear benefits in aerobic capacity (VO_2Max), whereas the outcomes of the walk tests have been more uniformly favorable after rehabilitation. A pre-and postrehabilitation testing program is essential to measuring outcomes and also to help plan an exercise program.

Dyspnea

Shortness of breath is uniformly improved in COPD by pulmonary rehabilitation. The research to support this benefit in other conditions also tends to support the relief of dyspnea in restrictive and pulmonary vascular disease as well. The relief of dyspnea in patients with COPD after rehabilitation has been demonstrated in several studies. The improvement of dyspnea is seen in both the performance of activities of daily living (ADLs) and with exercise testing. The benefit of decreased dyspnea can then be sustained over time with a maintenance program. There are several mechanisms that may improve dyspnea. Possible mechanisms include (1) improved efficiency with less effort required for all activities, (2) decreased ventilation with given activities, and (3) desensitization with less subjective dyspnea for a given amount of ventilation. Although the measurement of dyspnea is a subjective–qualitative measure, the improvement in this symptom makes it an index that needs to be closely followed; therefore, it has become one of the standard measures of success in pulmonary rehabilitation. Dyspnea is either directly measured on a self-reported scale or is indirectly measured based on evaluation of selective activities. The commonly used scales for dyspnea and quality of life are outlined in Table 1.

Quality of Life

Quality of life (QOL) is improved in most of the studies of pulmonary rehabilitation, with good subjective improvement in symptoms. With valid instruments for QOL assessment, the most recent studies have shown benefits and are being undertaken even now. Table 1 has a list of some of these instruments and their areas of validity.

Overall, pulmonary rehabilitation does show good clinical improvements in COPD, and by extension should also benefit other forms of lung disease. A comprehensive program will have the greatest impact on QOL. The specific parts of a program for pulmonary rehabilitation apply particularly to outpatient rehabilitation, but portions also apply to inpatient rehabilitation.

Components of a Pulmonary Rehabilitation Program

Smoking Cessation

In any individual with lung disease, smoking cessation is essential. Cigarette smoking has been shown to be as addictive as alcohol or narcotic

Table 1
Dyspnea and QOL Instruments

Measure	*Direct/ Indirect*	*Validity and correlates*	*Description*
• Borg Scale of Percieved Breathlessness	Direct	High for dyspnea, correlates with VE, VO_2, VAS	Modification of Borg scale of percieved exertion. 10-point scale.
• Visual Analogue Scale (VAS)	Direct	High for dyspnea, correlates with VE, VO_2, VAS	VAS of 100 cm length. Subject indicates dyspnea by choosing a point on the line. Good correlation with Borg Scale.
• Chronic Respiratory Disease Questionnaire (CRQ)	Indirect	Has good clinical validity for dyspnea, has individualized dyspnea scale that makes comparisons difficult	20-item self-reported test, interviewer administered. Measures four dimensions: dyspnea, fatigue, emotional function, mastery of breathing. Evaluates five usual activities.
• St. George's Respiratory Questionnaire (SGRQ)	Indirect	Fair for dyspnea, better for QOL. Good test–retest reliability and good clinical correlation	Self-administered QOL questionnaire with 53 questions. Measures three areas: symptoms, activity, impact on ADL.
• Sickness impact profile	General	Multiple domains assessed, Good validity. Not disease specific.	30-minute self-administered. Covers many areas of function: social, ADL, mobility, vocational, communication, cognition, hygiene, emotional status.
• Medical Outcomes Study—Short Form-36 (SF-36)	General	Multiple domains assessed, Good validity. Not disease-specific.	10-minute self-administered. Covers multiple areas of function: role functioning, pain, health, vitality, social, mental health.

ADL, activities of daily living; QOL, quality of life; VE, minute ventilation; VO_2, volume of oxygen consumed.

agents. The addictive power of tobacco explains the tendency of individuals to continue to smoke even in the face of pulmonary disease. Quitting smoking is clearly in the patient's interest, and direct confrontation and insistence on the cessation of smoking by the entire staff may be required. The involvement of the primary physician is important because the physician's counseling and warning are important indicators of compliance with the program. A usual requirement to start a program of pulmonary rehabilitation is to either stop smoking or commit to cessation during the rehabilitation program. The rehabilitation role then becomes one of support and education for the patient and the family through (1) support of the initiation of smoking cessation, (2) support of the continuation of smoking cessation, (3) integration of smoking cessation with the rehabilitation program, and (4) education of the patient and his or her family in maintaining a smoke-free environment.

Education

Education is central to the pulmonary rehabilitation program. Educational program components should include a review of medications, oxygen equipment, mechanics of the disease, lifestyle modifications, and energy conservation. In COPD, education has been shown to decrease hospitalizations and ameliorate exacerbations. Education alone does not provide the same benefits as education combined with a rehabilitation program. There are seven essential portions of the education program.

Energy Conservation

The basic principle to impart is that individuals with pulmonary disease do not have a normal exercise tolerance and, thus, need to be aware of ways in which to be efficient in activities, preserving energy in every possible way. A helpful analogy for individuals with lung disease is to compare their energy state to an electronic device with impaired batteries. They do not have sufficient energy to achieve all tasks at full speed, and need to consider carefully how they will use the "charge" that is available to them. Through being more "energy smart," they can achieve more in the course of a normal day. Examples of energy conservation techniques are included in Table 2. Combined with improved capacity for work form endurance training, energy efficiency is a major component of the benefits seen in these patients after a program of rehabilitation.

Medications

Medication education is an important part of the program of a patient in pulmonary rehabilitation. Unfortunately, many patients do not fully understand the medication regimens they are on, often not using their inhaled

Table 2
Goals and Methods of Pulmonary Rehabilitation

Prevention

Goals	*Methods*
• Smoking cessation	▪ Enroll in a cessation program, emotional support; monitor abstinence
• Immunization compliance	▪ Assure proper immunizations; communicate with primary physician
• Prevent exacerbations	▪ Self-assessment skills taught ▪ Self-intervention taught ▪ Instruct on accessing private physician
• Appropriate medication use	▪ Review medications and dosing schedules ▪ Review interactions and side effects ▪ Review appropriate use of inhalers and nebulizers
• Pulmonary toilet	▪ Review bronchial hygiene ▪ Teach proper cough techniques ▪ Use of chest physiotherapy, as needed ▪ Teach chest physiotherapy techniques to family, as appropriate
• Appropriate use of oxygen therapy	▪ Teach use with exertion ▪ Review self-monitoring ▪ Review use of equipment ▪ Encourage acceptance of the need for O_2 ▪ Review importance of use and consequences of failure to use oxygen
• Nutritional counseling	▪ Counseling to achieve ideal body weight ▪ Counseling to avoid high-carbohydrate diet ▪ Instruction in avoidance of high-sodium diets ▪ Encourage balanced nutrition with avoidance of fad diets
• Family training	▪ Teaching regarding: • COPD • Pulmonary toilet • Medication use • Oxygen use ▪ Family support group ▪ Counseling as needed

Dyspnea relief: exercise training

Goals	*Methods*
• Exercise	▪ Multifaceted program individualized to each patient's needs
▪ Strengthening	▪ Emphasis on gradual increase in strength • Focus on proximal muscle groups • Avoid injury to weakened musculoteninous structures • Focus more on high-repetition, low-intensity training

Continued

Table 2 *(Continued)*

Dyspnea relief: exercise training (Continued)	
Goals	*Methods*
▪ Conditioning	▪ Work to gradually increase exercise tolerance • Cross-training program • Emphasis on the development of an independent training program • Increase ambulation endurance with gait training • Appropriate oxygen titration during exercise
▪ Respiratory muscle training	▪ Inspiratory and expiratory muscle training • Isocapnic hyperpnea • Inspiratory resistance training • Inspiratory threshold training
▪ Upper extremity training	• Increase strength • Increase capacity for sustained work • Improve shoulder girdle strength
▪ ADL training	▪ Energy conservation techniques ▪ Adaptive techniques ▪ Relieve anxiety and stress ▪ Encourage pacing in activities
• Breathing retraining	▪ Pursed lip breathing ▪ Diaphragmatic breathing
• Anxiety reduction	▪ Stress relaxation techniques: • Paced breathing • Autohypnosis • Visualization ▪ Medications as needed: • Treat anxiety • Treat depression
• Improve confidence	▪ Build compensatory techniques ▪ Build confidence in ability to exercise

Disease management		
Goals	*Methods*	
• Disease acceptance	▪ Education regarding disease process ▪ Reassurance about aggressive treatment	
• Coping skills	▪ Support group ▪ Treat depression, as needed	▪ Psychology and social work intervention, as needed
• Quality-of-life improvement	▪ Improve ADL tolerance ▪ Improve disease management	▪ Improve coping skills
• Advance directives review	▪ Counseling regarding ▪ Help in preparing paperwork	• Health care proxy • Resuscitation orders
• Encouragement	▪ Support group ▪ Psychological support	▪ Social work support
• Continuing compliance	▪ Team encouragement ▪ Involve primary care physician in plan	▪ Physician counseling ▪ Family education

COPD, chronic obstructive lung disease; ADL, activities of daily living.

medications properly. The education should include discussions of commonly used medications, drug interactions (especially interactions with over-the-counter medications), review of the use of inhaled medications, and family education in the use and side effects of the medications. By maximizing the involvement of the patient and his or her family in the management of medications, a better therapeutic relationship is established, helping to assure adequate adherence to the prescribed regimen and helping to assess the efficacy of treatments.

Oxygen Therapy

Oxygen therapy education is unique to pulmonary disease, and the proper use of oxygen can help to save patients from illness and disability. Oxygen therapy, used correctly, can have a direct effect on improving survival in end-stage lung disease. Survival is improved through the prevention of pulmonary hypertension and polycythemia. Oxygen education is a combination of didactic and individual settings to assure that the individual patient has a good understanding of their oxygen equipment and of safety and medical issues. Hands-on training under the guidance of the therapists is essential. Topics for discussion include travel requirements, emergency procedures, and options for oxygen delivery. Oxygen needs during exercise are titrated on a one-to-one basis. This allows patients to titrate their oxygen independently to avoid hypoxemia while not using more oxygen than required. Patients need to keep their oxygen saturation well above 85% or a PO_2 of 60 mmHg because this is on the shoulder of the steep portion of the oxygen saturation curve. Certain individuals with severe shunts from congenital heart disease with subsequent pulmonary vascular disease may be exceptions to these rules, but are determined on a case-by-case basis. Both the maintenance of safety and maximizing the subject's independence are central goals of oxygen education.

Nutritional Counseling

Managing the nutritional requirements of individuals with lung disease is an essential component of their treatment. Either a nutritionist or another member of the rehabilitation team can do the nutritional teaching. Depending on the nutritional needs of the patient, the intensity of the intervention can range from group education to one-on-one intervention for the patient with either severely increased or decreased weight.

The individual with COPD has an increased basal metabolic demand that may be related to both a higher energy cost of breathing at rest, as well as with activities. Associated with the lower lean body mass, both functional capacity and survival decrease independent of the forced expiratory volume in 1 second or other pulmonary indices. There may be a role for the use of anabolic steroids and growth hormones in combination with exercise, but full evaluation of the safety of these interventions has not been completed. Also, there appears to be an effect only on the repletion of lean body mass and no effect on functional outcomes. In fact, there may be excess risk, as a large prospective study of growth hormone in Europe was stopped early because of excess mortality. Weight loss in obesity is clearly beneficial, but has to be done carefully to assure that there is no further loss of lean body mass. Dietary substrate utilization is also important, especially in COPD. Because the metabolism of fats and proteins yields a lower CO_2 load per unit of energy than carbohydrates, fats and proteins are a preferred source of energy in individuals with CO_2 retention. Appropriate intake of vitamins, trace minerals, potassium, magnesium, phosphate, and calcium has to also be assured in order to maintain optimal health.

Individuals with pulmonary vascular disease often have to avoid excessive salt and fluid loads because they have difficulty managing intravascular fluid shift. Individuals with restrictive lung disease have limitations that are based on poor tolerance of increased metabolic load, and have lean body mass loss. A diet of frequent small meals with a high protein intake is often preferred for this population.

Disease-Specific Education

Education about the specific issues of a patient's specific disease are essential to the pulmonary rehabilitation process. Nearly every review, study, or discussion of a comprehensive rehabilitation program emphasizes the importance of the disease-specific education component of the program. A comprehensive rehabilitation program must include a disease-specific educational component.The education usually includes both a didactic portion and a series of handouts or a textbook that the patient can refer to in order to reinforce the didactic materials. Our own program has adapted materials from a number of programs into a loose-leaf binder that is added to during the course of the pulmonary rehabilitation program. In this fashion, as didactic sessions take place, the most up-to-date information can be passed on to the patient and can reinforce the lesson presented. In addition, textbooks can provide a further basis for the individual's education.

Stress Management

Stress management does not change the course of pulmonary disease, but it may allow a patient to function better with the disease. Anxiety, depression, and fear are commonly seen in patients with severe pulmonary disease. Stress education has been shown to improve a patient's function through allowing better coping with their limiations. A meta analysis of psychosocial interventions in COPD demonstrated that relaxation training was most beneficial in the areas of subjective dyspnea and psychological well-being with a decrease in utilization of hospital services and improved independence. This may be a result of improved relaxation leading to less need for unnecessary utilization of emergency services. It is a clinical observation that the use of anxiolytic medications declines with stress relaxation, but this has not been formally studied.

The form of relaxation technique used is often a matter of staff ability and familiarity, and no single type of relaxation technique has clearly been proved superior. Additionally, each individual patient will respond differently to a different treatment regimen. Common techniques include hypnosis and autohypnosis, meditation, visualization, timed breathing, and relaxation audiotapes and videos. The goal of relaxation is to allow the individual to find a tool that decreases anxiety and can be used during times of exacerbations to help prevent panic. Once relaxation training has been achieved, the skill must be maintained with regular use. Techniques are commonly used for all types of lung disease and are not disease-specific.

Pulmonary Toilet

Secretions in lung disease can range from absent to a life-threatening problem in individuals with a severe bronchitic component to their disease. Pulmonary rehabilitation can provide teaching to help manage secretions on an individual basis and should include caregivers, to carry the treatment on after completion of the pulmonary rehabilitation program. The techniques of chest physical therapy are well-described in other sources and will not be reviewed in detail here. They include percussion, postural drainage, and can also include suctioning and insufflation/exsufflation in selected patients. Any increase in sputum production or change in the quality of the sputum should be aggressively medically treated to prevent a severe pulmonary infection. The utility of respiratory muscle training has not been established, but may be considered on a case-by-case basis in individuals with ventilatory muscle weakness.

Design of a Pulmonary Rehabilitation Program

The ideal location for a pulmonary rehabilitation program is in either a hospital-based outpatient setting with availability of multiple resources, or in a well-supported satellite program. The program needs to be comprehensive with a multidisciplinary approach. The composition of the team can be made to fit the demands of the patient population, the resources of the institution, the limits of reimbursement, and staff expertise. In smaller settings, many tasks are provided by one or two individuals. Pulmonary rehabilitation specialists are often physical therapists, respiratory therapists, or nurses who have an interest in pulmonary disease. The most important issue is to have a cohesive and enthusiastic team with a unified vision of providing excellent patient care. This then provides the patients and their families with a cohesive and organized program.

The program should have a comprehensive guidebook with instructional materials a comprehensive schedule, and a set of clear and uncluttered guidelines. A program that meets three times a week often provides a sufficient degree of interaction and can be accommodated by most patients. Compliance during and after the pulmonary rehabilitation program is often enhanced by close contact with the primary physcian. This also assists in maximizing the medical management of the patient, titrating oxygen requirements, establishing inhaler dosing schedules, and adjusting parenteral steroids during the course of rehabilitation.

Support groups allow the patients to continue the lifelong program of pulmonary health management. The groups can be made general, especially in smaller programs, or can be made for specific disease groups in larger programs. Smoking cessation support groups may also be established if smoking cessation is a primary goal of the rehabilitation program. Often, social outings and events centered around the support groups can improve the socialization of this very ill group of patients and strengthen their links to the program. This will also help to improve the patient's adherence to his or her independent exercise program. Special lectures on areas of interest to individuals with lung disease by members of the team also help to keep patients involved.

For patients who are to undergo surgery or transplant, a program of preparation for the perioperative period is helpful. This includes education in secretion mobilization, familiarization with early postoperative mobilization, and introduction to the physical therapy staff who will participate in the early care after surgery. This introduction can make early mobilization easier because a therapeutic alliance can be formed to facilitate early mobilization. Education about surgery also helps reduce patient anxiety. An outline of the goals and methods of the rehabilitation program are in Table 2.

The rehabilitation program design includes the following features:

1. Patient screening: This is essentially the selection of individuals for pulmonary rehabilitation. The initial evaluation is by the referring physician, followed by an intake evaluation to assess specific needs. A schedule is then created to meet the patient's needs. If an individual has good conditioning at their evaluation, the program may be done at a higher level,

with emphasis on the educational components of the program. Individuals with cognitive issues may need greater family involvement, and any medical issues that are unclear can be clarified with the referring physician. Regular rehabilitation team meetings allow the rehabilitation staff to bring new issues forward, and allow a modification of the medical management or goals for the patient.

2. Exercise testing: Ideally this should be performed on all subjects before the initiation of training, as a symptom-limited VO_2 maximum determination will allow for an aggressive training program that starts at 60% of the maximum exercise capacity and is progressively increased. Safety parameters and therapist confidence can be established, which allows a consistent approach in rehabilitation. Six-minute walk testing with oxygen titration is also useful to help document oxygen needs and assess progress.
3. Exercise prescription: An exercise prescription should include clear demographic data, as well as clear indication of the contact numbers of the prescribing physician. As with all rehabilitation prescription, it requires four elements:
   a. Diagnosis: This has to be accurate in order to help the team understand the patient's needs. This should also include any planned transplant or lung surgery.
   b. Specific prescription: The prescription should describe, in detail, the rehabilitation program, including the educational, psychosocial and nutritional needs of the patient. The exercise portion needs to specify both upper and lower extremity exercises and include both strengthening and conditioning exercises. The prescription should also state if exercise is to be done with supplemental oxygen. A symptom-limited exercise test is helpful, allowing the physician to specifically state a starting point and oxygen requirements for an aggressive rehabilitation program. The prescription should include the intensity, duration, and goals of the program.
   c. Frequency: The frequency of the patient attendance in the program needs to be specified, and is usually ordered in times per week. For most patients, four or five times a week is too strenuous and is impractical. A three-times-a-week program is common. Modifications may be required owing to debility, travel distance, scheduling, or other factors.
   d. Duration: The planned length of the program should also be specified. The goal is to allow an individual to have 18 to 24 sessions of rehabilitation, usually over 6–8 weeks. Maximal response to a conditioning program takes a longer time, but the realities of limited reimbursement makes 3- to 4-month programs undoable.
   e. Precautions: These need to be very detailed in individuals who are this fragile. Safe vital sign parameters need to be specified, as well

as the lower limits of oxygen saturation. Once again, the symptom-limited exercise test allows for a greater degree of confidence in prescribing these limits.

The specific components of a rehabilitation program are as follows:

1. Upper extremity exercises, including strengthening and conditioning exercises. These are typically done with upper body ergometers and with therabands and free weights.
2. Lower extremity exercises, including strengthening and conditioning exercises. These are typically done with bicycle ergometers, treadmill exercise, and, less frequently, with rowing machines or other equipment. The strength training is usually done and with therabands, free weights, and circuit training. The program should usually use the simplest equipment possible to allow the patient to develop an independent program that they can continue after completion of their training.
3. Educational components need to cover all the areas discussed in the Heading entitled "Education." It is important that the staff be well versed in pulmonary diseases so that they can allay patient anxieties and address specific questions.
4. Psychological/social interventions also need to be specific to the individual patient needs. Depression and anxiety need active treatment and will often respond well to a combined supportive and pharmacological treatment.

Perioperative Rehabilitation Program for Individuals After Lung Surgery

The perioperative program essentially consists of rapid mobilization and getting out of bed and to a chair on the first postoperative day. On the following days up to discharge, the goal is ambulation and avoidance of complications. Ambulation should be started as soon as is possible from a point of medical stability. Chest tubes are not a limiting factor for mobilization, and even on suction, portable suction devices can be used to allow for ambulation when air leaks in the chest tubes are a problem. Pain control is essential, and should be adequate to allow pulmonary toilet and ambulation. Usually an individual should be able to do all of their basic ADLs and ambulate independently within 5–7 days after an uncomplicated surgery. In individuals where complications or severe debility do not allow for rapid mobilization, inpatient acute rehabilitation may be helpful. The outcomes on an inpatient rehabilitation unit are usually very good, with stays of 7–10 days able to allow for independence in all but the most debilitated individuals.

Pulmonary toilet after surgery is essential to prevent postoperative pneumonia. Chest physical therapy should be aggressively provided by the nursing staff and by the therapy staff to keep secretions well managed. The time devoted to pulmonary toilet should not detract from the time spent on patient mobilization. In the case of transplantation, education is also started in the first few postoperative days, focusing on medications, immunosuppression, and rejection. In a situation of a patient or family crisis, social work and psychosocial interventions may be needed as well. However, if a comprehensive preoperative rehabilitation program was done, the need for intensive social, educational, or psychosocial services should be limited.

The perioperative mobilization program should ideally have two sessions a day, and take place 7 days a week to maximize recovery. In reality, 6 days a week and an average of 1.5 sessions is usually all that can be attained. Designated therapists should provide these services because the confidence of experienced staff will allow faster and more aggressive mobilization. All patients need close monitoring of oxygen saturation, and in the case of cardiac arrhythmias or suspected ischemia, telemetric monitoring may also be necessary. The focus of this acute hospital-based program is on ambulation and regaining ADL independence. The main exercises include ambulation training, treadmill training, and bicycle ergometry. As soon as a patient has recovered sufficiently to transfer safely, a bedside bicycle ergometer is advised to allow for independent endurance training.

Postoperative Rehabilitation Program

The outpatient program is reinitiated as soon as possible after the patient returns home. Because of complications or a prolonged recovery, selected patients will require inpatient rehabilitation before returning home. For individuals who require a prolonged wean from a ventilator, inpatient rehabilitation at a center that can provide ventilator weaning is necessary. Otherwise, inpatient rehabilitation should be done at a center with experience in treating severe cardiac and pulmonary disease. Often, a center performing a great deal of cardiothoracic surgery or with a large population of pulmonary patients will have relationships with rehabilitation programs. It is important to be sure that the inpatient rehabilitation takes place in an acute rehabilitation center because failure to be aggressive early on can lead to a prolonged course with potentially increased complications.

The outpatient program is essentially the same as before surgery. Often, the exercise program is shorter and may be done on once to twice a week, as the educational components have been covered and supervised exercise is the main goal. Establishment of independence in the exercise program is now a primary goal, and emphasis on adherence to exercise has to be emphasized. Patients need to be aware that failure to adhere to the exercise regimen will lead to a loss of functional capacity.

Maintenance

After any rehabilitation program is completed, the patient is discharged from rehabilitation and is expected to continue to maintain their previous level of functional gains. This is when most of the failure in rehabilitation comes because many individuals do not continue their exercises. The family, primary care physician, and other support groups are essential to create an environment that will encourage exercise compliance. Attendance at support groups after completion of the rehabilitation program is helpful. A support group also allows current patients to meet graduates of the program. Wellness centers, where an ex-patient can come for a nominal fee and exercise under a lowered level of supervision in the rehabilitation setting, are popular with patients and rehabilitation programs. The ongoing participation can help to increase compliance. Overall, the establishment of an effective maintenance program for exercise conditioning is the greatest challenge faced in the rehabilitation of the patient with lung disease. A successful solution to this dilemma will be one of the most important future developments in pulmonary rehabilitation.

Conclusion

Pulmonary rehabilitation helps to maximize the QOL and the functional ability of the individual with lung disease. In the case of the patient undergoing lung surgery, rehabilitation has an important role in the preparation and maximization of recovery form surgery. In lung volume reduction surgery, a combination of exercise and surgery have been shown to provide the greatest benefit for patients with severe emphysema, well above the effects of either one of the interventions alone. There is still a great need for further research into the exact contributions of pulmonary rehabilitation in transplant, pneumonectomy, and other surgical procedures, as well as in interstitial and pulmonary vascular conditions. In the interest of providing the best care to all of our patients with severe lung disease, we should provide intensive pulmonary rehabilitation for all of them. Familiarity with the various lung conditions seen in severe pulmonary disease, and recognition that exercise is safe within reasonable parameters will allow more rehabilitation physicians to become involved with this large group of patients.

Mechanical Ventilation in Rehabilitation

Mechanical ventilatory support is an important part of the management of a subset of patients in the rehabilitation practice. The patient populations that require this support usually have motor neuron disease, neuromuscular disease, or high-level spinal cord injury. There is usually little or no primary pulmonary disease. The advances in ventilatory management have largely come from the ability to now offer non-invasive ventilation and improved technology to make portable ventilatory support possible. The patient on chronic ventilatory support is often referred to as a ventilator-assisted individual (VAI), and the ACCP has established guidelines and achieved consensus on the appropriate approaches to the management of these individuals.

New advances in ventilator management include smaller ventilators, portable units, and noninvasive ventilator management. With improved management of the acute events and anticipatory management of ventilatory failure in progressive neuromuscular disease, the numbers of patients on ventilatory management have increased. These advances have also led the ability to increase the number of VAIs who are now managed in nonacute settings and at home. Obviously, the increase in independence of patients on ventilatory support is to be seen as a goal, and the physiatrist can provide help in returning to the community.

Criteria for Long-Term Mechanical Ventilation

Patients who have lost the ability to maintain adequate ventilation without support are candidates for long-term ventilatory support, and fall into several main areas. Patients may lack central ventilatory drive from a neurological event, may have ventilatory muscle failure, or have severe pulmonary disease (Table 3). The first two groups are of primary interest to the physiatrist.

The criteria for evaluation of the need to initiate ventilatory support depends on the observation of criteria for inability to ventilate adequately on one's own. In some situations, the ventilatory support is only needed during a part of the day (e.g., at night) and in this group, noninvasive ventilatory support (NIV) is the best option, whereas in cases with total ventilatory failure, unless close, full-time supervision is available, tracheostomy and permanent positive pressure ventilation may be needed. The individual needs of each patient will dictate the level of support.

The indications for ventilatory support are in Table 4.

Evaluation

In many patients with high-level spinal cord injury, central nervous system involvement, advanced neuromuscular disease, or clear ventilatory failure, the documentation for the need for support is straightforward. In cases where the level of nocturnal hypoventilation may not be clear, or in what may be borderline cases, polysomnography with documentation of level of ventilation and hypoxemia/hypercarbia can help to establish eligible individuals. In individuals with only nocturnal ventilatory insufficiency,

Table 3
Conditions Requiring Mechanical Ventilation

Central hypoventilation	*Respiratory muscle failure*	*Chronic respiratory disorders*	*Other*
Intracranial hemorrhage, Arnold chiari malformation, CNS trauma, congenital and central failure of control of breathing, myelomeningocele, high SCI, stroke	ALS, congenital myopathies, botulism, muscular dystrophies, myasthenia gravis, phrenicnerve paralysis, polio/postpolio, SMA, myotonic dystrophy	COPD, BPD, CF, ILD	CHF, congenital heart disease, tracheomalacia, vocal cord paralysis, Pierre-Robin syndrome
Central alveolar hypoventilation		Kyphoscoliosis, thoracic wall deformities, thoracoplasty	

CNS, central nervous system; ADL, activities of daily living; SCI, spinal cord injury; ALS, amyotrophic lateral sclerosis; SMA, spinal muscular atrophy; COPD, chronic obstructive pulmonary disease; BPD, bronchopulmonary dysplasia; CF, cystic fibrosis; ILD, interstitial lung disease; CHF, congestive heart failure.

Table 4
Indications for Ventilatory Support

Clinical syndrome of ventilatory failure	*Medical conditions have been maximally managed*	*Following diagnoses present*	*Indications for invasive ventilation (trach)*
Significant daytime CO_2 retention (>50 mmHg) with normalized pH	Optimal medical treatment	Neuromuscular disease	Uncontrollable airway secretions
Mild daytime or nocturnal CO_2 retention (45–50 mmHg) with symptoms of hypoventilation	Patient can handle secretions and protect airway	Chest wall deformity	Chronic aspiration and repeated pneumonias
Significant nocturnal hypoventilation or hypoxemia	Reversible contributing factors have been treated	Central hypoventilation or obesity hypoventilation	Failure of trial of NIV
		OSA with failure to improve with CPAP	24-hour support needed; poor supports or inability to manage NIV
		COPD with severe hypoventilation	Patient preference

NIV, noninvasive ventilatory support; OSA, obstructive sleep apnea; CPAP, continuous positive airway pressure; COPD, chronic obstructive pulmonary disease.

a trial of nasal continuous positive airway pressure may be sufficient to restore ventilatory function to safe levels. Management of comorbidities also needs to be sufficient to assure that congestive heart failure, electrolyte abnormalities, or other issues are not causing the ventilatory insufficiency.

Location for Management of VAIs

Patient independence has to be measured against safety and available resources in the determination of the best setting for the management of VAI's. Ideally, home management should be the goal for all patients with ventilatory failure, but the reality is that often these patients end up in long-term care facilities because the burden of care is too high for caregivers or the support needed in the home setting is not available. Often, the initiation of ventilatory support is done in an acute care facility, and then the patient's transition through a rehabilitation facility to either a long-term facility or home. In the case of chronically progressive diseases, such as amyotrophic lateral sclerosis or muscular dystrophy, the initiation and management may all be done as an outpatient program, as the patient and caregivers are educated and become familiar with the safe use of the noninvasive support. Invasive support requires acute hospitalization for the establishment of the tracheostomy and the initiation of the ventilatory support. Rehabilitation hospital admissions for individuals with acute ventilatory failure leading to VAI often benefit from an acute inpatient rehabilitation stay in order to facilitate reentry into the community.

Outcomes of Ventilatory Management

There is significant mortality associated with long-term ventilatory support. The severity of illness and the underlying disease associated with the respiratory failure seem to be the single greatest factor associated with mortality. The underlying morbidity and mortality of the underlying condition, especially a neuromuscular condition, is often the issue that will decide the eventual prognosis.

Noninvasive Versus Invasive Ventilatory Support

Chronic ventilatory support can be broken into two main categories: invasive and noninvasive support. There are advantages and disadvantages to both types of ventilation. The current consensus among rehabilitation specialists is to attempt to achieve a program of NIV if possible because this is most likely to give patients the best outcomes with respect to function and outcomes. The types of ventilatory support with their benefits and issues are listed in Table 5.

Table 5
Types of Noninvasive Ventilatory Support

Noninvasive support	*Benefits*	*Issues*	*Comments*
• Noninvasive positive pressure ventilation	• No tracheostomy • Best used nocturnally • Often can be done with only a nasal attachment • Maintains full ability to speak • Maintains ability to swallow normally	• Cannot have close monitoring • May not be well tolerated • Not useful for full 24-hour respiratory support	• Often done in assist control method at night • Relaxed daytime setting • Use settings slightly below spontaneous breathing rate to allow for spontaneous breathing to occur • Start with low volumes and pressures initially in order to allow patient to tolerate better • Full support in the 12- to 24-cm H_2O range • Assure adequate support by monitoring $etPCO_2$, $PaCO_2$, and O_2 saturations
• Negative pressure ventilation (iron lung classically), also cuirass, body wrap	• Most physiological • Pneumobelt is a useful daytime adjunctive device	• Often poorly tolerated • Bulky and cumbersome • Difficult to maintain a good fit over time • Bulky and expensive • May develop skin breakdown	• Wraps are less efficient (smaller surface area affected) • Positioning difficult, and fitting has to be good to allow good functioning • Can be bulky to apply
• Pneumobelt and rocking bed	• Physiological • Useful daytime adjunctive device	• Rocking bed needs an attendant, very mobility- and independence-limiting • May develop skin breakdown	

Continued

Table 5 *(Continued)*

Noninvasive support	*Benefits*	*Issues*	*Comments*
• Diaphragm pacing	• Very physiological • Good outcomes in selected patients (high SCI or central apnea)	• Very limited applicability • Requires invasive procedure to place • No system alarms • Issues of possible sleep apnea	• Requires periodic surgical replacement of parts • Very costly initially
• Glossopharyngeal breathing	• Useful to extend time off ventilator support for individuals with nocturnal ventilation	• Limited to adjunct use only • Training required • Usually ineffective in patients with obstruction, decreased chest wall compliance and severely weakened upper airway muscles	
Noninvasive aids for secretion clearance	*Benefits*	*Issues*	*Comments*
• Manually assisted cough	• Generates good cough • Simple • No devices needed	• Needs good cooperation between the caregiver and the patient • Needs cooperative and able patient	• Needs to be done on an empty stomach • Must have frequent application • Avoid in osteoporosis • Need to preceed with insufflation in patients with VC < 1500 cc
• Mechanical insufflation–exsufflation	• Used where manually assisted cough fails • Has ability to be repeated to clear secretions	• Cannot be used with bullous disease or situation where barotraumas may be an issue	• Mechanical device generates 30–40 cm H_2O inflation with abrupt decrease to –30 to –50 cm H_2O • Usually done in five-cycle groups

Continued

Table 5 *(Continued)*

Noninvasive Aids for Secretion Clearance	*Benefits*	*Issues*	*Comments*
• Mechanical oscillation	• Benefits mucocilliary transport • Helpful with airflow limitation or chest wall disease • Can be used along with chest PT	• May not be of any greater benefit than manually assisted cough • Needs further study	• High frequency oscillators, assist mucocilliary transport
Invasive positive pressure ventilation	*Benefits*	*Issues*	*Comments*
• Tracheostomy tubes	• Best in patients with 24-hour dependence • Failure of NIV • Rapidly progressive ventilation • Use with aspiration • Helpful in patients unable to protect airways	• Lower quality of life than NIV • Has more complications • Tracheal = malacia • Infections • Increased and more severe bronchitis and pneumonia • Barotraumas	• Use standard tidal volumes • Use sufficient pressures to assure adequate ventilation • May need O_2 supplementation • Avoid SIMV mode (increased work of breathing) • Need adequate disconnection alarm system • Need backup power system and ventilator in patients who cannot breathe on their own for 4 hours

VC, vital capacity; PT, physical therapy; SCI, spinal cord injury; SIMV, synchronized intermittent mandatory ventilation; NIV, noninvasive ventilatory support.

Discharge Criteria for VAIs to Various Levels of Care

Ideally, all patients will be able to be discharged to the lowest level of care possible. The level of cooperation and comfort with the ventilatory support of the patient and the patient's family is the most important factor in deciding the level of care on discharge. Other issues include medical support, nursing care, respiratory therapy service availability, and equipment.

To go to a long-term care facility, a patient should be on less than 40% supplemental oxygen, have positive-end expiratory pressure of less than 5 cm H_2O, can perform some ventilator-free breathing (essential in NIV), and have been stable for 1–2 weeks with these settings. For home discharge, all of the above need to be met, but the stability should be there for 3–4 weeks, and there should be family or personal care attendants available. The patient has to be able to supervise and participate in directing caregivers, participate in his or her medical regimen, have no major affective disorders, have a stable home and family setting, have willing and available caregivers, have a home environment suitable for a ventilator, and have adequate financial support to allow for care at home. The specific needs in the home environment are covered in the literature and are not be reviewed here.

In conclusion, in all cases where possible, NIV is preferred over invasive ventilatory support. Unfortunately, there are often issues that arise to make home discharge difficult, but with a dedicated team, often these obstacles can be overcome and NIV in a home environment may offer the best functional and best QOL for individuals needing chronic ventilatory support. Physiatric involvement is essential in patients with ventilatory failure and neuromuscular, central, or other cases of muscular failure. Familiarity with the types of ventilatory support and with the needs of patients is an essential part of that care.

Key References and Suggested Additional Reading

American Thoracic Society. Cigarette smoking and health: official statement of the American Thoracic Society. Am J Respir Crit Care Med 1996; 153: 861–865.

Anonymous. Guidelines for the management of chronic obstructive pulmonary disease. Working Group of the South African Pulmonology Society (see comments). S Afr Med J 1998; 88:999–1002, 1004, 1006–1110.

Anonymous. Pulmonary rehabilitation: joint ACCP/AACVPR evidence-based guidelines. ACCP/AACVPR Pulmonary Rehabilitation Guidelines Panel. American College of Chest Physicians. American Association of Cardiovascular and Pulmonary Rehabilitation (see comments). Chest 1997; 112:1363–1396.

Atkins BJ, Kaplan RM, Timms RM, et al. Behavioral exercise programs in the management of chronic obstructive pulmonary disease. J Consult Clin Psychol 1984; 52:591–602.

Bach JR. Mechanical exsufflation, noninvasive ventilation, and new strategies for pulmonary rehabilitation and sleep disordered breathing. Bull NY Acad Med 1992; 68:321–340.

Bach JR, Moldover JR. Cardiovascular, pulmonary, and cancer rehabilitation. 2. Pulmonary rehabilitation. Arch Phys Med Rehabil 1996; 77:S45–S51.

Blake RL, Jr., Vandiver TA, Braun S, Bertuso DD, Straub V. A randomized controlled evaluation of a psychosocial intervention in adults with chronic lung disease. Fam Med 1990; 22:365–370.

Burdet L, de Muralt B, Schutz Y, Pichard C, Fitting JW. Administration of growth hormone to underweight patients with chronic obstructive pulmonary disease. A prospective, randomized, controlled study. Am J Respir Crit Care Med 1997; 156:1800–1806.

Carrieri-Kohlman V, Douglas MK, Gormley JM, et al. Desxensitization and guided mastery: treatment approaches for the management of dyspnea. Heart Lung 1993; 22:226–234.

Celli BR. Current thoughts regarding treatment of chronic obstructive pulmonary disease. Med Clin N Am 1996; 80:589–609.

Celli BR, Snider GL, Heffner J, et al. Standards for the diagnoisis and care of patients with COPD. Am J Respir Crit Care Med 1995; 152(Suppl 5):S78–S121.

Cox NJ, Hendricks JC, Binkhorst RA, van Herwaarden CL. A pulmonary rehabilitation program for patients with asthma and mild chronic obstructive pulmonary diseases (COPD). Lung 1993; 171:235–244.

Creutzberg EC, Schols AM, Bothmer-Quaedvlieg FC, Wouters EF. Prevalence of an elevated resting energy expenditure in patients with chronic obstructive pulmonary disease in relation to body composition and lung function. Eur J Clin Nutr 1998; 52:396–401.

Dekhuijzen PN, Folgering HT, van Herwaarden CL. Target-flow inspiratory muscle training at home and during pulmonary rehabilitation in COPD patients with a ventilatory limitation during exercise. Lung 1990; 168:502–508.

Devine EC, Pearcy J. Meta-analysis of the effects of psychoeducational care in adults with chronic obstructive pulmonary disease. Patient Educ Couns 1996; 29:167–178.

Ferreira IM, Verreschi IT, Nery LE, et al. The influence of 6 months of oral anabolic steroids on body mass and respiratory muscles in undernourished COPD patients. Chest 1998; 114:19–28.

Fishman AP, Pulmonary rehabilitation research NIH Workshop Summary. Am J Respir Crit Care Med 1994; 149:825–833.

Gilmartin ME. Pulmonary rehabilitation. Patient and family education. Clin Chest Med 1986; 7:619–627.

Goldstein RS. Candidate evaluation. In: Casaburi R, Petty TL, eds. Principles and Practice of Pulmonary Rehabilitaion. Philadelphia: WB Saunders, 1993; 317–321.

Herningfield JE, Nemeth-Coslet R. Nicotine dependence. tnterference between tobacco and tobacco related disease. Chest 1988; 93: 375–380.

Mahler DA. Pulmonary rehabilitation. Chest 1998; 113:263S–268S.

Make BJ. Collaborative Self-management strategies for patients with respirtatory disease. Respir Care 1994; 39: 566–569.

Make BJ, Hill NS, Goldberg AI, et al. Mechanical ventilation beyond the intensive care unit: Report of a consensus conference of the American College of Chest Physicians. Chest 1998; 113:289s–344s.

Maltais F, LeBlanc P, Simard C, et al. Skeletal Muscle adaptation to endurance training in patients with chonic obstructive pulmonary disease. Am J Respir Crit Care Med 1996; 154:442–447.

Medical Research Council Working Party: Long-term domiciliary oxygen therapy in chronic hypoxic cor pulmonale complicating chronic bronchitis and emphysema. Lancet. 1981; 1:681–685.

Milani RV, Lavie CJ. Disparate effects of out-patient cardiac and pulmonary rehabilitation programs on work efficiency and peak aerobic capacity in patients with coronary disease or severe obstructive pulmonary disease. J Cardiopulm Rehabil 1998; 18:17–22.

Moy ML, Ingenito EP, Mentzer SJ, Evans RB, Reilly JJ, Jr. Health-related quality of life improves following pulmonary rehabilitation and lung volume reduction surgery. Chest 1999; 115:383–389.

Nocturnal oxygen therapy trial group: continuous or nocturnal oxygen therapy in hypoxemic chronic obstructive airways disease: a clinical trial. Ann Intern Med. 1980; 93:391–398.

Ojanen M, Lahdensuo A, Laitinen J, Karvonen J. Psychosocial changes in patients participating in a chronic obstructive pulmonary disease rehabilitation program. Respiration 1993; 60:96–102.

Owens MW, Markewitz BA, Payne DK. Outpatient management of chronic obstructive pulmonary disease. Am J Med Sci 1999; 318:79–83.

Petty TL. Thye worldwide epidemiology of chronic obstructive pulmonary disease. Curr Opin Pulmon Med 1996; 2:84–89.

Reardon J, Awad E, Normandin E, Vale F, Clark B, ZuWallack RL. The effect of comprehensive outpatient pulmonary rehabilitation on dyspnea. Chest 1994; 105:1046–1052.

Reis AL. Preventing COPD: you can make a difference. J Respir Dis 1993; 14: 739–749.

Reis AL, Kaplan RM, Limberg TM, Prewitt LM. Effects of pulmonary rehabilitation on physiologic and psychosocial outcomes in patients with chronic obstructive pulmonary disease. Ann Intern Med 1995; 122:823–832.

Resnikoff PM, Reis AL. Maximizing functional capacity. Pulmonary rehabilitation and adjunctive measures. Respir Care Clin N Am 1998; 4:475–492.

San Pedro GS. Pulmonary rehabilitation for the patient with severe chronic obstructive pulmonary disease. Am J Med Sci 1999; 318:99–102.

Sassi-Dambron DE, Eakin EG, Ries AL, Kaplan RM. Treatment of dyspnea in COPD. A controlled clinical trial of dyspnea management strategies (see comments). Chest 1995; 107:724–729.

Schols AM, Mostert R, Soeters PB, Wouters EF. Body composition and exercise performance in patients with chronic obstructive pulmonary disease (see comments). Thorax 1991; 46:695–699.

Schols AM, Slangen J, Volovics L, Wouters EF. Weight loss is a reversible factor in the prognosis of chronic obstructive pulmonary disease. Am J Respir Crit Care Med 1998; 157:1791–1797.

Schols AM, Soeters PB, Dingemans AM, Mostert R, Frantzen PJ, Wouters EF. Prevalence and characteristics of nutritional depletion in patients with stable COPD eligible for pulmonary rehabilitation. Am Rev Respir Dis 1993; 147:1151–1156.

Sin DD, McAlister FA, Man SF, Anthonisen NR. Contemporary management of chronic obstructive pulmonary disease: scientific review. JAMA. 2003; 290:2301–2312.

Strijbos JH, Postma DS, van Altena R, Gimeno F, Koeter GH. A comparison between an outpatient hospital-based pulmonary rehabilitation program and a home-care pulmonary rehabilitation program in patients with COPD. A follow-up of 18 months (see comments). Chest 1996; 109:366–372.

Toshima M, Kaplan RM, Reis AL. Experimental evaluation of rehabilitation in chronic obstructive pulmonary disease: short term effects on exercise endurance and health status. Health Psychol 1990; 9:237–252.

White B, Andrews JL, Jr., Mogan JJ, Downes-Vogel P. Pulmonary rehabilitation in an ambulatory group practice setting. Med Clin N Am 1979; 63: 379–390.

Wijkstra PJ, van der Mark TW, Kraan J, van Altena R, Koeter GH, Postma DS. Long-term effects of home rehabilitation on physical performance in chronic obstructive pulmonary disease. Am J Respir Crit Care Med 1996; 153:1234–1241.

7 Pediatric Rehabilitation

Jilda N. Vargus-Adams

Introduction

Pediatric rehabilitation medicine is a small but far-reaching field. This chapter aims to introduce the reader to the common diagnoses encountered in pediatric rehabilitation and to review common therapies and complications. Many of the diagnoses are best managed by intradisciplinary treatment teams, including a pediatric physiatrist and other appropriate professionals (pediatric therapists, neurologists, neurosurgeons, orthopedic surgeons, urologists, psychologists, orthotists, educators, developmental pediatricians, social workers, nurses, etc.).

Growth and Development

Children change rapidly during the first few years of life. Pediatric physiatrists may participate in the diagnosis and treatment of developmental delays. Table 1 includes many of the major milestones of child development.

Assessments for Children

To understand the current functioning of patients or to assess changes over time, the pediatric physiatrist may employ specific measures or instruments. Many of these tools have been designed specifically for use with children.

In the rehabilitation unit, the Functional Independence Measure for Children (WeeFIM) is commonly used to follow patients' progress during

From: *Essential Physical Medicine and Rehabilitation*
Edited by: G. Cooper © Humana Press Inc., Totowa, NJ

Table 1
Developmental Milestones

Age	*Gross motor skills*	*Fine motor skills/self-care skills*	*Communication/Cognition*
6 months	• Rolls over • Sits with support • Bears weight when held erect	• Reaches for objects • Transfers objects hand-to-hand	• Reciprocal voalization • Looks for dropped object • Turns to sounds
12 months	• Creeps on all fours • Pulls to stand • Cruises	• Pincer grasp • Self-feed finger foods	• Single words or word-like utterances • Follows commands • Object permanence
18 months	• Walks well • Climbs steps with hand held • Seats self in chair	• Uses spoon • Imitates household tasks • Stacks two blocks	• Intelligible single words (at least 6) • Points to named objects
24 months	• Ascends and descends stairs • Runs • Kicks ball	• Uses fork • Doffs clothing • Establishes handedness • Draws • Stacks six blocks	• More than 50 words • Two-word sentences • Follows two-step commands
36 months	• Jumps • Single-limb stance • Uses pedal toy	• Dons clothing • Usually toilet trained • Throws ball overhand • Stacks eight blocks • Draws single line	• Uses pronouns, adjectives, adverbs, negatives, and plurals • Longer sentences • Knows full name and colors

their stay. The WeeFIM measures functioning, ranging from "dependent" to "independent" in mobility, self-care, cognition, and communication domains. Many other assessment tools may be used for various outcomes of concern. Several of these are listed in Table 2.

A large number of additional measures are available to the physician, therapist, or psychologist when necessary. Comprehensive neuropsychological evaluation is often warranted for children with impairments. This evaluation, conducted by a pediatric neuropsychologist, may include several different and specific instruments to best describe a child's functioning. The neuropsychologist will also make recommendations for educational strategies and ongoing management.

Pediatric Therapy and Equipment

Physical, occupational, or speech therapy is frequently provided to children with developmental delay, injury, or other concerns. Publicly funded early intervention programs ensure that therapy is available to children from birth to 3 years of age if a physician expresses concerns about development (mandated by the Individuals with Disabilities Education Act). Thereafter, children may qualify for public developmental preschool or therapy in a school setting. Services provided in schools must contribute to the child's ability to participate in the educational process; thus, life skills or athletic endeavors that are not necessary in the school environment may not be appropriate goals for school therapy. Additional outpatient services may also be warranted.

Pediatric therapy has various theoretical backgrounds. The most common is neurodevelopmental therapy (NDT). NDT, also known as the Bobath approach, emphasizes the role of neurological dysfunction in impeding typical postural control and motor development. Furthermore, normal motor skills are the aim of therapy. NDT focuses on inhibiting primitive reflexes, spasticity, and abnormal movement patterns, and emphasis is placed on the quality of movement and functional activities. Many other treatment approaches may be incorporated into a child's treatment plan. Very little robust research has addressed what types of therapy are best for children with special needs. Questions about frequency, duration, and timing of therapy are also unanswered.

Newer therapies for children include the use of constraint-induced movement therapy (for hemiplegia, drawing on experience in adult stroke), plyometrics and dynamic neuromuscular training (particularly for adolescent female athletes), and strengthening programs for children with neurological diseases, such as cerebral palsy. The evidence base for some of

Table 2
Outcome Measures in Pediatric Rehabilitation

Development	*Adaptive and/or physical functioning*	*Cognition*	*Quality of life/behavior*
• Battelle Developmental Inventory (BDI)	• Vineland Adaptive Behavior Scales: *rates functioning in daily activities, interaction*	• Wechsler Intelligence Scale for Children (WISC): *provides verbal, performance, and full-scale IQ, ages 6 and up*	• Child Health Questionnaire: *widely used measure of health-related quality of life (like the SF-36 for adults)*
• Bayley Scales of Infant Development: *comprehensive evaluation of cognition, motor and behavior*	• Pediatric Evaluation of Disability Inventory (PEDI): *evaluates self-care, mobility, and social function*	• Stanford-Binet Intelligence Scale: *IQ measurement age 2 and up*	• Child Behavior Checklist (CBC): *parental report of behavior issues*
• Denver Developmental Screening Test/Denver II: *a screening test for developmental delay in first few years*	• Functional Independence Measure for Children (WeeFIM): *assesses function in six domains, like the FIM* • Gross Motor Function Measure (GMFM): *rates gross motor skills, especially in cerebral palsy* • Peabody Developmental Motor Scales: *comprehensive evaluation of fine and gross motor skills*	• Kaufman Assessment Battery for Children (K-ARC): *intelligence and achievement measure for ages 2–12* • Woodcock Johnson Psycho-Educational Battery (WJ-R): *cognitive and achievement test for ages 3 years and up.*	• Connor's Rating Scales (CRS-R): *method to assess symptoms of ADHD*

SF-36, Short-Form 36; ADHA, attention deficit hyperactivity disorder.

these interventions is growing. A large variety of alternative and complementary therapy approaches are suggested. Many of these interventions are either poorly studied (patterning, Therasuit) or not helpful (hyperbaric oxygen therapy), whereas others may have some supportive evidence (therapeutic horse riding, aquatic therapy).

Orthoses are frequently employed for children with special needs. Ankle–foot orthoses may be used to provide better foot and ankle positioning for patients with high tone (cerebral palsy, stroke) or low tone (Down syndrome, myelomeningocele) feet. Gait trainers and walkers (often used in a reverse position with the walker behind the child) are appropriate for many young children with gross motor concerns. More expensive and technically complicated equipment is usually prescribed by a specialist. These items would include augmentative communication devices, powered mobility (for children as young as 2 years of age), and long leg braces of any sort.

Cerebral Palsy

Cerebral palsy (CP) is the most common disability of childhood. CP is defined as a disorder of movement or posture resulting from an injury to the developing brain. The brain injury is nonprogressive (sometimes called "static encephalopathy"), but the associated impairments and functional status may change with growth and development.

CP affects about 1 in 500 live births, and the incidence is stable to increasing in the United States. Most cases of CP do not have an identifiable etiology, although prematurity is the largest single associated factor. Other risk factors for CP include small for gestational age, low birth weight (<2500 g), prenatal infection, prenatal stroke, maternal risk factors, or postnatal infection or trauma. Severe birth asphyxia is the cause of less than 10% of CP. In premature infants, intraventricular hemorrhage can lead to periventricular leukomalacia, which often results in spastic diparetic CP. Diffuse insults to the brain, such as hypoxia/ischemia, may result in spastic quadriparetic CP, whereas kernicterus (bilirubin encephalopathy), which preferentially affects the basal ganglia, may cause athetoid CP. Hemiparetic CP is usually the result of an *in utero* vascular event (frequently the middle cerebral artery distribution) of unknown etiology.

CP is classified by type of movement disorder and part of body affected (*see* Table 3).

The diagnosis of CP is difficult before 4 to 6 months of age. Warning signs include motor delay or deviance (hand preference before 1 year, fisted hand, bunny-hop crawl), abnormal findings on neurological examination

Table 3
Classification of Cerebral Palsy

Type	*Incidence*	*Presentation*
Spastic (80% total)		• Spasticity, hyperreflexia, abnormal reflexes
• Hemiparetic	20–30%	• One side, usually arm more affected than leg • Usually develop equinus as toddlers
• Diparetic	18–33%	• Legs more affected than arms • Delayed gross motor skills • Often "commando crawl" and scissor
• Quadriparetic	25–35%	• Total body involvement, may have hypotonic trunk • Frequent comorbidities (mental retardation, dysphagia, epilepsy)
Mixed spastic/ dyskinetic	10–20%	• Usually quadriparetic with additional movement disorder
Dyskinetic	Rare	• May have choreiform, athetoid, choreoathetoid, or dystonic movement
Hypotonic or ataxic	Very rare	• Merit investigation for other diagnosis

(tone abnormalities, asymmetry, movement disorders), and persistent primitive reflexes (obligatory asymmetric tonic neck reflex, persistent startle or grasp reflexes). Brain imaging, preferably magnetic resonance imaging, is important in the diagnosis of CP. Although CP is quite common, other diagnoses must be considered, including neurodegenerative disorders, spinal cord lesions, neuromuscular diseases, inborn errors of metabolism, and cognitive disability.

Parents frequently ask if their children with CP will walk. Children with spastic hemiparetic CP usually walk at 12 to 18 months. Children with spastic diparetic CP mostly walk in some fashion by 4 years. A minority of children with spastic quadriparetic CP walk, and 25% of these children are dependent for all activities. Walking is most likely in children who sit independently by 2 years and least likely in children who cannot sit by 4 years.

Problems associated with CP include sensory deficits (vision problems, such as strabismus or field cuts, and somatosensory disruption), speech and language issues (dysarthria, dysphagia), epilepsy, cognitive limitation, and osteoporosis. Motor issues typically include abnormal tone, weakness, and diminished selective control. Management of CP often requires attention to musculoskeletal complications of spasticity. Equinus foot deformities, hip

Table 4
Spasticity Treatment in Children

Interventions	*Therapy*	*Medical*	*Surgical*
Localized	• Range of motion • Bracing • Modalities (ice, heat)	• Nerve blocks with phenol or botulinum toxin	• Orthopedic procedures
Systemic		• Oral medications (baclofen, dantrolene, tizanidine, diazepam) • Intrathecal baclofen	• Selective dorsal rhizotomy

subluxation and dislocation, and scoliosis all may require intervention with anti-spasticity measures and/or orthopedic or neurosurgical procedures.

Spasticity

Spasticity is a disorder of muscle tone that manifests as a resistance to passive movement that is greater with higher speeds of movement. Spasticity is common in CP and other upper motor neuron (UMN) disorders, such as brain injury or spinal cord injury (SCI). Myriad interventions for spasticity (Table 4) permit the pediatric physiatrist to markedly reduce the impact of spasticity on the comfort and function of children with disabilities. Unfortunately, treating spasticity does not usually resolve all issues for the child, as related impairments (weakness, poor selective motor control) and other problems (cognitive dysfunction) will persist.

Therapists can work on spasticity with range-of-motion (ROM) exercises. Frequently, bracing is used to hold joints in positions of relative stretch or in more functional positions when spasticity is an issue. For most children, flexion is prominent, so stretching and bracing helps maintain or improve extension.

For more significant spasticity, therapy measures may be insufficient to maintain ROM and promote function. If spasticity is focal (such as in just the plantar flexor muscles or a biceps and pronator), localized interventions should be considered. In children, botulinum toxin injections are widely employed in such situations. Botulinum toxin binds presynaptically at the neuromuscular junction and prevents acetylcholine release—resulting in muscle weakness that persists for 3 to 5 months. It is administered by intramuscular injection, either using only anatomical landmarks or with assistance via electrical stimulation, electromyography (EMG) guidance, ultrasound, or computed tomography guidance. Children usually require anesthesia or sedation for any injections that are done with guidance or EMG.

Phenol nerve blocks also may be used for focal spasticity. These blocks are accomplished by injecting a neurolytic (phenol or sometimes alcohol) very near the targeted nerve to chemically damage the nerve. Electrical stimulation allows the physiatrist to locate the nerve or motor point accurately. This option is usually less expensive than botulinum toxin and may have a longer effect. The primary risk of nerve blocks is sensory dysesthesia when a mixed nerve is targeted. Nerves commonly treated include the obturator nerve (to reduce adductor tone), the sciatic nerve, and the tibial nerve.

Orthopedic surgery may be helpful for focal spasticity. Soft-tissue procedures include tendon lengthening or release and more complicated procedures, including tendon transfers and osteotomies. Because the underlying neurological problems remain after surgery, some children may have progressive deformity or resurgent spasticity with time or growth.

Systemic spasticity treatment usually begins with medications. Baclofen, which acts at central nervous system γ-aminobutyric acid receptors, is often the first-choice drug, but it may cause sedation even at low doses, and there is a risk of withdrawal symptoms if baclofen is stopped suddenly. Dantrolene sodium works at the level of the muscle to decrease calcium release at the sarcoplasmic reticulum. Some patients experience weakness on dantrolene, and liver function must be followed closely because of potential hepatotoxicity. Tizanidine is a newer agent that works centrally and may cause sedation or liver problems. Diazepam has been widely used for spasticity, but may be most appropriate for short-term use, such as following surgery, owing to cognitive issues and development of tolerance.

For a subset of children with spasticity, enteral medications are insufficient, either because of lack of effect or severity of side effects. For these children, surgical interventions should be considered. Sometimes multiple level orthopedic procedures are helpful, and it is recommended that these be done simultaneously, if possible. Selective dorsal rhizotomy involves severing dorsal roots in the cauda equina to reduce excitatory inputs. The procedure is performed via laminectomy and is typically employed for young children (4–10 years of age) with moderate impairment, especially spastic diparetic CP. Intrathecal baclofen (ITB) is administered via an implanted pump placed in the abdomen with a catheter running to the intrathecal space. Very low doses of baclofen may result in significant reduction in spasticity when administered in this fashion. The risk of withdrawal is higher with ITB than with enteral therapy, and complications with the drug delivery mechanism may occur; however, ITB has been a very popular treatment for children with severe spasticity.

Spina Bifida and Pediatric SCI

Spina bifida is the second most common childhood disability. Spina bifida includes all neural tube deficits that result during embryonic development, usually occurring in the first few weeks. Risk factors for spina bifida include low socioeconomic status, maternal factors, and inadequate folic acid intake. The incidence of spina bifida has been decreasing, attributed in large part to folate supplementation.

Spina bifida is usually recognized on fetal ultrasound, but may present at birth with an open area of the dorsal spine and herniation of the meninges and nervous tissue (also called "myelomeningocele"). If only the meninges are involved, it is a meningocele. Neurosurgical repair is recommended in the first few days of life. Depending on the level of involvement and the degree to which the spinal cord is damaged, children with spina bifida may have a wide range of deficits. Most motor impairments are related to the level of injury and involve weakness or paralysis, hyporeflexia, and hypotonia (lower motor neuron). Sensory impairment is generally below the level of injury as well. The most common level of injury is lumbar or lumbosacral, although thoracic spina bifida accounts for a significant minority.

Spina bifida occulta is a spinal deformity affecting the vertebrae where there is no neurological involvement. This entity may be identified after investigation of a sacral pigmented or hirsute patch or dimple or as an incidental finding on radiological exam. It is a common deformity (up to 8% of the population) and only rarely has associated neurological deficits.

Spina bifida is associated with Arnold Chiari malformation type II in the majority of cases, and other central nervous system malformations may also occur. Hydrocephalus is common and typically requires ventriculoperitoneal shunting in infancy. Shunt malfunctions are common and result in multiple revisions. Tethered cord may occur initially or as the child grows. If a child with spina bifida shows deterioration in function, including loss of strength or sensation, pain, or UMN signs, imaging should be performed to look for syringomyelia or tethered cord. Most children with spina bifida have neurogenic bowel and bladder. Bladder management includes use of intermittent catheterization as retention becomes a problem. Children may begin a bowel program at 2 to 3 years of age and may begin learning catheterization skills when they reach school age. Other associated problems include scoliosis/kyphosis, lower extremity orthopedic deformities, cognitive deficits, precocious puberty, latex allergy, and osteoporosis.

Thoracic level spina bifida results in paraplegia, whereas lower levels of spina bifida usually have greater lower extremity strength and control. With appropriate bracing and equipment, many children with spina bifida are able to achieve some form of upright mobility. Low thoracic- and lumbar-level lesions necessitate use of high-control devices, such as a reciprocal gait orthoses, although crutch walking is achievable for some children. Many children eventually choose to use wheelchairs owing to increased energy cost and need for assistance in ambulation. Children with low lumbar spina bifida will stand and cruise by 1 year, and progress to community ambulation, sometimes with the aid of ankle–foot orthoses. Children with sacral spina bifida are all expected to achieve community-level ambulation.

Acquired SCIs in children are less common than spina bifida and are usually caused by motor vehicle collisions, falls, sports injuries, or penetrating trauma. In young children, high cervical lesions are more common, probably because of the relatively larger and heavier head. In past years, it was reported that children frequently had SCI without obvious radiological abnormality, but with better magnetic resonance imaging, SCI without obvious radiological abnormality is far less common. Pediatric SCI is classified with the same American Spinal Cord Injury Association system used in adults. Also similar to adults, children with SCI may receive high-dose steroids after injury and/or spinal stabilization surgery. Prophylaxis for deep venous thrombosis, however, is not as widely employed in children, especially for those that have not yet reached puberty. Immobilization hypercalcemia occurs most frequently in adolescent boys with complete quadriplegia in the first few months after SCI. It presents with gastrointestinal complaints, fatigue, and behavior changes and should be treated with fluid, mobilization, and other medications, if refractory.

Management of neurogenic bladder begins with resolution of spinal shock and development of detrusor sphincter dyssynergia. Children should receive appropriate urodynamic studies and clean intermittent catheterization. Self-catheterization should be taught whenever possible. Other SCI issues are also common between children and adults: skin integrity, autonomic dysreflexia, spasticity, osteoporosis, use of adaptive equipment and wheelchairs, etc. Contractures, hip subluxation, and scoliosis may become more important issues for children because of the contribution of growth.

Pediatric Acquired Brain Injury

Traumatic brain injury (TBI) is the leading cause of acquired disability in children and a leading cause of death. Most TBIs are the result of motor

Table 5
Glasgow Coma Scale for Young Children

Score	*Eye opening*	*Best motor response*	*Best verbal response*
6		• Obeys commands	
5		• Localizes to painful stimulus	• Smiles, oriented to sound, follows objects, interacts
4	• Spontaneous	• Withdraws to painful stimulus	• Cries but consolable, interacts appropriately
3	• In response to verbal command	• Abnormal flexion posture to painful stimulus	• Cries but is inconsistently consolable, moaning
2	• In response to pain	• Extensor posture to painful stimulus	• Inconsolable crying, irritable
1	• No opening	• No response	• No response

vehicle collisions, but falls, other nonintentional mechanisms, and assault also contribute. TBI is classified as mild (Glasgow Coma Scale [GCS] score >12, no abnormality on brain imaging), moderate (GCS score 9–12 or abnormal imaging), or severe (GCS score <9). An adapted GCS is used for young children (Table 5). Most TBIs are mild, but moderate and severe injuries cause the most morbidity, mortality, and expense.

Children with TBI may have cognitive, sensory, and/or motor deficits. Cognitive issues are felt to be the most significant cause of disability after TBI. These problems are wide-ranging and include behavior issues, agitation, poor arousal or attention, poor memory, impaired judgment, and poor social and emotional skills. Sensory impairments are likely to result from cranial nerve injuries altering smell, hearing, or vision, although somatosensory deficits may also occur. Motor impairments are quite variable depending on the injury.

In the acute phase of severe TBI, complications may include storming (or central autonomic dysfunction), wherein the child has fever, hypertension, tachycardia, diaphoresis, and posturing, or heterotopic ossification wherein bone is formed in soft tissues, especially in adolescents with fractures. A unique late complication in children is the advent of precocious puberty, particularly for girls. Other potential complications are posttraumatic epilepsy, dysphagia, spasticity, and hydrocephalus.

Although it was once thought that the plasticity of an immature brain would help children with TBI have better recovery, infants and toddlers appear to have worse outcomes than older children. Mild TBI seldom results in long-term deficits, and children with mild TBI appear the same as control children 1 year after injury. Poorer outcomes have been noted for intentional injury. All children with TBI should receive long-term follow-up because cognitive deficits may not be apparent until the child is older.

Anoxic brain injury occurs when the brain is subjected to hypoxia and ischemia. In children, the mechanism is often near drowning, although cardiac events are also implicated. In cases of submersion, additional problems may be encountered because of lung injury. Events in cold water may have a better outcome owing to the protective effects of hypothermia. It can be very difficult to predict the outcome of acute anoxic brain injury although prolonged cardiopulmonary resuscitation, metabolic acidosis, and delay in resuscitation are all associated with poor outcome. The specificity of these risk factors is not perfect because some children who present with asystole, apnea, and acidosis have good recovery. Long-term follow-up demonstrates that children with anoxic brain injury frequently have poorer outcomes than those with TBI, with higher rates of prolonged coma and vegetative state.

Unlike many conditions encountered in pediatric physiatry, acquired brain injury is highly preventable. All efforts to promote safe transport of children (appropriate car seats, use of the back seat until 12 years), adequate supervision, and the use of helmets should be encouraged.

Pediatric Limb Deficiency

Congenital limb deficiency occurs in around 1 per 2500 live births. Several classification systems exist, but the most accepted terminology categorizes deficiencies as transverse (no structures distal to level) or longitudinal (some degree of distal structure), with further definition explaining the most distal intact segment (for transverse) or the absent or atypical bones (for longitudinal). The most common deficiency is a left terminal transradial deficiency (limb is absent distal to somewhere in the forearm). Upper extremity deficiencies are far more common than lower extremity deficiencies. Congenital limb deficiencies may occur as a result of altered embryological development in the first trimester. Most congenital limb deficiencies occur as isolated anomalies, although craniofacial deformities and genetic syndromes are occasional comorbidities.

For upper limb transradial deficiencies, a passive mitt prosthesis is provided at around 6 months of age (when the child sits), a prosthesis with terminal device is provided around 1 year of age (when the child walks), and the child can use all types of prosthetic components by 4 to 5 years old.

Lower limb prostheses should be provided when the child is ready to pull to stand, but knee joints are not provided until preschool age.

Acquired limb deficiency is less common than congenital deficiency in children and is usually the result of trauma, although tumors and other disorders are also causative factors. Following amputation, children's long bones may develop terminal overgrowth. This uniquely pediatric complication, occurring at the bony apophysis, may require surgery.

Orthopedic and Rheumatic Disorders

Orthopedic problems are not uncommon in the young child. Club foot, or talipes equinovarus, is a congenital deformity that includes equinus (plantar flexion of the ankle), varus (inversion at the heel), and varus of the forefoot (inversion of the forefoot), which occurs in 1 per 400 live births and is usually treated with casting, although some children require surgery. Developmental dysplasia of the hip (DDH) may include subluxation, dislocation, or an altered acetabulum, and has a similar incidence to club foot. DDH may result in significant hip problems if not detected and appropriately treated in infancy. Testing for DDH includes the Galeazzi test (a dislocated hip is evident when the baby's knees are flexed in a supine position and one knee appears lower than the other), the Barlow test (a hip can be dislocated by flexion and adduction while the femur is pushed outward— and usually reduces into place with subsequent abduction), and the Ortolani test (reduction of a dislocated hip can be accomplished by abducting the hip while pushing anteriorly on the greater trochanter). Ultrasound imaging is indicated if any abnormalities are detected on physical exam of an infant's hip. Early orthopedic management of DDH is imperative to prevent future disability.

Congenital torticollis is usually the result of fibrosis of the sternocleidomastoid muscle, although hemivertebrae or other anatomic anomalies may also be causative. After radiological evaluation, stretching should be initiated, but some children require additional interventions. Pulling on the arm of a young child may result in nursemaid's elbow (radial head subluxation), which becomes evident when the child refuses to move the arm but will use the hand. A nursemaid's elbow can usually be reduced with supination and flexion.

Normal development includes initial genu varum (bow legs) in infancy, genu valgum (knock knees) in toddler years, and reversal to minimal genu valgum by school age.

Active adolescents may develop Osgood-Schlatter's disease and complain of anterior lower knee pain with activity. Because of inflammation at the tibial tubercle and the attachment of the patella tendon, these adolescents have pain and tenderness that often resolves if athletic endeavors are restricted for several weeks. Spondylolisthesis (slippage of one vertebra anterior to the one below it) in children results from dysplastic or bony abnormalities at L5–S1 or L4–L5 and results in back pain. Spondylolisthesis is especially common in female gymnasts. If the slip increases, it can progress to spondylolysis, which may require surgery. Scoliosis is usually idiopathic and may benefit from conscientious bracing while growth is ongoing. If curves exceed 40 to 50°, surgical correction is considered. Neuromuscular (associated with CP, spina bifida, or neuromuscular disease) or congenital scoliosis is not typically responsive to bracing.

When a child develops a limp that is the result of hip pain, the differential diagnosis includes transient synovitis of the hip, avascular necrosis of the femoral head (Legg-Calve-Perthes disease), and slipped capital femoral epiphysis. Transient synovitis is the more common cause, and presents in young children with limp and poor hip internal rotation. With rest and anti-inflammatory medication, most children improve in a few days. Avascular necrosis occurs in school-age children who complain of groin and thigh pain and are found to have poor hip mobility in most planes. Treatment is usually rest and bracing, with better outcomes in younger children and those with less involvement. Slipped capital femoral epiphysis is highly associated with obesity and occurs in young adolescent children. This disorder typically requires surgical intervention and may result in chronic hip problems.

Juvenile rheumatoid arthritis (JRA) is the most common rheumatological disorder of childhood. JRA has many types and presentations and its cause is not understood. All types involve joint inflammation that lasts several weeks or longer. The most common is pauciarticular JRA (fewer than five joints affected), which is highly associated with iridocyclitis, necessitating regular eye examinations. Polyarticular JRA affects more than four joints and is more common in girls. When associated with a positive rheumatoid factor, polyarticular JRA can be particularly severe and disabling. Systemic JRA has acute onset of illness with fever, organomegaly, lymphadenopathy, and arthritis. JRA may be treated with nonsteroidal anti-inflammatory drugs, corticosteroids, or a wide range of other anti-rheumatic drugs or biologics. Rehabilitative management focuses on avoiding contracture and providing appropriate orthoses and adaptive equipment. Joints of particular concern include the cervical spine, temporomanidibular joint, wrist, hip, and knee.

Systemic lupus erythematosis (SLE) occurs in children and adolescents as a multiorgan autoimmune disorder with vasculitis. Girls are more commonly affected. Nephritis, encephalopathy, and cytopenia are serious manifestations of SLE. Juvenile dermatomyositis is another systemic disorder with unknown etiology. Vasculitis, weakness, and high creatine phosphokinase are typical presentations in school-age girls, but a vast range of symptoms may develop. Therapy for SLE and juvenile dermatomyositis is largely symptomatic and should be guided by a pediatric rheumatologist.

Spondyloarthropathies occur in children in association with human leukocyte antigen-B27. Ankylosing spondylitis presents with spine or sacroiliac joint complaints in adolescent boys. Associated findings include enthesitis (pain at tendon insertion sites), uveitis, and other joint involvement. Psoriatic arthritis is an arthritis that accompanies psoriasis with uveitis. A minority of children with Crohn's disease or ulcerative colitis have associated arthritis. Reiter's syndrome, also more common in boys, consists of arthritis, urethritis, and conjunctivitis, and may occur following infection.

Brachial Plexus Injury

Congenital injury to the brachial plexus occurs in up to 1 in 200 live births. Risk factors include shoulder dystocia, large size of the infant, multiple births, breech position, instrumented delivery, and maternal diabetes. The cause of most birth brachial plexus injury is traction of the plexus during delivery.

Injury to the brachial plexus can occur at any of the roots, trunks, or divisions, although the upper trunk is the most common location. Upper trunk (C5, C6) injuries result in an Erb's palsy, with shoulder adduction and internal rotation, elbow extension, forearm pronation, and wrist flexion, and are the most common. Total plexus injuries (C5–T1) result in a flaccid, insensate upper limb. Horner's syndrome (ptosis, pupillary miosis, and facial anhidrosis) is associated with injury at C8 and T1. Many brachial plexus injuries have various degrees of damage at various nerves, so the presentation may be unique.

Infants suspected of brachial plexus injury should be carefully evaluated to determine motor and sensory functioning and ROM. UMN signs, such as spasticity or hyperreflexia, should prompt the clinician to investigate for other causes including hemiparesis. Imaging of the shoulder and EMG may aid in diagnosis and understanding the cause and extent of injury.

Brachial plexus injuries should be treated with physical and/or occupational therapy including stretching, efforts to increase awareness and strength, and sometimes bracing or electrical stimulation. For the majority of children, considerable recovery occurs spontaneously. Infants with Erb's palsy can be expected to fully recover if they have biceps and deltoid activity at 3 months. For total plexus injuries, if the impairments are severe, recovery is far less likely and early intervention is warranted. As children grow and age, surgery may be recommended if recovery is incomplete, especially by age 4 to 6 months. Surgical procedures range from nerve grafts or transfers in young infants to muscle transfers or bony procedures in older children.

See Chapter 8 for information about neuromuscular conditions seen in pediatric rehabilitation.

Key References and Suggested Additional Reading

Alexander M, Molnar G, eds. Pediatric rehabilitation. PM&R State of the Art Reviews, Vol. 14, No 2, Philadelphia: Hanley & Belfus; 2000.

Koman LA, Smith BP, Shilt JS. Cerebral palsy. Lancet 2004; 363: 1619–1631.

Molnar G. and Alexander M, eds. Pediatric Rehabilitation, 3rd ed. Philadelphia: Hanley and Belfus; 1999.

Rosenbaum PL, Walter SD, Hanna SE, et al. Prognosis for gross motor function in cerebral palsy: creation of motor development curves. JAMA 2002; 288:1357–1363.

8 Neuromuscular Rehabilitation

Nancy E. Strauss, Shikha Sethi, and Stanley J. Myers

Introduction

Neuromuscular disease refers to any genetic, metabolic, or acquired dysfunction intrinsic to nerve or muscle. A motor unit (Fig. 1) is the smallest functional unit of the motor system and consists of a motor neuron, its axon, and all the muscle fibers innervated by the axon. Neuromuscular disease can be organized as the study of pathologies affecting one of the following four parts of the anatomic nerve–muscle cascade:

1. Diseases of the motor neuron.
2. Diseases of peripheral nerves (peripheral neuropathies).
3. Neuromuscular junction disorders.
4. Disorders of muscle (myopathies).

If the end role of the dysfunctional anatomic structure or biochemical pathway is known, then the deficits to expect in a patient with such a lesion can be anticipated.

Anterior Horn Cell Disorders

The anterior horn cell is the lower motor neuron (LMN) that is needed to keep the motor axon functioning. It is located in the spinal cord and transmits messages from the upper motor neuron (UMN) through the anterior root, which becomes the motor nerve. A lesion or loss and degeneration of the anterior horn cell may cause weakness, atrophy, hyporeflexia or areflexia, hypotonia, fasciculations (nonvolitional random contraction of a group of muscle fibers representing a whole or part of a motor unit), and

From: *Essential Physical Medicine and Rehabilitation*
Edited by: G. Cooper © Humana Press Inc., Totowa, NJ

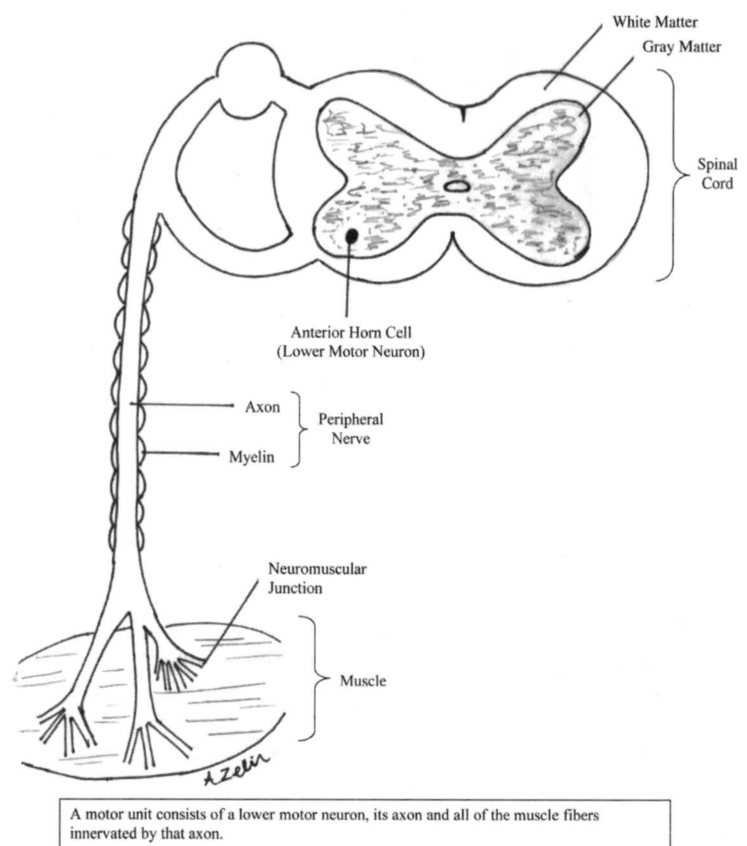

Fig. 1. The motor unit.

denervation (interruption of the nerve connection). Sensation should be normal because the sensory pathway is not affected. The exact distribution of abnormal findings will depend on which motor neurons are degenerated or diseased. Motor neuron disease can be inherited with onset in infancy or childhood, as in spinal muscular atrophy. Poliomyelitis is a motor neuron disease affecting the neurons in the spinal cord and brain stem that is acquired from a viral etiology. Amyotrophic lateral sclerosis (ALS; Lou Gehrig's disease) is idiopathic and involves UMNs, as well as LMNs, with degeneration and loss of motor neurons in the spinal cord, brainstem, and motor cortex.

Peripheral Neuropathies

The deficits found in neuropathies depend on which fibers are dysfunctional. Pure motor neuropathies may cause weakness, atrophy, hypo- or areflexia, denervation, and may present similarly to anterior horn cell disease. Pure sensory neuropathies may cause impairments of light touch, proprioception, pain, and/or temperature depending on which fibers are affected. Sensorimotor neuropathies have both motor and sensory involvement. Neuropathic weakness is usually more prominent distally (distal extremities) and sensory abnormalities are usually in a stocking-glove distribution. The pattern may be symmetric or asymmetric. When autonomic nerve fibers are affected, internal physiological homeostasis is not maintained and may result in skin changes, abnormal sweating, orthostatic hypotension, cardiac arrythmias, heat intolerance, constipation/diarrhea, incontinence, sexual dysfunction, dry eyes, dry mouth, loss of visual accommodation, and pupillary irregularities. Efficient nerve transmission requires intact axons and myelin; thus, neuropathies can either be the result of axonal degeneration, demyelinization, or a combination of the two. Nerve transmission may fail because of axonal degeneration (axonal neuropathy), demyelinization (causing conduction slowing or failure of transmission), deposition of extracellular material between nerve fibers (as in amyloidosis), or as a result of compromise of the vascular supply to nerves. Hereditary neuropathies (such as Charcot-Marie-Tooth disease [CMT; hereditary motor sensory neuropathy]) are usually more uniform lesions. Acquired neuropathies (such as Guillain-Barre Syndrome [acute inflammatory demyelinating polyneuropathy]) are usually more patchy or nonuniform.

Neuromuscular Junction Disorders

Diseases of the neuromuscular junction affect synaptic transmission between motor nerves and muscles and can either be presynaptic or postsynaptic. A functioning neuromuscular junction is required for efficient and effective transfer of impulses from the motor nerve to the muscle itself. Presynaptic dysfunction (as in myasthenic syndrome/Eaton Lambert syndrome) results from a defect in release of acetylcholine from the nerve terminal of the motor axon. A postsynaptic dysfunction (as in myasthenia gravis) results from antibodies to acetylcholine receptors on the postsynaptic muscle membrane. The abnormal finding is weakness with no sensory abnormality. Weakness may be fluctuating and varies depending on the time of day or activity. There is easy fatigue or frank paralysis from blocked neuromuscular junction transmission. Botulinum toxin (Botox®) injections work by blocking the release of acetylcholine from presynaptic motor nerve terminals.

Disorders of Muscle

When the dysfunction is in the muscle itself, abnormalities include weakness, hyporeflexia, and hypotonia with normal sensation. If the nature of the condition is inflammatory (polymyositis, dermatomyositis), then muscle tenderness may be present. Myotonia, a phenomenon in which there is a delay in muscle relaxation after contraction, is characteristic of several disorders. Weakness in myopathies is usually more prominent in a proximal distribution (trunk, hips, shoulder girdle). A myopathy is a primary disorder of muscle that may be static or nonprogressive; however, a dystrophy is a destructive, progressive muscle disease. Myopathies can be inherited (congenital, metabolic) or acquired (toxic, endocrine).

Inherited Versus Acquired

Acquired conditions can be idiopathic with no known cause or secondary to a known insult to the neuromuscular system. Causes of acquired diseases may include toxins, endocrine abnormalities, infections, inflammatory processes, acquired metabolic abnormalities, or autoimmune dysfunctions. Knowledge of genetic transmission of hereditary neuromuscular disorders reveals that diseases may be inherited with different inheritance patterns. In autosomal-dominant conditions, there is a 50% chance of the affected person passing it on to their offspring, although expression of the condition can be quite variable. Usually there is a strong family history with grandparents, parents, aunts, uncles, and others, of either sex being affected. In autosomal-recessive conditions, there is a 50% chance of passing the gene on to offspring and a 25% chance of the offspring having the condition if both parents are carriers. Thus, grandparents and parents are not clinically involved, although siblings may be. In X-linked conditions, there is a 50% chance that the male offspring will have the condition and a 50% chance that the female offspring will be a carrier. There is a group of mitochondrial myopathies that do not follow the Mendelian genetic pattern. Breakthroughs in genetic research have led to the identification of chromosome location in many of the inherited disorders. Once a defective gene is found, scientists can identify the gene product (protein) and determine if it is absent, defective, or low in quantity, and use this information for researching treatments and cures.

Investigating to Find the Correct Diagnosis

Neuromuscular disorders include a large spectrum of conditions with varying age of onset, etiology, time course (acute, chronic or variable), severity, distribution of symptoms, and prognosis. Some are extremely mild in presentation and are often misdiagnosed or undiagnosed. Others are severe in presentation and are aggressive in their degenerative course. It is extremely important to establish the "correct" diagnosis so that the appropriate treatment, counseling, and overall medical care can occur. The physiatrist should carefully review medical records and suspect a neuromuscular disorder, especially when complaints do not seem to respond to treatment. One should not presume that the referring diagnosis is always the correct one. For example, a patient with the diagnosis of fibromyalgia who presents with muscle tenderness, fatigue, and poor endurance may, in fact, have polymyositis. The patient with chronic foot deformity, instability, and foot pain may, in fact, have a hereditary neuropathy. A child who is referred for just being slightly clumsy with borderline delayed motor milestones may actually have a congenital myopathy. The physiatrist should never hesitate to call on a neurologist to work together on the diagnostic work-up. Because many of these conditions are rare, a referral to a medical center with a comprehensive meuromuscular center is often necessary to establish the correct diagnosis. If the diagnosis is incorrect, then there is tremendous potential for poor quality of care in every aspect of the patient's life. Neuromuscular diseases have associated medical problems which can only be anticipated if the correct diagnosis is made.

History

Subjective Symptoms

When a person develops muscle weakness, it is usually perceived as "fatigue," which is often the chief complaint. Because this highly nonspecific complaint can result from many disease processes, it is not always very helpful in diagnosis. "Endurance" is usually reduced before patients identify a reduction of absolute strength. Another common complaint is "clumsiness," rather than the complaint of weakness. Patients may complain of specific tasks that are difficult. With proximal muscle weakness, it may be difficulty rising from a chair, walking up an incline, or raising arms above the head. Difficulty with small motor hand function (such as buttoning) or distal lower extremity motor function (such as tripping) may indicate distal weakness. Extraocular muscle weakness leads to complaints of blurry vision or diplopia. Difficulty holding the head upright can indicate neck muscle weakness. New onset of choking may indicate palatal weakness or trouble chewing may be a result of weakness of the masseter and temporalis muscles. Facial muscle weakness can result in the inability to whistle or close eyes fully. Weakness of respiratory muscles causing a restrictive pulmonary pattern may present as fatigue, shortness of breath, sleepiness, or decreased concentration. Complaints of impaired sensation or numbness may be nonspecific and described as a tightness or a choking or burning feeling. Complaints of dyesthesias, hypersensitivity, or hyposensitivity may be present. Neuropathic pain may be reported as stinging, burning, stabbing, or lancinating. Some patients report that they feels as if they are walking on sharp pebbles. Others report that they cannot even tolerate the feeling of their top bedsheet resting on their feet.

Past Medical and Surgical History

Important clues as to neuromuscular pathology can be elicited by obtaining a thorough past medical and surgical history. This should include a prenatal and birth history, which may reveal decreased fetal movements, breech presentation, congenital hip dislocation, scoliosis, or other orthopedic abnormalities associated with muscle disease. Timing of motor milestones aids in recognition of a delay in motor development. A history of problems with general anesthesia may be the first clue that a muscle disease is present. A history of metabolic endocrine abnormalities (including diabetes or thyroid disease), exposure to toxins, nutritional deficits (ethanol use), or prior infections may point to an etiology.

Family History

Because many neuromuscular diseases are hereditary and may have variable expression, a good family history can be revealing. A family member may be so mildly affected that it is never formally diagnosed and is attributed to being "nonathletic" or "just clumsy." This is not uncommon in the congenital myopathies and hereditary neuropathies, where the effects are often minimal and nonprogressive. Family history must not only include a history of the particular disease but also a history of any of the associated signs and symptoms or related problems. Examining a family member may also be helpful in the investigation.

Social and Functional History

Marital status, number of children, educational background, employment, habits, and recreational activities is information that may not aid in the diagnosis, but will aid in developing goals in the rehabilitation plan. Functional history includes level of independence for various activities of daily living and mobility, assistive devices used, and architectural layout of home, job and school, if applicable.

Physical Examination

An important part of the physical examination is ensuring that the patient is disrobed adequately so that the examiner can properly *inspect and observe* the patient's body posture, positions, and movements. The degree and location of muscle atrophy, as well as the presence of fasciculations, are important findings. If the patient is covered with clothing, it is impossible to do an adequate physical examination.

A comprehensive physical examination with particular detail to the neuromusculoskeletal system is essential. Significant loss of muscle strength must be present before it can be detected on manual muscle testing (usually at least 50%); thus, the examiner must not rely on manual muscle testing alone, but must use other assessments to detect weakness. Inspection and observation of the patient's posture, body alignment, and movement through space are revealing. Myopathic patients may show atrophy or pseudohypertrophy with weakness out of proportion to the degree of muscle wasting. Pseudohypertrophic muscles appear larger; however, this is the result of replacement with fibrous tissue rather than actual muscle hypertrophy. It is commonly seen in the calves and often the quadriceps and deltoids of boys with Duchenne's muscular dystrophy. Body alignment changes to correct for muscle weakness include hyperlordosis as a compensation for weak hip extensors, and genu recurvatum (knee hyperextension) to compensate for weak quadriceps musculature. In muscle diseases, we expect strength to be more diminished proximally. However, there are exceptions to every rule, and there are "distal" myopathies. Gait analysis may reveal a Trendelenberg/waddling gait if gluteus medius weakness is present. Toe walking will increase the knee extensor moment, and may be a compensation for knee extensor weakness. Inspection of the spine while sitting may reveal a scoliotic curve that is not obvious when prone in a patient with a myopathic, collapsible scoliosis. Inspection in multiple positions is essential. Functional testing and observation of the patient performing activities, such as running, hopping, jumping, heel walking, toe walking, and ascending and descending stairs, will aid the examiner in assessing strength, endurance, biomechanics, and compensatory mechanisms. Weakness of the trunk and proximal lower extremities may result in patients using the Gower's maneuver while attempting to rise from the floor, with patients placing their hands on their lower extremities and using upper extremity support to climb up their legs to achieve upright posture. In neuropathies, weakness is usually more prominent distally; thus, intrinsic wasting of the small muscles of the hands and feet along with weakness of grip strength, foot, and toe extensors is common. Gait analysis may reveal a steppage gait, where the patient may need to raise his or her leg to clear the floor secondary to weak dorsiflexors and toe extensors. In diseases of the neuromuscular junction, the weakness may be in the facial, as well as proximal, muscles. Distribution of weakness in motor neuron diseases depends on the extent and location of the motor neuron loss. Palpation of the muscles is important and may reveal a stranded, atrophic type of wasting more commonly seen in neuropathies or denervating conditions or one of rubbery pseudohypertrophy more common in some myopathies. In end-stage muscle diseases, muscles have a fibrous, stranded texture. Inflammatory myopathies may reveal tenderness upon muscle palpation. Percussion of the muscle may reveal myotonia (delayed relaxation after contraction). Sensory testing is essential, as this should be normal in purely myopathic processes, but impaired in neuropathic processes with sensory involvement. Deep tendon reflexes may be reduced in LMN disorders; however, because ALS has aspects of both UMN and LMN dysfunction, there may also be hyperreflexia in this condition. Strength of the trunk and muscles of respiration can be observed by asking the patient to give a strong cough. Nasal flaring and low-volume nasal voice may indicate weakness of respiratory musculature. Repeating an activity several times may elicit weakness by exhausting muscle reserve and revealing poor endurance. Decreased muscle tone can be demonstrated by passively moving the extremities. When evaluating an infant, holding the infant in space and observing control of their head and extremities may reveal hypotonia, as seen in the "floppy infant." When examining range of motion (ROM) of the extremities, restrictions may indicate muscle imbalance as the result of weakness. When muscle imbalance is present, contractures usually develop. Contractures and muscle imbalances are usually found in the larger joints in myopathic conditions, and in the smaller joints in neuropathic conditions. Muscles that cross two joints are more prone to contracture. Gastrocsoleus (plantar flexion) contractures, as well as hip flexor and iliotibial band tightness, are common lower extremity contractures in the myopathic/dystrophic patient. Restriction of ankle ROM with plantar flexion contractures often results from dorsiflexion weakness out of proportion to plantar flexion weakness.

Diagnostic Testing

The physician has a wide spectrum of tests to aid in the diagnosis of neuromuscular diseases. Laboratory tests are important to help search for etiologies of acquired disorders. Blood and urine analysis can measure various enzymes that are characteristically abnormal in certain disease states. Creatine phosphokinase (CPK), a protein normally present in high concentration in healthy muscle and not present in significant quantity in the blood, will spill into the blood and be elevated in muscle destructive disease. This is evident early in Duchenne's or Becker's muscular dystrophy, when muscle mass is still good and symptoms of weakness have not even become apparent. In later stages, when muscle mass is extremely reduced, the value lowers, with little CPK left to leak into the serum. Electrodiagnosis, which is discussed in more detail in Chapter 12, is of considerable value for evaluating the physiology (and function) of peripheral nerves, neuromuscular junction and muscle. Analysis of electrical potentials gives valuable information about motor unit activity and can aid in locating the site of the lesion, differentiating a neuropathic process from a myopathic process and help determine prognosis. Serum CPK may transiently rise following needle insertion and should not be measured for at least 24 hours following an electromyography (EMG) exam. A muscle biopsy should not be done on a muscle that was recently tested with needle EMG because needle-induced inflammation and damage can lead to erroneous findings on pathology. Both nerve and muscle biopsies are helpful in the diagnostic work-up. Genetic testing is the gold standard for establishing a diagnosis.

Rehabilitation Approach

It is important that the physiatrist have a good knowledge of the specific disease process in terms of distribution of neurological deficit, disease course, prognosis, and associated medical problems. Before formulating the rehabilitation plan, the patient's impairment should be determined. *Impairment* refers to the abnormal physical finding. An example is shoulder girdle weakness. If there is an impairment, did it cause a disability? A *disability* is the functional limitation owing to the impairment, such as the patient's inability to raise their arms above his or her head. The *handicap* is the social disadvantage secondary to the disability, such as a teacher who is unable to write on a blackboard and teach a class. By knowing the functional limitations, the physiatrist can set goals for the patient.

Descriptions of Selected Diseases of the Motor Neuron

Amyotrophic Lateral Sclerosis

ALS is the most common adult-onset motor neuron disease. It is a fatal, progressive disease with an average survival of 3 to 5 years from time of diagnosis. ALS is idiopathic and remains a diagnosis of exclusion. Because the prognosis is poor, ALS is a diagnosis that should be made only after all other causes of weakness and atrophy have been ruled out.

ALS results from progressive destruction of motor neurons seen in the cortical Betz cells, corticospinal tracts, in certain cranial motor neurons in the brainstem, and in the ventral horns of the spinal cord. The process of denervation and reinervation with disease progression results in both UMN and LMN involvement, causing spasticity, weakness, cramps, fasciculations, and atrophy. The percentage of UMN versus LMN symptoms will vary in individual patients.

ALS often presents as a focal, distal, asymmetric weakness usually initially involving the feet. The patient may complain of tripping, difficulty negotiating curbs, difficulty buttoning clothes, turning keys, or twisting off jar caps. Weakness spreads to adjacent areas and may eventually involve respiratory muscles and frank respiratory failure. Extraocular muscles, bowel and bladder sphincters, sensation, and cognition are generally spared in ALS. In some patients, the initial findings may involve the distal upper extremity muscles, whereas other patients may present with nasal speech, dysarthria, and dysphagia.

Bulbar involvement in ALS may start with subtle speech changes and mild dysphagia that progresses to sialorrhea, hypophonia, dysarthria, and advanced dysphagia. A pseudobulbar affect with loss of emotional control and sustained weeping or laughing may be amenable to pharmacological treatment with lithium or levodopa. Clinically definite ALS, as defined by the 1998 El Escorial criteria, requires the presence of UMN and LMN signs in the bulbar region and at least two spinal regions, or UMN signs in two spinal regions and LMN signs in three spinal regions. Approximately 90% of ALS cases are sporadic, whereas a small number have a familial, usually autosomal-dominant, inheritance.

Spinal Muscular Atrophy

Originally described by Werdnig in 1891, spinal muscular atrophy (SMA) is an autosomal-recessive disorder that affects all races equally. It is a single disease entity linked to abnormality or absence of the survival motor neuron (*SMN*) gene at chromosome 5, although multiple genes may be involved. The disease presents with a range of severity.

SMA is a classic motor neuron disease presenting as diffuse weakness from muscle denervation owing to atrophy of the ventral nerve roots. The disease is symmetric and affects the trunk and limbs with greater proximal than distal involvement. In general, central nervous system (CNS) or organ involvement is limited, there is no sensory involvement, and the eyes and face are spared. Given the CNS sparing, it is typical to see SMA children that are very bright.

SMA is generally divided into three types depending on age of onset and severity. SMA1, also known as Werdnig-Hoffman disease, is defined by weakness manifesting before 6 months of age and an inability to maintain a sitting position at any time in life. Infants usually have bright faces and communicative eyes but are unable to lift arms or legs against gravity. Toes and fingers may move. The chest assumes the shape of a bell because of weakness of intercostal muscles, but relative sparing of the diaphragm. With time, bulbar muscles become weaker and infants have difficulty sucking, swallowing, and eventually maintaining the airway and clearing infections. Mortality by 2 years of age is common.

SMA2 is a relatively milder form of the disease defined by an inability to stand. Onset is generally between 6 and 18 months of age. The course and prognosis vary depending on the severity of the disease.

Individuals with SMA3, also known as Kugelberg-Welander disease, typically can stand and walk, but still manifest symmetric weakness. These individuals may be wheelchair users by 20 or 30 years old. Some may have near normal life expectancy.

Post-Polio Syndrome

Poliomyelitis is an infection of the polio virus in the anterior horn cells of the spinal cord. Destruction of the anterior horn cells during acute polio left many polio survivors with residual motor weakness, most common in the lower extremities. With the advent of the Salk and Sabin vaccine in 1961, polio infection was largely eradicated worldwide.

In post-polio syndrome (PPS), individuals asymptomatic from polio infection decades ago present with new-onset weakness or pain in previously affected muscles or at the border zone of previously infected and normal muscles. Initial complaints include fatigue, weakness, joint pains, muscle pains, and dysphagia. The more severe the initial polio infection, the more severe the complaints in PPS tend to be.

There is no widely accepted theory for the etiology of PPS. Current theories propose either normal aging and cell drop-out in the context of fewer anterior horn cells owing to past polio destruction, exhaustion of the large LMN unit that has been working over its capacity for years, or new inflammation. Musculoskeletal overuse injuries are common. These individuals are often using their maximal energy for daily activities with little or no functional reserve.

Descriptions of Selected Diseases of Nerve

Charcot-Marie-Tooth Disease

Up to 20% of all neuropathies have a confirmed or suggested inherited basis. Of these, CMT disease accounts for almost all of the genetically based neuropathies. CMT disease, also known as hereditary motor and sensory neuropathy or peroneal muscular atrophy, is a broad classification of clinically related conditions. More than 300 genetic mutations contribute to the family of conditions classified as CMT disease, so variations in clinical presentation are common. In addition, variable penetrance is common, even within a single family. The diagnosis of CMT disease is based on history and physical examination and EMG. In some subtle cases, a nerve biopsy may be used to reinforce the diagnosis. Genetic testing is available for determining some of the diseases in the CMT disease spectrum (1A, X-linked, etc.) Once the diagnosis is made, other family members may be examined for evidence of the disease. Because the most common forms of CMT disease are autosomal-dominant, genetic counseling for family planning is often indicated.

The disease is a painless, chronic, symmetric distal neuropathy. It affects the longest nerve fibers and has a predilection for muscles innervated by the peroneal nerve. Onset is usually in late adolescence or early adulthood. Patients often present with a high arched foot with the toes flexed at the interphalangeal joints (hammer toes). The metacarpophalangeal joint may be dorsiflexed, creating prominence of the ball of the foot. The deformities may be reducible or flexible at first, but as they become rigid, the metatarsal heads may become painful with walking. Initially, the patient may develop a clumsy walk with tripping and repeated sprained ankles. Symptoms can progress to involve weakness and "stork" or "champagne bottle" deformities of the legs caused by atrophy of muscles below the knee, with sparing of muscles above the knee, difficulty with fine movements of the hands, claw hands, and atrophy and weakness in intrinsic hand muscles. Deep tendon reflexes are usually lost as the disease progresses. In its late stages, when the diagnosis is already well known, pain, paresthesias, numbness, burning, and a stocking-and-glove vibratory loss may be present. In the mildest forms of CMT disease, patients may not even know they have the disease unless a family member is diagnosed with a more severe form. In most cases, CMT disease is not fatal and patients can expect a normal life expectancy.

Several forms of CMT disease are usually distinguished. The principal types include CMT1, CMT2, CMT3, CMT4, and CMTX. CMT1 and CMT2 are the most common forms and are phenotypically similar, both autosomal-dominant with variable penetrance. CMT1 is demyelinating and more frequent. On physical exam, hypertrophic nerves owing to thickened myelin sheaths may be palpated. CMT2 shows axonal degeneration, and often has more severe distal weakness but less sensory or upper extremity involvement than CMT1. CMT3, or Dejerine-Sotas disease, is a rare, severe, autosomal-recessive or -dominant, demyelinating neuropathy that begins in infancy. Infants have severe muscle atrophy, weakness, and sensory problems. CMT4 is a name for several subtypes of autosomal-recessive demyelinating motor and sensory neuropathies. Each neuropathy subtype is caused by a different mutation, may affect a particular ethnic group, and produces distinct disease. CMTX is an X-linked-dominant or -recessive disease with more severe manifestations in males.

Hereditary Neuropathy With Predisposition to Pressure Palsy

Hereditary neuropathy with predisposition to pressure palsy is genetically similar to CMT1 with a deletion in the peripheral myelin protein (*PMP*) gene rather than a duplication. Recurrent mononeuropathies at sites prone to nerve compression, such as the elbow, fibular head, carpal tunnel, and the brachial and lumbar plexus, are seen. Eventually, the disease may progress to a generalized demyelinating neuropathy.

Acute Inflammatory Demyelinating Polyneuropathy

Acute inflammatory demyelinating polyneuropathy (AIDP), or Guillian-Barre Syndrome, causes acute, generalized weakness. AIDP manifests over a few days, with initial symptoms of symmetric numbness and tingling in the arms or legs progressing to hypo- or areflexia, and progressive limb weakness. Symptoms classically start in the lower legs and then appear in the hands in an "ascending paralysis," although symptoms may start in the arms or face. Approximately 30% of patients will have respiratory failure and up to two-thirds will manifest autonomic dysfunction, such as hyper- or hypotension, arrythymias, and bladder or bowel dysfunction. Patients may complain of acute pain in the limbs or back, although actual sensory findings of reduced sensation are usually not present. Patients often report a history of a viral illness 2 to 3 weeks before the onset of weakness. Viral precipitants for AIDP include Epstein Barr virus, cytomegalovirus, HIV, and *Campylobacter jejuni* enteritis. In many cases, no specific viral etiology can be determined. Most patients will reach their worst point within 1 month and then start to improve. Patients who are not severely involved with extensive denervation usually make a good recovery.

Cerebrospinal fluid of patients with AIDP shows increased protein and reduced cell counts with an albumino-cytological dissociation. Classic EMG/nerve conduction study findings include prolonged or absent F waves with normal sural sensory studies. The earliest severe damage in AIDP is to the proximal nerve roots, accounting for the abnormality in F waves early in the disease. This is followed by a brisk inflammatory response and segmental demyelination. More severe cases also manifest axonal degeneration. Histologically, a lymphocytic and macrophage infiltrate of the nerves is seen. Medical management includes monitoring for respiratory or autonomic dysfunction, plasma exchange, and intravenous immunoglobulin (IVIG).

Chronic Inflammatory Demyelinating Polyneuropathy

As opposed to the rapid onset of AIDP, chronic inflammatory demyelinating polyneuropathy (CIDP) manifests over months with a generally symmetrical progressive, stepwise, or relapsing weakness. Patients complain of a loss of balance, numbness, and tingling, and may have painful paresthesias. Reflexes are usually diminished or absent. Cerebrospinal fluid findings are similar to AIDP. No specific cause for CIDP has been identified, but prednisone or other immunosuppressive oral therapy may help ameliorate symptoms. Plasma exchange and IVIG may be used if oral therapy fails. Relapses are common but under treatment, the disease can be modulated. Differentiation from other chronic, symmetric, mixed sensorimotor polyneuropathies is important because CIDP responds to steroid treatment, whereas others may not. For example, an idiopathic, chronic, length-dependent axonal neuropathy separate from CIDP may account for up to one-quarter of chronic neuropathic complaints in adults. The course is stable, but no treatment has yet been identified.

Diabetic Polyneuropathy

Diabetic patients may present with a variety of neuropathic complaints. The most common diabetic polyneuropathy is a distal, symmetric sensory neuropathy causing decreased sensation, painful paresthesias, and vibratory loss in a stocking-and-glove distribution. Diabetic feet with sensory loss are at risk for burns, cuts, and skin breakdown with poorly fitting shoes. Because of impaired microvascular blood supply to the extremities, small cuts can develop into frank ulceration, leading to gangrene and the common scenario of toe, foot, and limb amputations.

Autonomic neuropathy in diabetic patients may manifest with orthostatic hypotension, resting tachycardia, loss of sinus rhythm, pupillary dysfunction with poor dark adaptation, bladder and bowel dysfunction, and impotence. Diabetic patients are also prone to compression mononeuropathies, plexopathies, cranial nerve abnormalities, and radiculopathies. Diabetic amyotrophy is a microvasculitis usually involving the lumbosacral plexus, which can start as sudden, severe, unilateral pain in the lower back or hips and spread to the anterior thigh. Weakness develops days to weeks later in the hip and thigh muscles and can lead to atrophy and wasting of the quadriceps. Patellar reflex is usually absent. Electrodiagnostic testing usually reveals denervation. Medical treatment includes good glycemic control. Patients exposed to high blood sugar levels over time are at greater risk of developing neuropathic, as well as retinal and renal complications of diabetes.

Toxic Neuropathies

In general, toxic neuropathies are caused by drug ingestion or industrial chemical exposure from the workplace or the environment. They most often present with distal, symmetric sensory changes, weakness, and hyporeflexia, although autonomic and CNS symptoms may occur. Toxins may be factors in neuropathies with uncertain etiologies. A detailed occupational and environmental history is warranted in patients in whom a cause of neuropathy is not evident.

Alcohol-Related Neuropathy

Whether the neuropathy seen in patients with chronic alcoholism is caused by a direct effect of alcohol toxicity or nutritional deficiency is still debated. The syndrome seen includes distal sensory loss, most commonly numbness of the soles, paresthesias progressing to neuropathic pain described as burning or lancinating, and/or distal weakness. Gait unsteadiness and ataxia can be caused by cerebellar degeneration, sensory ataxia, or distal weakness. Alcohol abstinence and good nutrition may help improve symptoms.

HIV Neuropathies

Neuromuscular complications in HIV infection are numerous and often related to the stage of the HIV disease process. Co-infection with other viruses, lymphoma, and drug toxicity from certain antiretroviral medications can cause neuropathy. Early in HIV—often at seroconversion—AIDP may manifest in an otherwise healthy-appearing individual. The course of AIDP is the same as for HIV-negative individuals, with respiratory failure being the most severe complication. CIDP may manifest at any time in the disease process with complaints of distal and proximal weakness. A distal, painful sensorimotor polyneuropathy is the most common HIV-associated peripheral neuropathy. Symptom severity inversely correlates with CD4 count. Direct infection of the dorsal root ganglia with HIV is seen in autopsies, but it is unknown if this is the sole cause of the neuropathy. Mononeuritis multiplex may be seen in HIV infection from vasculitis or a viral infectious etiology. In late stages of HIV infection, a progressive polyradiculopathy from cytomegalovirus infection can be rapidly fatal.

Descriptions of Selected Diseases of the Neuromuscular Junction

In normal neuromuscular junction (NMJ) transmission, a motor nerve action potential arriving at the nerve terminal initiates calcium influx into the nerve cell that helps facilitate exocytosis of acetylcholine vesicles. At the postsynaptic membrane acetylcholine binds acetylcholine receptors, initiating sodium influx into the muscle cell. End-plate potentials generated by sodium influx reach threshold and generate a muscle fiber action potential that induces excitation–contraction coupling and muscle contraction. Normally, more acetylcholine than is needed is released into the synaptic cleft with a normal motor nerve action potential. The extra acetylcholine either diffuses away or is rapidly hydrolyzed by acetylcholinesterase.

Myasthenia Gravis

Myasthenia gravis (MG) is an autoimmune disorder that affects postsynaptic NMJ transmission. It is most frequently seen in women in their 30s or men in their 50s.

In MG, autoantibodies to the acetylcholine receptor at the postsynaptic membrane cause immunolysis of receptors resulting in fewer functioning acetylcholine receptors. Resulting NMJ transmission can be slowed or fail. Increased concentration of acetylcholine at the postsynaptic membrane can help overcome some of the deficit. Clinically, this is accomplished by inhibiting acetylcholinesterase with medication, i.e., pyridostigmine (Mestinon).

The clinical scenario in MG is a result of slowed or failing NMJ transmission. The patient experiences easy fatigability and weakness of ocular, bulbar, truncal, or proximal limb muscles. The disease can be fatal if respiratory muscles are weakened sufficiently to cause respiratory failure. To monitor respiratory function, patients often have forced vital capacity checked daily during acute illness. Early symptoms of MG may be subtle, with double vision or mild ptosis. If ocular symptoms do not progress for 2 to 3 years to involve any other muscles of trunk or limbs, the patient may be diagnosed with ocular MG. If symptoms do progress, it is likely that the maximal state of weakness during an exacerbation will be in the first 3 years. After this time period, the disease is still likely to recur, but not be much worse than the nadir already experienced.

Typical findings include a facial snarl caused by weakness of facial muscles, ptosis, a tendency for the head to flop forward owing to weakness of neck extensors (so that the patient props up the head with his or her hand), and use the hands to help open and close the mouth to chew. As the patient talks, his or her voice and enunciation will be clear at first, but can be lost as the patient continues speaking and fatigues the muscles involved. If the patient gazes upward for a period of time, ptosis may set in as muscles tire.

Congenital Myopathies

Congenital myopathies present at birth as hypotonia (floppy infant) and are usually nonprogressive or slowly progressive. The diagnosis is made primarily by muscle biopsy, which reveals characteristic histological pathology. Central core myopathy, nemaline rod myopathy, and centronuclear (myotubular) myopathy are the most common of the congenital myopathies.

Rehabilitation Tools

The goals set in neuromuscular rehabilitation are usually to maintain or improve ROM and mobility, endurance, strength, balance, and gait. Independence in activities of daily living is to be optimized and facilitated. The deleterious effects of deconditioning and immobility are to be minimized. Educating the patient and family is vital because rehabilitation ideally takes place daily and involves participation of family and caregivers, as well as therapists. Patient motivation and participation is essential.

The physiatrist should utilize all professionals who can offer expertise in restoring or maintaining function. The following team members may be involved in the rehabilitation program: physical therapist, occupational therapist, speech therapist, recreational therapist, vocational counselor, rehabilitation nurse, psychologist or psychotherapist, social worker, orthotist, and respiratory therapist. School staff, employers, architectural staff, and insurance company personnel may also have an impact on rehabilitation. Ideally, the physiatrist works closely with the neurologist, orthopedist, pulmonologist, internist, cardiologist, and nutritionist as needed.

Providing a rehabilitation program that is easily accessible to the patient, with staff experienced in neuromuscular disease, is optimal. Therapy can be hospital-, outpatient facility-, home-, or school-based. Because endurance is usually limited in this patient population, it is important to provide the therapy in a setting that is easiest for the patient. The therapy prescription should include diagnosis, frequency, duration, description of treatments requested, goals, and precautions. Training the patient and family or caregivers in a home exercise program is usually necessary to ensure continuity and carry over.

Exercise

Exercises can facilitate many of the rehabilitation goals by maintaining or improving strength, endurance, balance, mobility, and ROM. Patients with neuromuscular weakness often require increased energy expenditure for a given task and have a decreased functional reserve; thus, energy conservation becomes essential. Strengthening exercises in a patient with neuromuscular disease should be done carefully and submaximally, while avoiding over-fatigue. Usually, eccentric contractions should be avoided. Overwork weakness is common in aggressive diseases of the motor unit. Thus, an overly intensive strengthening program should be avoided. Endurance can be addressed by low-intensity exercises with frequent repetitions or simply by doing a task repeatedly. Improving endurance for standing, walking, or propelling a manual wheelchair are examples of goals. Balance exercises are helpful because strategies are planned to aid the patient in remaining upright. Exercises for mobility, including techniques to improve balance, may be facilitated by assistive devices or orthoses. Contractures of joints that develop secondary to muscle imbalance require active, active-assistive, and passive ROM exercises. These must be done frequently and may be supplemented by bracing.

Bracing

A brace (orthosis) is an external device that is often helpful in stabilizing a joint or providing external support needed to substitute for a weak muscle or unstable bony structure. Orthoses are described in Chapter 4. When ordering a brace for ambulation, it is important to do an adequate biomechanical assessment to ensure that by adding the external device, the patient does not lose compensatory biomechanical adjustments. For example, a patient with quadriceps (knee extensor) weakness may compensate by plantar flexing of the ankle, thus increasing the knee extension moment. An ankle–foot orthosis that limits this compensation may actually make ambulation difficult or impossible. Resting splints are often used to help stretch tight structures; an example is a dynamic ankle–foot orthosis for providing a slow steady stretch to the heel cord. The weight of the brace must be considered because patients with muscle weakness may not use an orthosis if they feel it is too heavy.

Standing and Mobility Aids

Positive effects (both psychological, as well as physiological) of standing and weight-bearing make efforts to keep patients with muscle weakness upright as long as possible highly desirable. Standers, such as parapodiums, provide external support. Mobility aids, such as canes, crutches, and walkers, offer increased support for walking. Often, the best way to determine which device, if any, is beneficial for the patient is by trying it during physical therapy and assessing the advantage.

Assistive Devices for Activities of Daily Living

Independence in activities of daily living has a direct impact on self-esteem and self-image. Occupational therapists and rehabilitation engineers have a wide array of devices available to assist and promote independence. For example, external devices that support and stabilize the upper extremity may aid in feeding, grooming and self-care. For patients who may not be able to bend down or reach up, long-handled reachers or related devices are valuable. Modifying the home with raised toilet seats, railings, and ramps are examples of external changes that may impact on independence.

Seated Mobility

When the energy cost utilized for walking becomes greater than the satisfaction of walking itself, or the frequency of falling with risk of injury increases, then the patient is often relieved when a wheelchair or scooter is prescribed for mobility. When standing balance is impaired to a level where falling is probable, then a wheelchair or scooter can become a welcome, safe option. When walking ceases, contractures develop at a more rapid pace and the deleterious effects of deconditioning occur. Manual wheelchairs are lighter, easier to transport, less expensive, and easier to maintain than motorized chairs. However, manual chairs require adequate upper extremity strength and endurance for independent propulsion. Motorized devices require cognitive and visual perceptual ability to be operated independently and safely. Occupational therapists and seating specialists aid in determining the specific custom modifications for each individualized wheelchair prescription.

Surgery for Correction of Orthopedic Deformity

When the musculoskeletal deformity is severe enough that ROM exercises and/or bracing is of limited value, then orthopedic surgical intervention can be considered. It also can be considered as a preventative measure when functionally limiting orthopedic deformity is expected as in progressive conditions with predictable courses. For example, muscle imbalance may result in plantar flexor, knee flexor, and hip flexor contractures. Surgical release may straighten the extremity; however, this does not restore muscle strength and may actually result in a weaker muscle. If contractures are responsible for loss of walking ability, surgery may prolong walking; however, the energy cost of ambulation will remain high with the associated muscle weakness and the energy expenditure may be too great to sustain ambulation. Spinal stabilization surgery is often performed in children with scoliosis secondary to neuromuscular weakness. Prevention of severe scoliosis is beneficial in limiting further pulmonary restriction, cosmetic deformity, sitting posture abnormalities, and related problems. After any orthopedic procedure, the patient's physical and occupational therapy programs must be carefully reevaluated and adjusted to ensure adequate therapy regimens to aid in adapting to their new biomechanics. As with all elective surgeries, the risk and the benefits of surgery must be carefully addressed. Anesthesiologists must be aware of the neuromuscular diagnosis and the increased risk of general anesthetic adverse reactions associated with neuromuscular disease. An example is malignant hypothermia (a potentially life-threatening reaction to certain general anesthetic agents), which is increased in certain patients with myopathy.

Pulmonary Rehabilitation

Pulmonary rehabilitation in the neuromuscular disease population is of utmost importance and is covered in Chapter 6. Restrictive pulmonary dysfunction secondary to muscle weakness may be further affected by scoliosis, which limits the space for expansion of the lungs. Noninvasive pulmonary management is often an essential treatment.

Speech Therapy

Speech and language pathologists assist patients with communication deficiencies secondary to muscle weakness by direct exercises or by providing external communication devices. When oropharyngeal muscle weakness impairs the swallowing mechanism, compensatory techniques are taught and dietary modifications offered. In cases where the risk of aspiration remains despite rehabilitative interventions, a gastroenterologist is consulted for alternative nutritional means.

Interventions for Neuropathic Pain

Painful peripheral neuropathies are usually best treated with a multifaceted approach. Pharmacological treatment options include antidepressants, membrane-stabilizing agents, and topical capcacin. Desensitization techniques led by a physical therapist or occupational therapist is of value. Transcutaneous electrical nerve stimulation is a pain relieving modality. Eliminating any aggravating sensory irritant (e.g., tight shoes, heavy bed covers) is helpful. Psychological pain-management techniques may be a useful supplement.

Key References and Suggested Additional Reading

Arezzo JC. New developments in the diagnosis of diabetic neuropathy. Am J Med 1999; 107: 9S–16S.

Bach JR. Guide to the Evaluation and Management of Neuromuscular Disease. Philadelphia: Hanley & Belfus, 1999.

Belsh JM. Diagnostic challenges in ALS. Neurology 1999; 53(Suppl 5):S26–S30.

Berciano J, Combarros O. Hereditary neuropathies. Curr Opin Neurol 2003; 16:613–622.

Brooke MH. A Clinician's View of Neuromuscular Diseases. Baltimore: Williams & Wilkins, 1977.

Dalakas MC, Rowland LP, DiMauro S. Inflammatory myopathies. In: Vinken PJ, Bruyn GW, Uchio E, eds. Handbook of Clinical Neurology, vol 18. New York: Elsevier Science, 1992, pp. 369–390.

Dick PJ, Thomas PK, eds. Peripheral Neuropathy. 3rd ed. Philadelphia: WB Saunders Co, 1993.

DiMauro S, Bonilla E, Hays AP. Skeletal muscle storage diseases: myopathies resulting from errors in carbohydrate and fatty acid metabolism. In: Mastalgia FL, Walton JN, eds. Skeletal Muscle Pathology, 2nd ed. Edinburgh: Churchill Livingstone, 1992:425–457.

Feldman RG. Occupational and Environmental Neurotoxicology. Philadelphia: Lippincott-Raven, 1999.

Gendelman HE, Lipton SA, Epstein L. The Neurology of AIDS. New York: Chapman & Hall, 1998.

Harper PS. Myotonic dystrophy: present management: future therapy. New York: Oxford University Press, 2004.

Hughes RA. Peripheral neuropathy. BMJ 2002; 324:466–469.

Jeha LE, Sila CA, Lederman RJ, Prayson RA, Isada CM, Gordon SM. West Nile virus infection: a new acute paralytic illness. Neurology 2003; 61: 55–59.

Kimura J. Electrodiagnosis in Diseases of Nerve and Muscle: Principles and Practice, 2nd ed. Philadelphia: FA Davis, 1989, pp. 149–162.

Kuncl RW. Motor neuron disease. New York: Saunders, 2002.

Luciano CA, Pardo CA, McArthur JC. Recent developments in the HIV neuropathies. Curr Opin Neurol 2003; 16:403–409.

Parry GJ. Management of diabetic neuropathy. Am J Med 1999; 107: 27S–33S

Said G, Saimont AG, Lacroix C. Neurological Complications of HIV and AIDS. Philadelphia: WB Saunders, 1998.

Sommer C. Painful neuropathies. Curr Opin Neurol 2003; 16:623–628.

Younger DS. Motor Disorders. Philadelphia: Lippincott, Williams & Wilkins, 1999.

9 Cancer Rehabilitation

Michael D. Stubblefield and Christian M. Custodio

Background

Cancer rehabilitation is the subspecialty of rehabilitation medicine concerned with the restoration of function and quality of life (QOL) to persons with cancer. As our treatments for the various forms of cancer improve, persons with cancer are surviving longer, and in many cases being cured of diseases that were once considered fatal. Cancer is becoming a chronic disease. A patient with prostate or breast cancer, for instance, even when it is metastatic, may have a better prognosis for survival at 5 years than a person with severe pulmonary or cardiac disease. The price of cure or increased survival is often high and may involve toxic chemotherapy, radiation therapy, or surgery.

The principles of cancer rehabilitation are similar to those in other fields of rehabilitation medicine. The major impairments to function encountered by the rehabilitation medicine physician working with a cancer population include pain, weakness, debility, and deformity.

Etiology

Cancer is now the leading cause of death in the United States for people younger than 85 years old. Although breast and prostate cancers are the most common, lung cancers cause the most deaths. This discrepancy has to do with the more indolent course of breast and prostate cancer, as well as the development of progressively more effective treatments. Disorders of function and pain in persons with cancer result not only from the underly-

From: *Essential Physical Medicine and Rehabilitation*
Edited by: G. Cooper © Humana Press Inc., Totowa, NJ

ing malignancy, but also importantly, from treatments that are often toxic. Such treatments include surgery, radiation therapy, and chemotherapy.

Pathogenesis

Disorders of pain, weakness, debility, deformity, and dysfunction in persons with cancer result from the direct and indirect effects of cancer or its treatment. Malignant and benign tumors can progress locally to involve vital structures including viscera and bone. Paraneoplastic phenomena, such as the Lambert-Eaton myasthenic syndrome (LEMS), although rare, can be a major source of weakness, autonomic nervous system dysfunction, and ataxia. Many types of chemotherapy are available and new drugs are constantly being developed. The toxicities of chemotherapy include nausea, vomiting, fatigue, malaise, myalgias, neutropenia, thrombocytopenia, anemia, osteoporosis, and neurotoxicity. Radiation therapy can damage any tissue including bone, ligament, tendon, muscle, nerve, blood and lymphatic vessels. Such damage may be acute or develop and progress many years after treatment. Surgery may result in medical debility, damage to the central or peripheral nervous systems, loss of limbs, and other musculoskeletal disorders.

Risk Factors

Many factors impact whether or not a patent with cancer will develop pain, weakness, debility, or deformity. The importance of pre-existing medical conditions that affect the joints, spine, nerves, heart, lungs, and other important organs must not be discounted because they can negatively impact patients' function and QOL as they progress through the stages of cancer and its treatment.

History

Detailed knowledge of a patient's medical history is important in correctly identifying the source of their pain or dysfunction, predicting their prognosis, and successfully treating them. An initial history should include the following:

1. *Referral source:* Most of the patients seen by the rehabilitation physician both in the clinic and in the hospital setting are referred from another physician. The referral source should always be identified with a written statement, such as, "The patient was seen and examined by me at the request of Dr. Smith in the orthopedic surgery service."
2. *Chief complaint:* Cancer patients are generally referred to the rehabilitation medicine service to address a specific question or issue. The reason

for the referral should be clearly and concisely stated in the "chief complaint" section of your note. As opposed to an emergency room, where the chief complaint is generally the first words uttered by the patient to the physician, i.e., "my back hurts," in the consult setting, the chief complaint should address the question or issue posed by the referral source, i.e., "Evaluation of progressive back pain and gait disorder."

3. *History of present illness (HPI):* The HPI should start with a list of the patient's major medical disorders that have the potential to impact pain and function. Such disorders should be listed concisely, chronologically, and in order of causality when known or possible. An expansion of past medical history will be more fully detailed in the past medical history section, as will current and past medical disorders not likely to impact rehabilitation, i.e., a hernia repair performed 40 years ago.
   a. *Example:* "The patient is a 68-year-old man with a history of hypertension, diabetes, hypercholesterolemia, and coronary artery disease complicated by a myocardial infarction in 1999 treated with coronary artery bypass surgery."

      The patient's cancer history should then be detailed in chronological order from the time of diagnosis until present and include initial symptoms, date of diagnosis, primary treatment (chemotherapy, radiation, and surgical history), recurrence date and location(s), secondary treatment(s), and any complications. The cancer type and stage should be listed. The start and stop dates for each chemotherapeutic agent used, the dates, location, and type of radiation therapy given, and the dates and details of all major surgical procedures should be included. Complications of disease and therapy must also be detailed, as should pertinent negatives. The patient's history should read in a concise but logical and chronological manner so that the patient's entire history of cancer can be fully appreciated.
   b. *Example:* "The patient was diagnosed with right-sided breast cancer on routine breast examination in 1998 and underwent a right-modified radical mastectomy with zero of five lymph nodes positive for cancer. Pathology confirmed invasive ductal carcinoma and the patient was treated with adriamycin and cytoxan from November 30, 2001 to February 4, 2002 followed by docetaxel from February 25, 2002 to April 29, 2002. No radiation was given. The patient was without evident disease until October of 2004 when she developed rapidly progressive low back and leg pain, as well as urinary incontinence. No weakness was noted on presentation. She presented to the urgent care center October 28, 2004 and a magnetic resonance imaging (MRI) of her spine demonstrated an L3 metastasis with circumferential epidural disease and high-grade spinal cord compression. She was placed on high-dose intravenous Solu-Medrol and underwent surgical decompression and reconstruction of the L3 vertebral body."

4. *Allergies:* All patient allergies should be listed, as well as any reported adverse drug reactions. The specifics of the allergic reaction should be detailed, i.e., rash versus anaphylactic shock. Keep in mind that patients often report adverse drug reactions, such as nausea and vomiting from codeine, as "allergies" when they are more correctly referred to as adverse reactions.
5. *Medications:* All current (at the time the history is elicited) patient medications, including over-the-counter medications, and nutritional and herbal supplements, should be listed including dose and dosing schedule. Any medications taken just prior to presentation may also be detailed where appropriate.
6. *Past medical and surgical history:* Expanded details of all current and past medical conditions and surgeries should be listed. Medical conditions that have already been adequately detailed in the HPI do not need to be reiterated.
7. *Social history:* The patient's complete social history, including home environment, marital status, number and ages of children, occupation, alcohol, drug, and smoking history, etc., should be detailed. Situations, such as lack of good social support, too many stairs to get into the home, lack of insurance or employment, and so on, often affect the rehabilitation medicine team's ability to restore patient function and independence. A good functional history, including a patient's ability to ambulate, perform activities of daily living, available adaptive equipment, and safety and judgment capabilities, is also important.
8. *Family history:* The patient's family history should be detailed.
9. *Review of systems:* A complete and detailed review of systems should be taken. The practitioner should elicit complaints concerning constitution, eyes, ears, nose, mouth, throat, cardiovascular system, respiratory system, blood and lymph circulation, skin, breasts, environmental allergies, psychological disorders, endocrine disorders, musculoskeletal disorders, and neurological disorders.

Physical Examination

The physical examination is absolutely crucial to the evaluation of pain and functional disorders. This importance cannot be overstated because the physical examination often yields more useful information than even the most sophisticated and sensitive imaging studies. A basic physical examination must detail weight, heart rate, blood pressure, respiration rate, constitutional signs, eyes, ears, nose, mouth, throat, cardiovascular system, respiratory system, gastrointestinal system, genitourinary system, skin, breasts, circulatory system, lymphatic system, musculoskeletal system, and gait. Neurological assessment should include cranial nerves II–XII, cerebellar testing, manual muscle testing, sensory testing (light touch, position

sensation, pin-prick sensation), and reflexes. A number of specialized and focused tests for the musculoskeletal system exist and are discussed extensively in other texts, such as *Physical Examination of the Spine and Extremities* by Stanley Hoppenfeld.

Diagnostic Evaluation

Perhaps the greatest challenges encountered in assessing pain and functional issues of persons with cancer is determining if these disorders are the result of cancer, cancer treatment, or benign conditions. Advances in imaging have helped to make this challenge somewhat easier, but the physician must be careful not to be misled by the studies. Imaging should be used in conjunction with a careful history and physical examination. Also, it is important to keep in mind that cancer in and of itself does not generally cause pain because most tumors are insensate. The cancer must directly or indirectly affect a pain-sensitive structure, such as the periosteum, soft tissues, muscles, or nerves. For instance, a small metastasis that is confined to the bone marrow of a vertebral body does not generally cause pain until it grows to compromise the bony cortex and periosteum, facet joints, spinal cord, nerve roots, or surrounding soft tissues.

Differential Diagnosis

Pain

The differential diagnosis of pain in cancer patients can be challenging. A practitioner must be careful not to assume that all pain in patients with cancer is related to the cancer. The stage, type, and location of metastases must be taken into account. Conditions as prevalent as osteoarthritis, spinal stenosis, and shoulder tendonitis can be very painful and are often exacerbated by the direct and indirect effects of cancer or cancer treatment. Multiple pain disorders may be present simultaneously in a patient. Correct determination of the cause or causes of pain is essential to its successful treatment.

The term *cancer pain* is very general and not particularly descriptive because it fails to take into account the pathophysiological basis of pain. Pain disorders are better categorized as somatic, neuropathic, or visceral. It is common for pain to have components of all three categories.

Somatic pain, also known as *nociceptive somatic* pain, is pain generated from activation of somatic nociceptors, and forms the basis of many musculoskeletal, traumatic, and cancer-related pain disorders. Neuropathic pain originates from neuronal activity at any level of the peripheral nervous system or central nervous system (CNS) from the small intradermal nerve fibers to the brain. Painful neuronal activity can originate from either physiological or spontaneous firing of the nerve. Neuropathic pain can be extremely difficult to treat. Common causes of neuropathic pain include radicular pain and neuropathy from neurotoxic chemotherapeutic agents. Visceral pain is mediated by nociceptors within the viscera, and is often called "nociceptive visceral" pain. The pain of gastrointestinal and renal colic, ischemic cardiac pain, and ischemic peripheral vascular pain are examples of visceral pain that can be seen in both the general and cancer population.

The details of the history and physical examination are instrumental in categorizing pain. Pain described in terms, such as "burning," "radiating," "lancinating," or "tingling," and accompanied by neurological deficits, such as weakness or sensory loss, often indicates a neuropathic origin. Pain that is "achy," "deep," "throbbing," exacerbated by activity, sharply localized, and reproducible with pressure is often somatic. Colicky pain in the abdomen that worsens with eating is likely to be visceral. There can be a great deal of overlap in a patient's description of their pain, as well as the signs and symptoms associated with it.

Weakness

Weakness is a very common complication of cancer and its treatment that can result from damage to the CNS, including the brain and spinal cord, the peripheral nervous system from the cauda equina to the neuromuscular junction, dysfunction of the neuromuscular junction in LEMS, or to the muscle itself. Cancer can cause weakness directly by impingement on a neural structure or indirectly through a paraneoplastic or metabolic mechanism. Cancer treatments including surgery, radiation, and chemotherapy can also damage the neuromuscular system.

Debility

Debility, or generalized fatigue and loss of vigor, is very common in cancer patients, especially during treatment and at the later stages of disease. Debility can result from the direct or indirect effects of cancer and cancer treatment. Surgery, for instance, places increased metabolic demand on the body resulting in fatigue that may persist for several weeks. Complications of surgery, such as infection or anemia, can further exacerbate low energy levels. Chemotherapy and radiotherapy have widespread metabolic effects that can result in anemia, poor cellular regeneration, anorexia, and fluid and electrolyte abnormalities. The effects on a patient's sense of overall well-being, energy levels, and even cognitive function can severely limit the patient's QOL.

Deformity

Deformity in cancer patients may result from surgery or radiation therapy. Deformity can have substantial cosmetic, as well as functional, implications. Surgery, for instance, can result in loss of an extremity, a breast, or even part of the head and face. Radiation therapy can damage any tissue included in the radiation field, and radiation-induced fibroses can progress for years after treatment, resulting in diminished function of the shoulder, neck, jaw, and other structures.

Treatment

Treatment of cancer-related impairments, such as pain, weakness, debility, and deformity, can be challenging. The basic principles of rehabilitation medicine continue to apply in the cancer setting. However, the practitioner must ground his or her application of those principles in an understanding of the underlying disease process, as well as past and anticipated future cancer treatments.

Treatment of pain disorders often involves a multimodality approach that may include physical or occupational therapy, medications, and interventional procedures. In the active cancer population, chemotherapy and radiation therapy may also be involved. Diagnostic accuracy in identifying the pathophysiological basis of the pain is important in choosing therapeutic modalities with maximum efficacy and minimal side effects.

Somatic pain, for instance, may be chronic osteoarthritic pain and respond well to simple analgesics, such as acetaminophen or nonsteroidal anti-inflammatory drugs (NSAIDs) and physical therapy. Rotator cuff tendonitis or adhesive capsulitis, disorders seen commonly in breast cancer patients, often require NSAIDs and physical therapy but may also benefit significantly from a subacromial corticosteroid injection and, potentially, a nerve-stabilizing agent (gabapentin, pregabalin, tricyclic antidepressants) if a superimposed cervical radicular component is contributing to the shoulder pain. A patient with a bony metastasis that is symptomatic may require radiation therapy, surgery, or both, as well as narcotic medications to control pain. It is common to use medications, such as the nerve-stabilizing agents and NSAIDs, adjunctively to help minimize the amount of narcotics used and their side effects.

Treatment of weakness is most effective when the cause of weakness is known. Weakness can be caused by CNS involvement by stroke, primary

Table 1
Orthotics

Joint	*Type*	*Indication*
Knee	• Knee immobilizer	▪ Knee buckling
	▪ Soft	▪ Immediate/temporary
	▪ Semi-ridged hinged	▪ Short-term
	▪ Custom hinged	▪ Long-term
Ankle	• Ankle–foot orthosis	
	▪ Posterior-leaf-spring orthosis	▪ DF weakness
	• Off-the-shelf	▪ Immediate/temporary
	• Custom	▪ Long-term
	▪ Hinged	▪ DF + PF weakness
	▪ Solid	▪ Spasticity, ankle pain
	• Doulble-metal upright	• Swelling, pain

DF, dorsiflexion; PF, plantar flexion.

brain tumor, metastasis, or epidural spinal cord compression. Weakness can also be a result of peripheral nervous system dysfunction, such as cauda equina syndrome, radiculopathy, plexopathy, neuropathy, disorders of neuromuscular transmission, such as LEMS, or myopathy.

Physical therapy can generally improve strength, endurance, energy conservation, joint and trunk range of motion, body mechanics, transfers, and gait. Therapists can train patients in the proper use of assistive devices, such as canes and walkers, when needed. Bracing is often beneficial in restoring function and QOL, but orthotic prescription must take into account the patient's overall medical status, functional potential, and prognosis. A list of commonly used lower extremity orthotics in the cancer population is listed in Table 1. Management of spasticity with medications, such as baclofen or botulinum toxin injections, may also help improve function.

Treatment of debility ultimately depends on the underlying cause. Patients with debility from prolonged hospitalization following a reversible illness generally improve, many to their baseline level of function. Emphasis on treating reversible contributing factors, such as anemia, metabolic abnormalities, and depression, ensuring proper nutrition, and promoting a safe and supportive environment in which to convalesce are important in hastening recovery. Physical and occupational therapy also play a key role in patients with a poor functional status. The debility associated with chemotherapy and radiation therapy usually dissipates over time if the underlying malignancy is successfully treated. Patients with end-stage disease will continue to decline functionally but often benefit from physical and occupational therapy, judicious use of appropriate bracing, and assistive devices.

Treatment of deformity may involve surgery, injections, physical or occupational therapy, and prescription of prosthetics. Breast reconstructive surgery is perhaps the most common form of reconstructive surgery in the cancer population and may involve myocutaneous flaps, saline implants, and a variety of other techniques. Reconstructive surgeries for craniofacial defects and following limb-salvage procedures are also common.

Limb amputations in the cancer population are often performed at very proximal levels. For instance, a lower extremity amputation may be at various levels of the foot or ankle, below the knee, above the knee, at the hip (hip disarticulation), or involve part of the pelvis (hemipelvectomy). Prosthetics can be designed to accommodate any level of amputation; however, the energy expenditure required on the part of the patient increases rapidly as the level of amputation proceeds proximally. Age and medical comorbidity also factor into energy expenditure. Therefore, an elderly and debilitated patient with an amputation at or above the thigh may not be a good prosthetic candidate, whereas a younger patient with a hip disarticulation may be. The general principles of prosthetic design and prescription apply to patients with cancer with two important caveats. First, patients who have had amputations with palliative intent as opposed to curative intent tend to have rapid recurrence or progression of their cancer depending on the type of malignancy, and may have a life expectancy of only a few weeks or months. In general, patients with a life expectancy thought to be less than 6 months are unlikely to benefit from prosthetic fitting because progression of disease and continued treatment of their malignancy is likely to make excessive demands on their time, strength, and energy reserves. Second, patients with longer life expectancies who are to continue on chemotherapy will have changes in overall health, energy level, and fluid volume that will impact directly on prosthetic fitting and training. Decisions on prosthetic fitting should be made with the patient, and every reasonable attempt at prosthetic fitting should be made if the patient expresses a strong desire to have and use the prosthesis.

Follow-Up

Outpatient follow-up of patients with cancer is variable and depends on what the rehabilitation physician is treating them for, as well as the stage of their disease. For instance, a patient with chronic stable lymphedema from treatment of breast cancer several years ago may only need evaluation every 6 months to 1 year. However, a patient with active cancer-related issues, such as a rapidly progressive neuropathy from chemotherapy or poorly controlled pain, may need evaluation weekly in the outpatient setting. Inpatient follow-up on the consult service should generally be done on a daily basis.

Complications

As one would expect, medical complications associated with cancer and cancer treatment range from insignificant to fatal. The rehabilitation physician should be familiar with the most common complications, how they impact a patient's function and QOL, and what treatments are available for them. Many of these complications were discussed previously, but will be discussed in more detail under the following subheadings.

Anemia

Anemia can result from blood loss, hemolysis, bone marrow infiltration by tumor, humoral effects of cancer and other chronic disease, iron or B_{12} deficiency, and chemotherapy. Mild anemia is a common source of debility, fatigue, dyspnea, light-headedness, angina, and poor wound healing. In general, mild anemias are not dangerous but may decrease a patient's exercise tolerance and ability to participate in meaningful therapy. Severe anemias, and even relatively mild anemia in some patients, can contribute to cardiac failure, coronary and peripheral vascular ischemia, cardiac arrhythmias, and even death.

In general, patients with anemias characterized by hemoglobin lower than 8 g/dL should not participate in physical or occupational therapy unless cleared to do so by a physician. The physician's decision to let a patient participate in therapy should be based on the relative risk and benefits anticipated as a result of participation in and the intensity of the therapy. Other factors to be considered by the physician include the chronicity of the anemia, the reversibility of the anemia, the patient's overall health, the patient's age, and the patient's cardiopulmonary status. Careful and frequent assessment of the patient's symptoms should be performed. Increases from a resting baseline of dyspnea, chest pain, palpitations, diaphoresis, nausea, vomiting, vertigo, and light-headedness may signal cardiac or cerebral ischemia and are often indicative of a presyncopal state. Blood pressure, heart rate, respiratory rate, and oxygen saturation should also be monitored, and therapy halted based on limits that are predefined by the physician for a given patient.

Thrombocytopenia

Low platelet counts, such as anemia, are also common in cancer patients. Thrombocytopenia most often results from decreased platelet production owing to tumor infiltration, chemotherapy, or radiation therapy. Increased peripheral platelet destruction from disseminated intravascular coagulation or sequestration in an enlarged liver may also cause thrombocytopenia in cancer patients.

In general, platelet counts in excess of 50,000/μL are not associated with significant bleeding. Patients with counts between 50,000 and 20,000 per μL can participate in therapy but not resistive exercises. Platelet counts less than 20,000/μL may cause spontaneous bleeding, including hemorrhagic stroke, hemarthrosis, and hematomas. Patients with platelet counts less than 20,000/μL should be evaluated and cleared by a physician before they are allowed to participate in physical or occupational therapy. As with anemia, the physician should consider the cause, chronicity, and reversibility of the thrombocytopenia, as well as the age, overall health, and prognosis of the patient. Patents with comorbid functional deficits that place them at a significant risk for falls should be confined to bed-level activities, especially when the thrombocytopenia is quickly reversible. Patients with chronic thrombocytopenia generally are at less risk for spontaneous bleeding and may tolerate lower platelet counts and participate in limited therapy with relative safety.

Neutropenia

Neutropenia is a common and anticipated result of myelosuppressive chemotherapy generally occurring 5 to 10 days following treatment. Absolute neutrophil counts less than 500 cells/mm places patients at risk for infection from bacteria, fungi, and certain types of viruses, such as herpes simplex virus. In patients who have undergone stem cell transplant or who have developed myelosuppressive infections, the duration of the neutropenia may be prolonged. Patients are placed on reverse isolation to minimize their exposure to nosocomial pathogens. Patients with neutropenia may participate in therapy, so long as strict reverse isolation protocols are adhered to and therapeutic activities do not place the patient at significant risk for fall or injury.

Thromboembolism

The term *thromboembolism* encompasses both deep vein thromboses (DVTs) and pulmonary emboli (PE). Cancer patients, particularly in the late stages of disease and those on treatments, such as tamoxifen, may be hypercoagulable and at risk for thromboembolism.

DVTs can cause painful erythematous swelling of the legs, arms, trunk, and even face. The clinician should have a very low threshold for ordering a duplex Doppler ultrasound evaluation of the affected extremity in any patient presenting with these signs and symptoms. Anticoagulation should be instituted as soon as a DVT is confirmed, unless there is a contraindication, such as recent neurological surgery. Low-molecular-weight heparinoids administered subcutaneously or unfractionated heparin administered intravenously should be used initially and gradually substituted by oral coumadin when possible. Anticoagulation is generally continued for several months but may be continued indefinitely if no reversible and treatable cause of hypercoagulability is found. If anticoagulation can not be instituted then an inferior vena cava (IVC) filter should be placed. IVC filters offer some, but not complete, protection from PEs, and do not prevent propagation of the DVT. Clot forming on the IVC filter can embolize to the lungs.

PEs are DVTs that have traveled to the lungs. PEs result in acute pulmonary vascular constriction with increased right heart pressures. This can cause dyspnea, pulmonary and cardiac ischemia, tachycardia, and other arrhythmias that may result in death. The sudden onset of chest pain accompanied by shortness of breath and tachycardia are suggestive of PE but are also characteristic of cardiac ischemia, gastroesophageal reflux, anxiety, and other disorders. Chest radiographs are usually normal, unless a pulmonary infarction has occurred. Electrocardiogram generally shows sinus tachycardia, although evidence of acute right heart strain (the "S1Q1T3" pattern) may be seen. A duplex Doppler ultrasound of the upper and lower extremities is not sufficient to rule out a PE because the entire thrombosis may have embolized, resulting in a negative study. A spiral computed tomography (CT) of the chest is rapidly replacing ventilation profusion scanning as the test of choice in the rapid diagnosis of PE. Anticoagulation is generally administered immediately upon suspicion of symptomatic PE and discontinued if testing is negative. There is a role for thrombolysis of PEs causing severe and life-threatening symptoms in selected patients.

Bone Metastases

Bone metastases can disrupt the normal architecture of bone causing bony weakness or instability, producing pain, and ultimately resulting in fracture. Whereas fractures of nonweight-bearing structures, such as the ribs, can cause pain, they do not usually present a significant risk to life or function. Fractures in weight-bearing long bones, such as the femur and humerus, can be life-threatening and can severely limit QOL and function. The presence of bony metastasis does not automatically mean that a patient is at risk for fracture. Many patients have diffuse metastases throughout their bony skeleton and have little or no pain and never experience a pathological fracture. The location of the metastasis, the type of cancer, and its activity, whether the bony lesions are lytic, sclerotic, or mixed, and the degree of cortical involvement by the tumor, contribute to the risk of pathological fracture.

Clinical determination of pathological fracture risk is a common problem encountered by the rehabilitation physician who treats cancer patients. Many systems designed to determine fracture risk have been designed, but none are completely accurate. In general, the presence of progressive pain and cortical involvement greater than 50% (only useful in long bones) are the best predictors of impending fracture.

Spinal Cord Compression

Spinal cord compression is a potentially devastating complication of cancer. Generally, spinal cord compression results from metastatic malignant epidural disease. Spinal cord compression resulting from epidural extension of a local primary tumor is less common. A known history of cancer is often, but not always present, especially in patients presenting with epidural spinal cord compression as a result of lung cancer. More than 90% of patients with epidural spinal cord compression have back or neck pain preceding the onset of weakness. The more severe the weakness at the time malignant spinal cord compression is identified and treated, the less likely the chance for a full functional recovery.

MRI of the entire spine is the test of choice to evaluate patients with suspected spinal cord compression. Plain films are of little value because they cannot adequately evaluate soft tissues. CT scan is also less sensitive than MRI in ruling out epidural spinal cord compression unless intrathecal contrast is given (CT myelogram).

In the setting of a patient with cancer, when any doubt as to the cause of back pain exists, an MRI of the entire spine should be ordered. Clinical clues that suggest a malignant cause of back pain include nocturnal pain, rapidly progressive pain, rapidly progressive neurological deficits not confined to a single root level, a palpable spinal mass, thoracic pain, and accompanying systemic symptoms, such as weight loss.

When epidural spinal cord compression is suspected, high-dose intravenous steroids may help protect the spinal cord and preserve strength and function. High-dose steroids should be started even before imaging is obtained in patients with known metastatic neoplasms. In patients without known cancer, however, high-dose steroids should not be given unless weakness is moderate, severe, or rapidly progressive because multiple myeloma and certain types of lymphomas (common causes of spinal cord compression in patients without known cancer) are extremely sensitive to steroids and may necrose making a diagnostic tissue biopsy impossible. Unnecessary treatment with steroids in this situation may delay the confirmation of tissue diagnosis for several months and potentially compromise curative treatment.

Lymphedema

Lymphedema is defined as the abnormal accumulation of lymphatic fluid, consisting of water and protein, in the skin and subcutaneous tissues. This results in swelling of a limb or occasionally other areas of the body. It is a common late complication of cancer therapy resulting from damage to the lymph nodes and lymphatic vessels, either from lymph node dissection surgery, radiation therapy, or both. Patients with lymphedema complain of pain, reduced range of motion, impaired cosmesis and disfigurement, psychological distress, and impaired activities of daily living; including difficulty with dressing, ambulation, and so on. Because lymphedema involves the skin, the affected area is more prone to infection and impaired wound healing. Because of pain and reduced range of motion, the involved limb is predisposed to complications associated with immobility, including DVT, deconditioning, and joint contracture.

Diagnosis is usually clinical, and diagnostic testing is used mainly to evaluate for other potential causes of limb swelling. An ultrasound is useful in excluding the presence of a DVT. CT scans and MRIs are useful in evaluating for the recurrence of tumor, and plain films or bone scans can help detect the presence of pathological fractures. Cellulitis can also present as a swollen limb and is usually associated with warmth, erythema, and possibly systemic symptoms, such as fevers and chills. Examination of the lymphedematous limb should include circumferential or volumetric measurements, noting the type of edema (pitting or nonpitting), description of skin consistency (soft, firm, fibrotic), and description of areas of discoloration or skin breakdown. Some special examination findings include Stemmer's sign (the inability to tent the skin over the second metacarpal or metatarsal; in lymphedema, an attempt to lift the skin results in lifting a lump of tissue, and the fact that lymphedema tends to spare the metatarsal-phalangeal joints.

There currently is no cure for lymphedema but there are ways to chronically manage it through nonpharmacological means. The mainstay of lymphedema treatment is complete decongestive therapy, which involves manual lymphatic drainage, graded compression using low-stretch bandages, exercise, and skin care. The goals of treatment are to provide education, reduce and prevent further swelling, prevent infection, and help patients cope with the psychological sequelae of lymphedema. Once limb volume has stabilized, chronic lifetime maintenance using self-massage, self-bandaging, and graded compression garments is required.

Key References and Suggested Additional Reading

Amata AA, Dumitru D. Acquired neuropathies. In: Dumitru D, Amata AA, and Zwarts MJ, eds. Electrodiagnostic Medicine, 2nd ed. Philadelphia: Hanley & Belfus; 2002:937–1041.

Bunting RW, Shea B. Bone metastasis and rehabilitation. Cancer 2001;92 (4 Suppl):1020–1028.

Cheville AL. Pain management in cancer rehabilitation. Arch Phys Med Rehabil 2001; 82(Suppl 1):S84–S87.

Cohen SR, Payne DK, Tunkel RS. Lymphedema: strategies for management. Cancer 2001; 92(4 Suppl):980–987.

Gillis TA, Cheville AL, Worsowicz GM. Cardiopulmonary rehabilitation and cancer rehabilitation. 4. Oncologic rehabilitation. Arch Phys Med Rehabil 2001;82(1 Suppl):S63–S68.

Gillis TA, Garden FH. Principles of cancer rehabilitation. In: Braddom RL, ed. Physical Medicine and Rehabilitation, 2nd ed. Philadelphia: WB Saunders; 2000, pp. 1305–1320.

Posner JB. Neurologic Complications of Cancer. Philadelphia: F. A. Davis; 1995.

10 Orthopedic Rehabilitation

C. David Lin

Hip Fractures

Background

Hip fractures are one of the most common injuries requiring hospital admission. In the United States, fractures of the hip result in hospitalization, disability, and loss of independence for more than 300,000 persons annually. The incidence of hip fractures is approximately 80 per 100,000, with the incidence increasing with age. Delayed recognition of hip fractures can result in increased morbidity and mortality. One-year mortality rates after a hip fracture are approximately 15 to 20%. Approximately 50% of patients who lived independently before injury are unable to reestablish an independent lifestyle.

Risk Factors

The incidence of hip fractures increases with age, doubling for each decade after 50 years of age. White women are two to three times more likely to sustain a fracture than non-white women. Other risk factors include sedentary lifestyle, excessive consumption of alcohol and caffeine, low body weight, smoking, and the use of psychotropic medications. Osteoporosis is also an important contributing factor because it decreases the bone's resistance to injury. Dizziness, stroke, polypharmacy, and peripheral neuropathies can disturb balance and predispose elderly patients to injury. Approximately 90% of hip fractures in the elderly result from a simple ground-level fall.

From: *Essential Physical Medicine and Rehabilitation*
Edited by: G. Cooper © Humana Press Inc., Totowa, NJ

History

Patients often report a fall followed by a decreased ability to ambulate. A characteristic symptom is groin or buttock pain that worsens with walking. Occasionally, the patient will complain of referred pain to the knee.

Clinical Examination

Patients with a displaced hip fracture usually lie with the limb externally rotated, abducted, and shortened. The typical patient is often an elderly female with dementia who sustains a fall and is unable to walk. The patient usually has localized tenderness over the hip and limited range of motion (ROM) of the affected limb during passive and active ROM of the hip. Patients with nondisplaced or stress fractures may have no obvious deformity.

Diagnostic Evaluation

In patients who report hip pain after a fall, hip fracture should be considered in the differential diagnosis until proven otherwise. An X-ray in an anteroposterior (AP) view obtained while the hip is internally rotated 15 to 20° will provide an optimal image of the femoral neck not evident in the standard AP view. If radiographs are normal and there is still high clinical suspicion of a hip fracture, a bone scan or magnetic resonance imaging (MRI) may be appropriate.

Classification

Hip fractures are classified according to anatomic location. They are typically separated into intracapsular (femoral neck fracture; *see* Table 1) or extracapsular (intertrochanteric [Table 2] or subtrochanteric fractures). Fractures that occur less than 5 cm below the top of the lesser trochanter are considered subtrochanteric fractures. Fractures distal to this are considered femoral shaft fractures.

Treatment

Most patients with hip fractures require surgical intervention. The surgical intervention chosen depends on the type of fracture, the preference of the surgeon, the severity of the injury, the age of the patient, and the prognosis for recovery. Femoral neck fractures can be treated by either internal fixation with multiple screws or prosthetic placement. Internal fixation is used in patients with nondisplaced or minimally displaced fractures, and occasionally in younger patients with displaced fractures. Displaced frac-

Table 1
Garden Classification for Femoral Neck Fractures

Type I	Incomplete, nondisplaced, or valgus impaction
Type II	Complete, nondisplaced
Type III	Complete, partial displacement
Type IV	Complete, total displacement

Table 2
Boyd and Griffin Classification for Intertrochanteric Fractures

Type I	Nondisplaced
Type II	Displaced
Type III	Reverse obliquity
Type IV	Subtrochanteric extension

tures have a higher incidence of nonunion and osteonecrosis. Therefore, prosthetic replacement is generally preferred in displaced fractures, especially in the older patients, to minimize complications. Intertrochanteric fractures are usually treated by internal fixation with a sliding hip screw or a trochanteric fixation nail. Subtrochanteric fractures are treated most commonly with intramedullary devices. The most common site of pathological femur fractures is in the subtrochanteric region.

Rehabilitation

Early ambulation and ROM is important to prevent the complications associated with immobilization. Rehabilitation should begin the first day after surgery with basic bed-to-chair transfers, along with deep breathing exercises. Chair-level exercises, such as active quadriceps exercises and ankle pumps, are utilized. The program should progress to consist of pregait activities, such as sit-to-stand transfers and static standing balance. Progression to walking with an assist device (parallel bars or walker) can usually be accomplished on the first or second postoperative day. If stable fixation of the fracture cannot be achieved, weight-bearing may be limited to avoid instrumentation failure.

During postoperative days 2 to 5, the patient should continue ambulation exercises, along with activities of daily living (ADLs) training with continued ROM and strengthening exercises. Advanced transfer techniques, such as car and tub transfers and stair training, usually begin by postoperative day 6. Once discharged, an outpatient or home physical therapy program typically continues for another 2 to 8 weeks. The primary goal of any rehabilitation program is to maximize function and, thus, allowing the patient to return to his or her prior level of activity.

Complications

The highest risk of mortality after a hip fracture occurs in the first 4 to 6 months, with an overall mortality rate of approximately 15 to 20% at 1 year.

Orthopedic complications after hip fractures include dislocations/subluxations, leg-length discrepancies, prosthetic loosening, heterotopic ossification, wound infections, nerve injuries, and hemorrhage. The peroneal portion of the sciatic nerve is the most common nerve injured in these fractures.

Heterotopic ossification is the deposition of bone in ectopic locations usually around the hip capsule, which results in loss of motion. Irradiation of the hip, use of nonsteroidal anti-inflammatory drugs, and use of etidronate with controlled ROM have been shown to be effective in the prophylaxis of heterotopic ossification.

Medical complications after hip fractures include urinary tract infections, pneumonia, atelectasis, deep vein thrombosis, skin breakdown, and delirium.

Total Hip Replacements

Background

Total hip replacement (THR) is surgically replacing the femoral head and acetabular surface of the hip. Hemiarthroplasty refers to the replacement of the femoral head only. The father of the modern-day hip replacement is Sir John Charnley, who, in 1961, developed the first low-friction arthroplasty. His success spawned the widespread use of hip replacements in the 1970s. Today, there are more than 300,000 THRs implanted worldwide annually.

Indications

Indications for THR are pain-limiting function secondary to osteoarthritis, rheumatoid arthritis, avascular necrosis, or congenital dysplasia of the hip. Sepsis of the involved joint is always an absolute contraindication.

Prosthetic Design

The prosthesis attempts to reproduce normal joint anatomy. The femoral component is usually made of a variety of materials, including titanium

Table 3
Weight-Bearing Precautions

Definitions	
• Nonweight-bearing:	No weight allowed
• Toe-touch weight-bearing:	Approximately 10% of normal weight
• Partial weight-bearing:	Less than 50% of normal weight allowed
• Weight-bearing as tolerated:	As much weight as the patient will allow
• Full weight-bearing:	100% Weight allowed

alloys, ceramics, and cobalt–chrome alloys. The acetabular component is usually composed of ultra-high-molecular-weight polyethylene. Fixation techniques include polymethylmethacrylate cement, porous coating, hydroxyapatite coating, and press-fit stabilization. Cement fixation is strongest immediately after curing, whereas cementless fixation is at its weakest immediately after insertion of the device. Micromotion should be avoided for at least 6 weeks in cementless systems. Studies have shown that cementless systems offer stronger long-term fixation and thus longer life of prosthesis before revision.

Rehabilitation

Education of the surgical process and outcomes are given to the patient before surgery. The patient should be instructed on total hip precautions (based on a posterior surgical approach), which are no hip flexion past 90°, no adduction of the leg past midline, and no internal rotation of the leg. With an anterior approach, the hip precautions are reversed, with limitations on extension past neutral, no external rotation, and no adduction of the leg past midline. An abduction pillow or a knee splint is often utilized to enforce total hip precautions, especially while the patient is in bed. Patients with a high risk of dislocation or with a history of recurrent dislocations are often treated with a hip brace to maintain hip precautions. With cemented THRs, the patient is immediately weight-bearing as tolerated (WBAT). *See* Table 3 for definitions of weight-bearing precautions. With bony ingrowth THRs, the patient is toe-touch weight-bearing for approximately 6 weeks, then advanced to WBAT.

On postoperative day 1, the patient should perform bedside exercises, such as ankle pumps, quadriceps sets, and gluteal sets. Bed mobility and transfer training should begin at this time. The patient should be reminded of their weight-bearing and total hip precautions. On postoperative day 2, the patient should initiate gait training with the use of an assistive device.

Functional transfer training should continue. Postoperative days 3 to 5 should include progression of ROM and strengthening exercises as tolerated. The patient should continue ambulation on level surfaces and progress to stairs. ADL techniques, such as using a long-handled reacher, a raised toilet seat, a sock aid, a dressing stick, and a long shoe horn, should be mastered. After postoperative day 5, the patient will continue aggressive strengthening and stretching exercises targeting the hip. Ambulation usually progresses from household distances to community distances. The patient should eventually be modified-independent in ADLs and achieve ambulation within the first few weeks.

At 6 weeks after the operation, most patients are walking with a cane (always using the cane on the side opposite the replaced hip). With advancing levels of independence, the patient may begin driving. Hip precautions should be maintained for a total of 3 to 6 months.

Results

Long-term retrospective studies show that most patients are completely pain free. Of all hip replacements, 90 to 95% are successful at the 10-year mark. The major long-term problems are loosening or wear. Loosening occurs because the cement crumbles or because the bone resorbs away from the cement. By 10 years, 25% of artificial hips will have evidence of aseptic loosening on an X-ray. A little less than half of these patients will have enough pain to require a revision of the implant. Over a prolonged period, wear can occur in the plastic acetabular socket. Wear particles can induce inflammation resulting in the thinning of the bone and thus, increase the risk for periprosthetic fracture.

Complications

Complications of THRs, like most orthopedic procedures, include aseptic loosening, infection, deep vein thrombosis (DVT), heterotopic bone formation, urinary tract infections, dislocations, and neurological deficits. Most surgeons opt for DVT prophylaxis after surgery because more than 50% of patients have DVT without intervention. Prophylactic regimens include warfarin, with international normalization ratio goals between 1.5 and 3.0, aspirin, low-molecular-weight heparin, or sequential compression devices.

Total Knee Replacements

Background

Total knee replacements (TKRs) are one of the most common procedures performed in orthopedic surgery today. TKR was introduced in the

1960s by Gunston, who realized the knee was not a single axis like a hinge, but rather the femoral condyles roll and glide on the tibia with multiple instant centers of rotation. Approximately 200,000 TKRs are performed annually in the United States alone.

Indications

Indications for TKRs are disabling pain and deformity secondary to osteoarthritis, rheumatoid arthritis, or traumatic arthritis. Sepsis of the knee joint is an absolute contraindication.

Prosthetic Design

Nonconstrained knee implants are the most common type of artificial knee. It is called nonconstrained because the artificial components inserted into the knee are not connected to each other, as it has no inherent stability. The system relies on the person's own ligaments and muscles for stability. The semiconstrained implant is a device that provides more stability for the knee. This type of knee prosthesis has some stability built into it. Constrained or hinged knee prostheses are not used as a first choice. The two components of the knee joint are linked together with a hinged mechanism. This type of knee replacement is used when the knee is unstable and the patient's own ligaments will not be able to support the other types of knee replacements. The fully constrained knee prosthesis is useful in treating severely damaged knees—especially in elderly people. A unicondylar knee replacement replaces only half of the knee joint. Although it is performed if the damage is limited to one side of the joint, many surgeons prefer performing a TKR on these patients.

Fixation of the joint is usually performed with a cemented procedure. Both the femoral and tibial components of the implant are fixed to the bone with polymethylmethacrylate. The cement allows the implants to have a perfect fit to the irregularities of the bone. The advantage is that the knee replacement is immediately stable. Noncemented hybrid designs are also available. Hybrid designs usually involve a noncemented femoral component, along with a cemented tibial component.

Rehabilitation

On the first two postoperative days, the patient is to begin transfer and ambulation activities. The patient begins quadriceps and hamstring isometric exercises and is placed in a continuous passive motion (CPM) machine. On postoperative days 3 to 5, the patient should being straight leg raises and strengthening and ROM exercises. The patient is taught basic ADL techniques, joint protection, energy conservation, and work simplification techniques. Resistive exercise should be avoided until full knee extension is present and as straight leg raises can be performed against gravity. In cemented prosthesis, the patient can begin WBAT immediately, whereas the patient is usually toe-touch weight-bearing or partial weight-bearing for 6 weeks for noncemented arthroplasties. The surgeon will usually obtain an X-ray approximately 5 to 6 weeks postoperatively to evaluate if the patient's weight-bearing status should be upgraded.

During the second week of rehabilitation, the patient should reach 90° of knee flexion. Ninety degrees of knee flexion is required for sitting and transferring into a car. Manipulation under anesthesia is considered when the knee ROM is severely compromised. During the fourth- to sixth-week postoperative period, the patient is usually advanced to a cane as tolerated. Progressive resistance exercises for the quadriceps/hamstrings and hip flexors continue during this period. Driving can usually be safe around the sixth week for right-sided total knee replacements.

The use of the CPM machine has been controversial. Studies have shown that with the CPM machine, 90° of knee flexion is gained faster and fewer manipulations are needed. However, in follow-up after discharge, there was no difference in ROM between patients with CPM and patients without CPM. Length of rehabilitation hospital days may be shorter with CPM. Using CPM machines 5 hours per day produces the same effect as 20 hours per day.

Results

Retrospective studies have shown 85 to 95% satisfactory results in 5- to 10-year studies. Noncemented prosthesis showed no difference in pain outcomes when compared with cemented prosthesis.

Complications

Complications of TKRs are similar to other orthopedic procedures. Common complications include aseptic loosening, joint sepsis, lack of flexion requiring manipulation, DVT, and extensor lag. The risk of DVT without prophylaxis is 55% for unilateral TKRs and 75% for bilateral TKRs. Aspirin, warfarin, or low-molecular-weight heparin are commonly used for DVT prophylaxis after TKRs.

Fractures of the Ankle

Background

Ankle fractures can be divided into three areas of injury: the lateral malleolus, the medial malleolus, and the posterior lip of the tibia (posterior malleolus). Stable fractures involve only one side, whereas unstable fractures involve at least two areas. They are classified as bimalleolar or trimalleolar (involving the posterior aspect of the tibia).

Clinical Examination

Patients may feel immediate pain and have difficulty walking. Swelling is often associated with ankle fractures, with marked tenderness over the fracture site. There may be some instability with passive ROM. Neurovascular status of the ankle should also be assessed.

Diagnostic Evaluation

AP and lateral radiographs should be obtained. A mortise view should also be obtained (15° internally rotated AP view), which will most clearly show the relationship of the fibula, tibia, and talus.

A Maisonneuve fracture, which is usually secondary to an external rotation injury of the ankle, is associated with a fracture of the proximal third of the fibula. On examination, the patient will not only have pain in the ankle but also in the area of the proximal fibula. Therefore, patients with tenderness over the proximal fibula associated with a twisting ankle injury should have AP and lateral views of the proximal fibula and tibia.

Treatment/Rehabilitation

Stable fractures of the distal fibula can be treated with a weight-bearing cast for approximately 4 to 6 weeks. Unstable, nondisplaced fractures require immobilization with a nonweight-bearing leg cast for 4 to 6 weeks. If proper healing occurs, these patients can be upgraded to a walking cast/boot for the next 2 weeks. In patients treated nonoperatively, follow-up radiographs must be obtained weekly for the first 2 to 3 weeks following the injury to rule out fracture displacement. Strengthening and ROM exercises can begin once fracture healing occurs. Patients with a displaced ankle fracture will require open or closed reduction. These patients will typically require immobilization and nonweight-bearing for 4 to 8 weeks following surgery.

Other Fractures of the Lower Extremity

Pelvic Fractures

Pelvic fractures can be divided into stable and unstable fractures. Stable fractures involve only one side of the pelvic ring, such as a unilateral fracture of the inferior and superior pubic ramus. Unstable fractures disrupt the pelvic ring at two sites. Treatment of stable pelvic fractures includes appropriate pain management, gait training that is usually WBAT, and appropriate DVT prophylaxis. Unstable pelvic and acetabular fractures usually require surgical intervention.

Femoral Shaft Fractures

The shaft of the femur is the portion between the subtrochanteric region and the distal supracondylar area of the knee. Fractures of the femoral shaft are most commonly caused by high-energy trauma. Adverse outcomes are usually associated with fat embolism, acute respiratory distress syndrome, and arterial injury secondary to the severity of the initial insult.

Knee Fractures

Knee fractures are classified as supracondylar, condylar (lateral or medial), or tibial plateau fractures. Older patients with osteoporosis can sustain fractures about the knee from low-energy trauma. In younger patients, these fractures usually involve high-energy force. Nonoperative treatment is usually indicated for nondisplaced fractures. Displaced fractures usually require open reduction and internal fixation.

Fractures of the Foot

The calcaneus is the most common fractured tarsal bone and usually occurs from falls onto the heel. Most fractures require surgery and may require nonweight-bearing for 8 to 12 weeks. Posttraumatic arthritis is common in these fractures. The talus is the only foot bone without muscular attachments. It also bears the most weight of all bones in the body. The talus has a tenuous blood supply and is predisposed to avascular necrosis and fracture nonunion. Surgery is commonly indicated in talar fractures, although certain nondisplaced fractures heal with a short leg cast for 12 weeks with nonweight-bearing, usually for the first 6 weeks.

Shoulder Instability

Background

The shoulder joint has great mobility secondary to its shallow glenoid fossa and loose capsule. Joint instability is most common at the shoulder joint. The most common direction of instability is anterior and multidirectional. Anterior instability can be described by the mneumonic TUBS—traumatic, unidirectional, Bankart lesion (a tear of the anterior glenoid labrum), often requiring surgery. Multidirectional instability can be described by the mneumonic AMBRI—atraumatic, multidirectional, bilateral, rehabilitation, and inferior capsular shift if surgery is necessary. Posterior dislocations occur less frequently, and are often secondary to a posteriorly directed force while the shoulder is in the adducted and internally rotated position.

Clinical Examination

After an acute dislocation, movement of the shoulder will cause considerable pain, limiting the physical examination. Anterior instability can be confirmed by the apprehension sign. The examiner places the arm in 90° of abduction and then externally rotates the arm. In a patient with anterior instability, there will be a sense of increased mobility and apprehension secondary to the pain. A posteriorly directed force by the examiner will decrease the apprehension and is therefore known as the relocation test. The sulcus sign is indicative of inferior laxity. The examiner applies an inferiorly directed traction to the shoulder. In patients with inferior laxity, this will cause inferior subluxation, seen as widening of the gap between the humeral head and the acromion. The neurovascular function of the upper extremities should be assessed before reduction. The axillary nerve is commonly involved in shoulder injuries.

Diagnostic Evaluation

AP and axillary X-ray views of the shoulder should be obtained. A common finding in anterior dislocations is a Hill-Sachs lesion, which is a compression fracture of the posterior humeral head. This occurs when the humeral head is compressed against the anterior edge of the glenoid. An MRI or shoulder arthrogram can also be ordered to assess the rotator cuff.

Treatment

Most shoulder dislocations should be reduced. Postreduction films should be obtained to confirm the reduction. The arm should be put in a sling after reduction.

Rehabilitation

Although the patient is immobilized in a sling, the patient should remove the sling and extend the elbow several times a day to prevent elbow contractures. Isometric exercises for the rotator cuff should begin almost immediately. Rehabilitation for the shoulder usually involves ROM restrictions the first several weeks. During the first 2 weeks, ROM is usually limited to 90° of forward flexion and 0° of external rotation. Strengthening exercises should begin around the second or third week mainly focusing on the external and internal rotators of the shoulder. ROM to 140° of forward flexion and 30° of external rotation usually occurs around the third week. At approximately 6 weeks, more vigorous exercises can be performed.

Rehabilitation for the shoulder can be divided into two phases: stretching and strengthening. In general, stretching exercises should begin first. Once ROM is restored, strengthening exercises are added.

Before stretching exercises, the patient should loosen up the shoulder by applying moist heat. Pain medications or nonsteroidal anti-inflammatory drugs should be taken approximately 30 minutes before the initiation of the exercise. Stretching of the shoulder usually begins with the pendulum (Codman's) technique. The patient leans forward and, while letting the arm hang freely, the patient uses his or her truncal muscles to cause a passive circular motion in the shoulder. Subsequently, passive stretching can be performed with a stick, a towel, or a pulley. It is important to hold the stretch for at least 5 seconds.

Exercises to strengthen the rotator cuff muscles can be performed easily with elastic bands that come in different degrees of resistance. Other strengthening exercises include the shoulder shrug to strengthen the trapezius, push-ups to strengthen the serratus anterior and rhomboids (and pectoralis muscles), and press-up exercises from a chair to strengthen the latissimus dorsi (and triceps).

Proximal Humerus Fractures

Background

Proximal humerus fractures can be divided into two general categories, the first being nondisplaced or minimally displaced, which occur in approximately 80% of cases. Nondisplaced proximal humerus fractures are usually secondary to low-energy insults in the older age group, especially in patients with osteoporotic bone. Displaced fractures occur in approximately 20% of cases, especially in the younger age group and usually from a high-energy trauma.

Clincial Examination

Swelling, ecchymosis, and discoloration in the shoulder and upper arm region are common. It is important to assess the function of the neurovascular structures, especially the radial and axillary nerves and the radial pulse.

Diagnostic Evaluation

Routine radiographs of the shoulder should be obtained. Axillary views are often helpful in making the diagnosis.

Treatment/Rehabilitation

Minimally displaced fractures (<1 cm) are usually treated with a sling and rehabilitation. After the first week, the patient can begin an exercise program consisting of pendulum exercises. After 3 weeks, the sling can be removed or worn part-time for comfort. Progressive stretching and then strengthening exercises should be aggressively performed after the third week.

Displaced fractures with greater than 1 cm separation require surgical intervention. Displaced four-part fractures disrupt blood supply to the humeral head and usually require prosthetic replacement of the humeral head, rather than an open reduction internal fixation.

Scaphoid Fractures

Background

The scaphoid is the most commonly injured carpal bone, accounting for 60 to 70% of all carpal fractures. If adequately treated, 90 to 95% will go on to union (thus, in 5–10% nonunion may occur in spite of treatment). Scaphoid fractures can be divided by anatomic location: distal pole, middle or waist, and proximal pole. The scaphoid receives its blood supply from branches of the radial artery. The blood supply to the scaphoid is tenuous because the major blood supply enters the bone in the distal third of the bone. Injuries proximal to the major blood supply may disrupt vascularity to the proximal scaphoid, resulting in nonunion and osteonecrosis.

Clinical Examination

Palpation over the anatomic snuffbox reveals tenderness. Pressure over the scaphoid tubercle on the palmar aspect of the wrist will produce pain. Pain can usually be elicited by wrist dorsiflexion and radial deviation. It is also important to assess the neurovascular integrity of the hand and wrist.

Diagnostic Evaluation

At the time of injury, a scaphoid fracture may not be visible on routine posteroanterior (PA) and lateral films of the wrist. It is often necessary to obtain a PA view with the wrist in ulnar deviation and an oblique view to further visualize a suspected scaphoid fracture. If the initial radiographs are normal, but the pain continues to persist, another PA and oblique view should be obtained in 2 to 3 weeks. A bone scan and MRI may be helpful if the diagnosis is in doubt.

Treatment/Rehabilitation

The wrist should be immobilized in the neutral position with a long-arm thumb spica cast for at least 6 weeks. If X-rays show a healing fracture after 6 weeks, the cast can be downgraded to a short-arm thumb spica cast. It should be noted that if a scaphoid fracture is suspected, the patient should be placed in a thumb spica splint, despite initial negative X-rays. Repeat X-rays should be ordered 2 to 3 weeks after the initial injury. If the radiographs are still normal and the patient continues with pain, a bone scan or MRI should be considered.

Healing times vary depending on the location of the scaphoid fracture. Nondisplaced fractures of the distal pole usually require 6 to 8 weeks, whereas fractures of the proximal pole can take as long as 3 to 6 months secondary to its poor vascularity. Fractures of the middle portion usually require 2 to 3 months for adequate healing. All patients with displaced fractures of the scaphoid will need *early* evaluation for possible surgical intervention. Furthermore, patients with nondisplaced fractures that have failed to heal after 2 months of immobilization will need surgical evaluation for possible intervention.

Other Fractures of the Upper Extremity

Humeral Shaft Fractures

Fractures of the humeral shaft often occur secondary to a traumatic insult. Most humeral shaft fractures can be treated non-operatively, with good union after closed reduction. Radial nerve injuries are often associated with this fracture. The radial nerve function can be quickly assessed by asking the patient to extend the wrist or fingers or by checking sensation on the dorsum of the wrist or posterior aspect of the forearm.

Most patients are prescribed a splint, followed by a fracture brace to the arm. ROM of the shoulder, elbow, and wrist should be encouraged while in the brace. The fracture brace is worn for at least 6 weeks until there is appropriate healing on X-ray.

Forearm Fractures

Isolated radial shaft fractures and both forearm bones (ulna and radius) require open reduction and internal fixation (ORIF). An undisplaced ulna shaft fracture can be treated with plaster immobilization. It is important to remember not to immobilize in a long arm cast or splint for more than 3 weeks. Usually the cast is set at 90° of flexion. If the fracture is aligned, the cast should be converted to a removable forearm brace around 2 weeks.

ROM should begin by this time. The extremity usually remains nonweight-bearing until approximately 6 weeks if adequate callus formation is present. A displaced ulna shaft fracture requires ORIF.

Two special types of forearm fractures, the Galeazzi and the Monteggia fracture usually require ORIF. A Galeazzi fracture is a distal radial shaft fracture that is associated with a distal radioulnar dislocation and is difficult to treat nonoperatively secondary to mechanical forces that tend to displace the distal radial fragment. A Monteggia fracture is a proximal ulna shaft fracture with dislocation of the radial head. Ulna shaft fractures should include radiographs of the elbow to rule out associated dislocations.

Wrist Fractures

Distal radial fractures are very common, especially after falls in adults. Colles fracture is the most common type with dorsal angulation of the distal fragment (silver fork deformity). A Smith fracture is the opposite of a Colles fracture, with the distal fragment angluating in the volar (downward) direction. The Barton fracture is an intra-articular fracture of the distal radius associated with dislocation/subluxation of the carpus. For nondisplaced and minimally displaced fractures, the wrist is immobilized with a sugar-tong splint followed by a short arm cast for a total of about 4 to 6 weeks. After the cast is removed, a removable splint should be worn for approximately 1 month. Shoulder and finger ROM should be performed to prevent stiffness. Displaced fractures are often unstable and require internal or external fixation. Weight-bearing is typically allowed at about 6 weeks if there is adequate callus formation.

Key References and Suggested Additional Reading

Brinker MR, Miller MD. Fundamentals of Orthopedics. Philadelphia: WB Saunders, 1999.

Brotzman SB, Wilk KE. Clinical Orthopedic Rehabilitation, 2nd ed. Philadelphia: Mosby, 2003.

Frontera WR, Silver JK. Essentials of Physical Medicine and Rehabilitation. Philadelphia: Hanley and Belfus, 2002.

Greene WB. Essentials of Musculoskeletal Care, 2nd ed. Rosemont, IL: American Academy of Orthopedic Surgeons, 2001.

Kibler WB, Herring SA. Functional Rehabilitation of Sports and Musculoskeletal Injuries. Gaithersburg, MD: Aspen Publishers, 1998.

Magee DJ. Orthopedic Physical Assessment, 4th ed. Philadelphia: Saunders, 2002.

11 Spine and Musculoskeletal Medicine

Grant Cooper, Yusuf Tatli, and Gregory E. Lutz

Axial Neck Pain

Background

Neck pain is a very common complaint, affecting up to 70% of the population at some point in their lives. This makes neck pain the second most common presenting musculoskeletal complaint (second only to low back pain). Any structure that receives innervation can be a likely pain generator in the neck. Potential causes of mechanical neck pain include muscle spasm, strain, osteoarthritis (OA), discogenic, and zygapophysial (Z)-joint disease.

Cervical strain is generally caused by mechanical postural disorders, overexertion, or injury especially flexion-extension injuries (whiplash). Axial neck pain is often accompanied by referral pain patterns in the head, back, and arms with a nondermatomal pattern. Referred pain is based on the principal of *convergence*, in which multiple anatomic sites utilize the same afferent pathway to communicate with the brain. The brain has difficulty distinguishing the original source of pain and so perceives pain in multiple areas. When patients have referred pain, they characteristically describe it as dull, aching, and difficult to localize.

The majority of neck pain is believed to resolve on its own. Because of this, aggressive diagnosis of acute axial mechanical neck pain (lasting <3 months) is often not necessary. When neck pain becomes chronic, it is much less likely to spontaneously resolve. The single most common cause of chronic neck pain is cervical Z-joint disease, accounting for approximately 50% of chronic neck pain in patients with a history of whiplash. The

From: *Essential Physical Medicine and Rehabilitation*
Edited by: G. Cooper © Humana Press Inc., Totowa, NJ

Z-joints are the facet joints in the cervical spine that articulate the superior articular processes of one vertebra with the inferior articular processes of the adjacent superior vertebrae.

History

The typical patient with chronic neck pain will report dull, aching pain in the neck that is accompanied by difficult-to-localize boring pain in the head, scapula, and/or arm. Often, these patients report a history of a motor vehicle accident either immediately precipitating the symptoms or else in the distant past. Other patients may report a history of more direct trauma, such as being hit in the head. A key component of the history is the *quality* of the pain. Axial neck pain and referral pain are not typically shooting, electric, or lancinating. Also, they are not accompanied by numbness, tingling, or weakness. These complaints warrant consideration of an alternate diagnosis, such as a cervical radiculopathy or radiculitis.

A boring, deep pain that is unrelieved by resting or associated fever, chills, recent weight loss, history of cancer, recent surgery, or night pain are red-flag symptoms and suggest a potential cancer or infection. Pain intensified by prolonged static posture, sitting, lifting, sneezing, and vibration exposure (e.g., riding in a car), flexion-extension, and axial loading is often discogenic or Z-joint because discogenic and Z-joint pain symptoms can vary according to changes in intradiscal pressure and Z-joint pressure, respectively.

Another important component to the history is the distribution of pain. Whereas referral pain is difficult to localize, pain from different Z-joints does follow characteristic patterns. For example, painful C5 and C6 Z-joints tend to refer pain into the shoulder and arm, whereas pain from C6 and C7 tends to refer pain to the medial scapula. This information will be particularly helpful if diagnostic and, potentially, therapeutic blocks of the joints are needed.

Physical Examination

The physical examination of axial neck pain includes inspection and palpation of the patient's neck. Observe for any muscle spasm or asymmetry. Palpate for any tender points or trigger points (trigger points are defined as tender points *with* a referral pain pattern when palpated).

Assess the patient's range of motion (ROM), which may be limited by pain. Also, assess the patient's strength of major neck movements (flexion, lateral flexion, rotation, and extension). When assessing the patient for potential Z-joint disease, there is no physical examination maneuver that has been shown to be diagnostic, including pain with extension and tenderness to palpation. The diagnosis of Z-joint disease ultimately relies on controlled diagnostic blocks of the nerves that innervate the putative painful joint(s).

Imaging and Diagnostic Procedures

Anterioposterior (AP) and lateral X-rays may be obtained to rule out a more serious underlying pathology, especially in patients with a history of trauma or those who are younger (<20 years) or older (>50 years). Anterior displacement of the pharyngeal air shadow indicates soft tissue swelling and possible disruption of the intervertebral disc or anterior longitudinal ligament. The width of the prevertebral soft tissue at the level of C3 should not exceed 7 mm in normal adults. It may be worthwhile to obtain flexion-extension lateral views to check for signs of instability that include more than 3.5 mm translation of a vertebral body and/or more than 11° of angulation of adjacent vertebrae. Magnetic resonance imaging (MRI) is also commonly used for this purpose.

To diagnose most cases of chronic neck pain, however, controlled diagnostic blocks of the medial branches of the cervical dorsal rami that innervate the suspected Z-joint(s) is necessary. Controlled blocks involve blocking the joint twice—once with a shorter acting and once with a longer acting anesthetic at different times. The patient (and ideally the physician) are blinded to which anesthetic was used. For the blocks to be positive, the patient must report complete (as in 100%) pain relief of at least a discrete portion of pain that lasts longer with the longer anesthetic than it did with the shorter acting anesthetic. The joints may also be blocked with intra-articular injections, although this is a more invasive procedure because it violates the joint capsule. All blocks are performed under fluoroscopic-guidance.

If the symptoms and physical findings are more suggestive of a chronic discogenic source, then discography should be used. Discography may help answer questions on choice of intervention, surgical versus nonsurgical management, and even possible outcomes.

Treatment

For cases of acute neck pain, treatment is generally conservative and includes rest, heat, nonsteroidal anti-inflammatory drugs (NSAIDs), and gentle ROM exercises. Flexibility, strengthening, and endurance exercises should be initiated as soon as pain becomes limited. Protection of the neck at night with a cervical pillow or orthosis may be helpful. Gradual return to full activity is encouraged. Education in proper body mechanics and exercise are vital for future pain prevention. Patients may also benefit from a cervical collar to be worn at night for a short time.

Patients who are found to have trigger points may benefit from trigger-point injections using anesthetic and corticosteroid. When the diagnosis of Z-joint disease is made, patients may be treated with radiofrequency neurotomy of the involved nerves. Radiofrequency neurotomy is a percutaneous procedure done under fluoroscopic guidance that serves to essentially sever the nerve with radiofrequency energy. Because the nerves may regenerate over time, the procedure may need to be periodically repeated. In chronic discogenic axial neck pain with positive discography results, recent literature demonstrates favorable cervical fusion results.

Cervical Radiculopathy

Background

Cervical radiculopathy is caused by ischemia, stretch, or compression of a nerve root. Cervical radiculopathy involves a neurological *loss*, such as loss of strength, sensation, and/or reflexes. This may manifest in the patient as weakness, numbness, tingling, or diminished reflexes. Cervical radicular pain is different from radiculopathy. Radicular pain is caused by compression of the dorsal root ganglion or inflammation of a nerve root—referred to as "cervical radiculitis." Radicular pain is characterized by patients as shooting, electric, and lancinating. Because radiculopathy is often associated with radicular pain, it is often confused and considered the same entity. However, it is important to keep in mind that they have different pathologies. Nevertheless, because they are often associated, the two entities are discussed together in this section as well.

History

Patients with radicular symptoms will complain of radiating, electric pain, numbness, and/or tingling that radiates into their arm and/or hand. Patients may also complain of weakness. Depending on the level of pathology, patients will complain of a characteristic distribution of symptoms. Recall that the nerve root in the cervical spine exits below the vertebra of the same number. For example, the C3 nerve root exits between the C3 and C4 vertebrae. Radicular symptoms may involve more than one level or be bilateral. A diffuse pattern of symptoms with bilateral numbness, weakness, and pain can be seen in central spinal stenosis. For a distribution of symptoms and accompanying nerve root level *see* Table 1.

Physical Examination

The physical examination includes assessing the cervical spine (as in the physical exam for neck pain) and assessing the upper extremity for neurological deficit: examine ROM and strength; biceps (C5), brachioradialis (C6), and triceps (C7) reflexes; sensation; and tone. After examining the neck, evaluate the patient's shoulder abduction (C5), wrist extension (C6), arm extension (C7), finger flexion (C8), and fifth digit abduction (T1). Also assess the patient's reflexes (biceps [C5], brachioradialis [C6], and triceps [C7]). Neck pain is a common symptom, and at times, can be dominating the radiculopathy. Radiculopathy is usually the result of a soft disc herniation or disc-space narrowing and arthrosis leading to foraminal stenosis. Patients may present with the "shoulder-abduction relief" sign with their shoulder abducted over their head, which decreases the neuormeningeal tension.

In unilateral radiculopathies, asymmetric hyporeflexia at a specific root level is common, whereas in centralized myelopathic processes, generalized symmetric hyperreflexia is often seen. Spurling's test may be performed to evaluate for foraminal encroachment on an irritated cervical nerve root and is an important diagnostic maneuver. This test is performed by rotating and laterally extending the neck (toward the symptomatic side), and applying *gentle* axial compression to the patient's head. This maneuver works by increasing the pressure on the exiting nerve root, and is positive if the patient experiences radicular symptoms. Reciprocally, flexing and laterally flexing the neck away from the symptomatic side and applying gentle traction to the patient's head should alleviate symptoms.

If there is any upper motor sign, such as a unilateral brisk reflex or spasticity, then checking for rapid alternating movements is essential. Hoffman's sign should also be assessed in patients with suspected radiculopathy. Rapid alternating movements can be assessed by evaluating the patient's speed and accuracy in tapping two fingers together on the same hand. If there is asymmetry or generalized difficulty, then the test is abnormal.

Hoffman's sign is assessed by stabilizing the proximal interphalangeal (IP) joint of the third digit in extension and briskly flicking the distal phalanx. A positive Hoffmann's sign is elicited if the patient's IP joint of the first digit or third distal IP joint of the same hand reflexively flexes.

Because the pain fibers are affected later than the vibration and position sense in radiculopathy, the sensory loss evaluation by pin-prick is not the most reliable test. However, vibration is generally not localized to one dermatome, so it is not useful in the setting of a radiculopathy.

Imaging and Diagnostic Procedures

AP, lateral, odontoid, and oblique X-rays of the cervical spine should be obtained to evaluate the bony structures and evaluate the foramina. MRI is also helpful to define the level and severity of the problem, particularly if epidural steroids or surgery is being considered. Diagnosis of cervical radiculopathy sometimes requires electrodiagnostic evaluation to differentiate from other causes (e.g., plexopathy, mononeuropathy, peripheral neuropathy), especially in "double crush phenomenon," which occurs when a nerve is compressed at two levels, such as can happen with a C5–C6 disc herniation and an ipsilateral carpal tunnel syndrome.

Treatment

The main treatment of cervical radicular symptoms is conservative and includes rest, ice, massage, NSAIDs, and physical therapy with an emphasis on ROM, strengthening exercises, and postural mechanics. Patients may also benefit from a cervical orthosis to be worn at night to avoid lateral bending and extension of the neck. Some patients may benefit from an oral steroid taper.

In patients with more severe symptoms or symptoms that do not respond to more conservative measures, fluoroscopically guided epidural steroid injections may be of benefit. The epidural steroid injection may be delivered using either an interlaminar or transforaminal approach. Indications for surgery include progressive neurological deficits and/or less commonly severe intractable pain that is not responding to aggressive nonsurgical care.

Shoulder Impingement Syndrome

Background

Shoulder pain is the third most common musculoskeletal symptom encountered in medical practice after back and neck pain. Impingement of the rotator cuff tendon in the subacromial space is a common source of shoulder pain. Causative factors of impingement syndrome could be classified into subacromial, intra-articular (anterior instability, superior labral tears, and biceps injury), and extra-articular nonsubacromial (muscle weakness/imbalance, scapular dyskinesis) categories. Impingement syndrome is typical of patients who participate in repetitive overhead activity and experience repetitive loading of the joint through activities, such as basketball, baseball, swimming, or painting.

History

The typical patient is a younger individual who presents with a complaint of sudden anterior shoulder pain that began following strenuous exertion involving overhead movement. Older patients may be more likely to present with a history of chronic anterior pain made worse with overhead movements, such as brushing hair. In some advanced cases, because of shoulder abduction and internal rotation weakness, patients may have difficulty removing the wallet from their back pocket. Patients may also report nighttime pain preventing sleep on the affected side. These patients may relate a history of treating themselves periodically with NSAIDs and rest.

Physical Examination

To assess the shoulder, first inspect it for any asymmetry in the muscle mass or scapular position. Palpate for tenderness or fullness at the acromioclavicular joint, supraclavicular fossa, biceps tendon, subacromial bursa, supraspinatus fossa, and infraspinatus fossa.

Next, assess ROM, strength, and reflexes. Active and passive ROM comparison helps on the differentials. For example, restricted-active ROM compared with passive ROM with a painful arc between 60° and 120° of abduction is common in rotator cuff dysfunction; however, adhesive capsulitis has both active and passive motion loss; glenohumeral arthritis has pain with any motion.

To specifically test for impingement syndrome, several specific tests exist. More important than the specific test selected is the understanding of the purpose of these tests—this is to put the shoulder into positions of impingment, reducing the subacromial space and irritating and eliciting pain in an already inflamed or irritable tendon. The impingement sign involves stabilizing the patient's scapula with one hand and internally rotating and flexing the patient's shoulder in the scapular plane with the other. This maneuver traps the supraspinatus tendon between the greater tuberosity and the acromion, irritating the tendon and eliciting pain in an already irritated tendon. Another impingement test is the Hawkins-Kennedy test. In this test, the patient's shoulder and the elbow are flexed to 90°, and the humerus is then put into internal rotation. Pain elicited with this test is indicative of rotator cuff tear or impingement syndrome.

Imaging and Diagnostic Procedures

In a patient with a positive impingment sign, a subacromial anesthetic injection may be given. Following the injection, the impingement maneuver is repeated and should not elicit pain. A positive impingement sign *before* a subacromial anesthetic injection but negative *after* the injection is strongly suggestive of impingment syndrome.

Other diagnostic tests may include impingement series radiographs that include AP and lateral views in internal and external rotation, scapular outlet view, and axillary view. On the scapular outlet view, the acromion is clearly visualized. Bigliani described three types of acomions: type I = flat, type II = curved (most common), and type III = hooked. Types II and III reduce the subacromial space and are most commonly associated with rotator cuff tear.

Treatment

Conservative treatment is generally sufficient and includes rest, activity modification, ice, and NSAIDs. Patients often also benefit from a subacromial injection of corticosteroid and anesthetic. There are many injection approaches to the subacromial space. The posterior approach, using a 22-gage needle, is often favored because it avoids the humeral head and easily accesses the space. If resistance to the injection is encountered, the needle is repositioned such that the injectate flows smoothly into the subacromial space.

In patients with presumed impingement syndrome found to have a calcification on radiographs, the treatment is similar to impingement syndrome. However, these patients may also benefit from ultrasound-guided aspiration and lavage of the calcification.

Rotator Cuff Tear

Background

The rotator cuff muscles are remembered by the mnemonic SITS—supraspinatus, infraspinatus, teres minor, subscapularis. A rotator cuff tear may occur in a patient with a history of impingement syndrome. Neer described three stages of subacromial impingment. In stage 1, repetitive microtrauma leads to edema and hemorrhage. In stage 2, the inflammation leads to fibrosis. Finally, in stage 3, the tendon fails and the rotator cuff tears. The majority of rotator cuff tears occur in the supraspinatus tendon. Less commonly, sudden trauma may also cause a rotator cuff tear. Partial tears generally involve less than 50% of the tendon thickness, and do not lead to retraction of the muscle.

History

Patients will often give a history of chronic impingement syndrome. They may describe this as anterior shoulder pain or subdeltoid pain that is worse with activity and refractory to NSAIDs and rest. The pain gradually worsens and the patient complains of weakness and stiffness limiting activities of daily living, such as carrying bags and lifting children. Weakness is not common in partial tears, but can be seen because of the pain, which is often greater than in full tears. Abrupt onset of weakness, especially in association with trauma, may indicate an acute tear.

Physical Examination

The physical examination includes inspection for shoulder girdle muscle atrophy, palpation to distinguish rotator cuff pain from bicipital tendonitis (tenderness over the anterior shoulder), subacromial bursitis, or acromioclavicular arthritic joint (point tenderness) pain. ROM and muscle testing is also performed. When evaluating strength, it is essential to keep in mind whether apparent weakness is secondary to loss of muscle or because of inhibition secondary to pain.

To specifically test the rotator cuff muscles, begin by testing abduction. This tests the supraspinatus muscle, which is primarily responsible for the first 30° of shoulder abduction. Bilateral comparison is useful. Testing internal rotation evaluates the subscapularis muscle. Another good test for internal rotation strength is the Gerber lift-off test. In this test, the patient puts the hand behind his or her back with the palm facing posteriorly and pushes against resistance. If the subscapularis is weak, the patient will not be able to push off the spine. Testing external rotation tests the infraspinatus and teres minor muscles. Patients should also be investigated for provocative and instability tests.

Imaging and Diagnostic Procedures

Impingement series (AP, outlet, and axillary views) radiographs should be obtained.

MRI should be obtained, and is the best imaging modality to assess the rotator cuff and surrounding soft tissues. It has sensitivity of close to 100% for a full tear. On imaging studies, measurement of the AP or mediolateral directions describes the severity of the lesion. One centimeter is classified as a small lesion, 1 to 3 cm is medium, 3 to 5 cm is large, and more than 5 cm is considered massive. Two tendon tears or more are considered massive as well. As an imaging study, ultrasound may also be utilized. However, it is less accurate in the detection of partial tears, with sensitivities ranging from 25 to 94%.

Treatment

Nonsurgical care may be used for partial thickness tears. NSAIDs, rest, ice, and physical therapy that emphasizes stretching and strengthening the rotator cuff and scapular stabilizers constitutes the cornerstone of initial management. In patients with a component of impingement syndrome causing pain, a subacromial anesthetic and corticosteroid injection may also be helpful. In partial thickness tears (<50%) that do not respond to conservative measures, arthroscopic debridement or subacromial decompression may be effective.

In tears with more than 50% involvement, surgical repair may be indicated. Prognostic factors for poor outcome are a tear size greater than 3 cm, and duration of symptoms for longer than 6 to 12 months. Following surgery, patients should begin early passive ROM and isometric exercises to prevent stiffness. After 6 weeks, therapy should progress to active and active-assistive ROM, with strengthening at 10 to 12 weeks postoperatively. Within 6 months following surgery, most patients may return to previous levels of activity.

Adhesive Capsulitis

Background

The pathophysiology of this common disorder is still not well understood. It is believed that inflammation leads to fibrosis, which results in stiffness. Diabetes mellitus is the most common risk factor. Patients with diabetes commonly have bilateral involvement, and may be resistive to treatment. Hypothyroidism, cerebral hemorrhage, herniated cervical disc, and Parkinson's disease are other risk factors.

History

Patients typically complain of vague shoulder pain that progressively increases in intensity and then slowly resolves. As the pain resolves, the patient complains of increasing stiffness.

Physical Examination

Decreased active and passive ROM is the hallmark physical examination finding. Early in the course of the disorder, patients may complain of pain at the ends of ROM. As the disorder progresses, ROM may become markedly impaired.

Imaging and Diagnostic Procedures

Adhesive capuslitis is largely a clinical diagnosis; however, radiographs of the shoulder may be obtained to rule out more serious underlying processes, such as OA, loose bodies, or tumors.

Treatment

Physical therapy that emphasizes ROM exercises, heat, NSAIDs, and ultrasound may be used for conservative care. Manipulation under anesthesia may be useful. In the early phase of the disorder, intra-articular and subacromial injections of anesthetic and corticosteroid may be helpful. Severe cases that are refractory to conservative care may require arthroscopic or open surgical capsular release.

Shoulder Instability

Background

The shoulder is the most commonly dislocated joint in the body. Glenohumeral dislocation is described as no articular surface contact between the glenoid and humeral head. A small degree of glenohumeral dislocation is called *subluxation*. Dynamic (cuff, biceps, deltoid, and scapular musculature) and static (labrum and glenohumeral capsule) complexes act as barriers and create normal glenohumeral stability. There are many classifications of glenohumeral instability, such as mechanism, direction, and degree. Anterior dislocation is the most common, and multidirectional dislocation is the second most common form of instability. Matson made acronyms to easily remember the differences between anterior and multidirectional instabilities. The mnemonic TUBS—traumatic, unidirectional, Bankart lesion (a concomitant tear of the anterior glenoid labrum), often requiring surgery—indicates anterior instability and the mnemonic AMBRII—atraumatic-onset, multidirectional, bilateral shoulders, rehabilitation (usually treated by rehabilitation), inferior capsular shift, and interval lesion (when rehab fails, then surgery for inferior capsular shift and interval lesion)—indicates multidirectional instabilities. The Bankart lesion is the most commonly seen culprit in first traumatic anterior dislocations. In some severe anterior dislocations, Bankart lesions may have a bony fragment. A Hill-Sachs lesion is a defect in the posterohumeral head because of glenoid rim impaction that also occurs in traumatic anterior dislocation.

History

Patients with first anterior shoulder dislocation usually describe a severe trauma history, such as a fall or major collision. These patients complain of significant pain. Patients with multidirectional instability have indistinguishable symptoms and are mostly activity related.

Physical Examination

A physical exam usually establishes the diagnosis of anterior shoulder dislocation. On inspection, the patient with anterior dislocation holds the arm in abduction and external rotation, whereas the posterior dislocation patient keeps the arm in adduction and internal rotation. Loss of the deltoid rounded contour, even a defect (Sulcus sign), can be seen. Palpation, ROM, strength, and neurovascular (particularly axillary vessels and nerve) evaluation of the limb should be performed.

The anterior apprehension test may be used for anterior instability. In this test, the patient's arm is flexed to 90°, and the shoulder is passively put into 90° of abduction. Using the forearm as a fulcrum, the shoulder is then slowly put into external rotation. In a positive sign, the patient will appear apprehensive as the shoulder rotates anteriorly. Posterior pressure to the anterior shoulder applied by the examiner secures the joint, relocates the shoulder, and should alleviate the patient's apprehension. Supine stress testing can also be used to judge the degree and direction of laxity.

Imaging and Diagnostic Procedures

Minimum plain radiographs should include true AP and either an axillary-lateral or a trans-scapular lateral (Y-view) views. The West Point view is performed to see the bony Bankart lesion, and Stryker's notch view is used to check a Hill-Sachs defect.

Computed tomography (CT) and MRI can be obtained for evaluation of associated fracture, labral and rotator cuff injury, and chronic pathologies.

Treatment

Early reduction of acute anterior dislocation is recommended. There is no best medication protocol for sedation/relaxation. There are many reduction techniques for anterior dislocations. However, the key factor is relaxation and gentle traction with slight abduction and rotation of the humerus. Duration of immobilization and surgery after the first anterior dislocation remains controversial. Recurrence is correlated with the age of the patient. The highest recurrence rate is seen in patients who are younger than 20 years of age. Patients more than 40 years of age have the lowest recurrence rates. However, these patients are at higher risk for associated rotator cuff tears.

Lateral Epicondylitis

Background

Also termed "tennis elbow," the name of this disorder may be a misnomer. Recent studies reveal that inflammation may not be the primary causative factor in the disorder, but rather tendinosis (fibrosis) is implicated. The tendon of the extensor carpi radialis brevis is most commonly involved; however, the tendons of the extensor carpi radialis longus, extensor digitorum communis, and extensor carpi ulnaris may also be involved.

Overuse, poor mechanics (especially in racquet sports [inappropriate grip size and too-tight racquet string tension]), and insufficient muscle conditioning are the important contributing factors in causing lateral epicondylitis. The 40s and 50s are the common years for patients to develop lateral epicondylitis. Dominant arm involvement is most common.

History

Patients will typically complain of lateral elbow pain with activities, such as shaking hands, playing tennis, plumbing, or any activity that requires repetitive forearm pronation and supination. The pain may limit the patient's ability to grasp objects, and therefore, the patient may complain of "weakness."

Physical Examination

Tenderness to palpation is elicited over or just distal to the lateral epicondylitis. Resisted wrist and finger extension will typically provoke pain. Cozen's test is used to specifically evaluate for lateral epicondylitis. In this test, the patient makes a fist, with the forearm in pronation and wrist radially deviated. Stabilizing the elbow with one hand, the examiner resists the patient's radial deviation with the other hand. When this maneuver produces pain, lateral epicondylitis is implicated. It is important to check the patient's ROM because patients with osteochondritis dissecans may have a loss of extension.

Imaging and Diagnostic Procedures

None are routinely indicated because this is primarily a clinical diagnosis.

Treatment

Lateral epicondylitis may be treated with a variety of effective conservative measures, including counterforce bracing designed to redistribute the stress away from the lateral epicondyle, stretching and strengthening exercises that emphasize eccentric contractions, ultrasound, ice, and NSAIDs. An anesthetic and corticosteroid injection may be helpful. In less than 5% of patients, surgical treatment in the form of release of the extensor origin or open debridement may be necessary.

Cubital Tunnel Syndrome

Background

This syndrome describes entrapment of the ulnar nerve as it passes the elbow joint. Often, the nerve is entrapped between the two heads of the flexor carpi ulnaris; however, there are multiple sites of potential entrapment. Cubital tunnel syndrome is the second most common peripheral neuropathy, and the elbow is the most common ulnar nerve compression site.

History

Patients typically complain of aching in the medial elbow and numbness and tingling in the fourth and fifth digits. If symptoms have been present for a long time, patients may complain of hand weakness and loss of fine motor control in the fourth and fifth digits. Patients will report worsening symptoms with elbow flexion. Proximal to the wrist, the ulnar nerve gives off a sensory branch to the dorsum of the fourth and fifth digits. Therefore, if the patient does not complain of symptoms in the dorsum of the fourth and fifth digits, the patient may have ulnar nerve compression in the tunnel of Guyon at the wrist and not at the elbow.

Physical Examination

Intrinsic hand muscle atrophy may be noted in long-standing disease. Tinel's sign may be used to elicit symptoms in patients with suspected cubital tunnel syndrome. In this sign, the patient's ulnar nerve is repetitively tapped as it passes through the fibro-osseous canal in the elbow. However, this is a nonspecific test, and will be positive in 25% of patients without cubital tunnel syndrome. Patients should also be tested for sensation in the ulnar nerve distribution and finger abduction and adduction strength. Numbness and/or weakness indicate an ulnar neuropathy. The nerve should also be palpated with the elbow in flexion and extension to rule out a subluxation.

Imaging and Diagnostic Procedures

Electrodiagnostic studies are used to confirm the diagnosis and establish extent of injury. However, patients with a high clinical suspicion and a negative routine ulnar nerve conduction study may mandate a segmental ulnar nerve study, which has a higher sensitivity.

Treatment

Elbow splinting at 45° of flexion, padding of the nerve, activity modification, NSAIDs, and ice are common first-line treatments. If electromyography is performed and is positive, steroid injections may be indicated. Surgical decompression and transposition may be performed, but are reserved for symptoms refractory to more conservative measures.

Carpal Tunnel Syndrome

Background

This is the most common peripheral neuropathy. The carpal tunnel is a rigid structure through which nine flexor tendons and the median nerves pass. Any increase in the pressure of the tunnel may compress the median nerve.

History

Patients usually report a hobby or job that involves repetitive wrist and finger flexion, including typing or knitting. Athletes who participate in grip-intensive activities, such as cycling, wheelchair sports, competitive racing, throwing sports, gymnastics, and lacrosse, are at high risk for developing carpal tunnel syndrome. Symptoms include tingling, burning, numbness, and/or pain in the first, second, third, and sometimes, medial half of the fourth digit. Nighttime symptoms that awaken the patient from sleep are classically associated with progression of the syndrome. Patients may describe nighttime pain with aggressive hand and wrist shaking to improve symptoms (Flick sign). Patients with longer standing carpal tunnel syndrome may also complain of hand weakness and/or "dropping things." Patients with a history of diabetes, hypothyroidism, or recent (or current) pregnancy have increased risk of developing carpal tunnel syndrome.

Physical Examination

Wasting of the thenar muscles is classic for advanced carpal tunnel syndrome. Sensation testing should be assessed. There are three clinical tests that are designed to evaluate for carpal tunnel syndrome. The compression test is the most sensitive test. In this test, the carpal tunnel is compressed by the examiner for 30 to 60 seconds. Tinel's sign is the most specific test. In this sign, the patient's median nerve is repetitively tapped as it passes through the carpal tunnel. In Phalen's test, the patient's wrists are flexed and held so that they appose one another. Any of these tests are positive if the maneuver elicits symptoms in the patient's median nerve distribution.

Imaging and Diagnostic Procedures

Carpal tunnel syndrome is often a clinical diagnosis. However, if the diagnosis is in doubt or surgery is being considered, electrodiagnostic studies may be performed. Electromyography can also be useful on co-existing or other pathologies (double-crush phenomenon). The primary damage to the nerve is a demyelinating lesion, but severe compression can cause axonal loss as well. A nerve conduction study may be helpful to check progression of the compression and to classify the degree of carpal tunnel syndrome.

Treatment

Splinting with the wrist in neutral position, ergonomic training, and activity modification is the cornerstone of conservative care. Splints may be worn at night and also during activities, such as typing (if typing or other exacerbating activities cannot be avoided). Splints may need to be worn 24 hours a day. Steroid and anesthetic injection may also be helpful. Surgical release of the carpal tunnel is reserved for severe symptoms unresponsive to more conservative treatment. Surgery may prevent further axonal loss.

De Quervain Tenosynovitis

Background

The dorsal aspect of the wrist contains six tunnels that transmit the tendons to the hand. In the first dorsal tunnel are the tendons of the abductor pollicus longus and extensor pollicis brevis muscles. Entrapment and inflammation of these tendons leads to de Quervain tenosynovitis. It is usually an overuse injury. Because of a required forceful grasp with excessive ulnar wrist deviation, it may occur in athletes who participate in fly-fishing, golf, and racquet sports.

History

Patients typically complain of radial wrist pain that is worsened by moving the wrist or thumb. Patients may also complain of radial wrist swelling.

Physical Examination

Finkelstein's test is used to evaluate for this disorder. In this test, the patient is instructed to form a fist around the thumb, and the patient's wrist is then put into ulnar deviation. This maneuver stretches the inflamed tendons. Pain with this maneuver indicates possible de Quervain tenosynovitis.

Imaging and Diagnostic Procedures

This is primarily a clinical diagnosis and no imaging studies are necessary. However, cases with a suspicion of carpometacarpal arthritis or history of trauma may require AP, lateral, or Robert's view X-ray studies.

Treatment

Activity modification may be sufficient for treatment. Thumb spica splinting and/or an anesthetic and corticosteroid injection may be useful. Surgical decompression is not generally necessary, but may be performed for severe, refractory symptoms.

Axial Low Back Pain

Background

Back pain is the most common musculoskeletal complaint, affecting as much as 80% of the population at some point in their lives. Few topics in musculoskeletal medicine have generated as much animated debate as the causes of low back pain. Part of this debate is owing to the fact that most cases of acute low back pain are believed to resolve spontaneously. In fact, the true picture of low back pain is more complicated. Many cases of low back pain may periodically remit and recur. Nevertheless, thanks in part to its reputation for spontaneous resolution, aggressive diagnosis of uncomplicated low back pain that lasts for less than 2 or 3 months is not often pursued. Potential causes of mechanical low back pain are numerous and include muscle spasm, muscle strain, discogenic pain, Z-joint pain, sacroiliac joint pain, and spondylolysis.

When low back pain lasts longer than 3 months, it is termed *chronic low back pain*. Chronic low back pain is much less likely to spontaneously resolve. Chronic low back pain has been more intensively investigated, and the common causes have been scientifically identified. The most common cause of chronic low back pain in middle-aged and older patients is discogenic pain, accounting for approximately 39% of cases. The second most common cause of chronic low back pain is Z-joint disease, accounting for approximately 15% of younger patients and as much as 40% of older patients with chronic low back pain. In younger patients (<30 years old), the posterior elements (spondylolysis, spondylolisthesis) are more common causes of low back pain.

History

Patients will typically complain of low back pain that is dull and aching. Some patients will report the onset of symptoms after lifting or bending, whereas other patients will not recall a history of trauma. Patients may also complain of buttock pain. Buttock pain is a common referral pain pattern for low back pain because both the buttock and lumbosacral spine are innervated by L4–S1. Referral pain patterns may also occur in the hip or leg. It is important to pay attention to the *quality* of pain because referral pain is deep, dull, and difficult to localize, whereas radicular pain is sharp, shooting, electric, lancinating, and band-like.

In any patient with low back pain it is always important to review for red-flag symptoms, which include any change in bowel or bladder habits, history of cancer, recent surgery, fever, chills, or night pain. Any of these red-flag symptoms should prompt a closer search for a more serious underlying pathology, such as cancer or infection. A younger male patient between the ages of 15 and 30 with prolonged morning low back pain and stiffness should be evaluated for ankylosing spondylitis.

Physical Examination

Inspection should note any asymmetry (e.g., kyphosis, scoliosis) or gait abnormalities. Palpation may reveal tender or trigger points. Percussion tenderness over bone suggests bone pain and warrants a closer evaluation for compression fracture, tumor, or infection. It is important to assess the patient's ROM in the lower extremities, in particular. Tight hamstrings, quadriceps, or tight iliotibial band may significantly contribute to a patient's low back pain. It is also important to check hip ROM to rule out the hip as the underlying cause of the patient's back pain.

Patients with pain with forward flexion may be more likely to have discogenic pain because forward flexion increases intradiscal pressure. Patients with pain with extension may be more likely to have Z-joint disease, stenosis, or spondylolysis because extension increases the pressure on the posterior elements. The Fabere or Patrick's test is used to evaluate for sacroiliac joint disease and hip pathology. In this test, the patient lies supine and the hip is flexed, abducted, and externally rotated as the examiner applies pressure onto the patient's bent knee and contralateral anterior superior iliac spine, forcing them into the examining table. When this maneuver elicits pain, the patient may have sacroiliac or hip joint pathology. Typically, patients with hip degenerative joint disease will have loss of flexion and internal rotation.

Imaging and Diagnostic Procedures

Standing AP and lateral X-rays may be obtained. If spondylolysis is suspected, an oblique X-ray may more easily demonstrate the abnormality. MRI may also be obtained to help rule out more serious pathologies. However, to precisely diagnose most cases of chronic low back pain, it may be necessary to perform a needle procedure.

To diagnose discogenic low back pain, a provocative discography with postdiscogram CT is performed (this test remains somewhat controversial).

This is a percutaneous procedure performed under fluoroscopic guidance in which dye is injected into the disc. When the patient's daily pain is provoked at one disc level but not at adjacent levels, the test is considered positive for discogenic pain. The test is presumed to work because in a diseased disc, the mechanical pressure and chemical irritation from the injectate of the already sensitized nerves in the annulus fibrosus of the disc results in pain. After the injection, the patient receives a CT scan to evaluate the extravasation, if any, of the dye. In a patient with discogenic pain, the pain originates from the nerve fibers that are located primarily in the outer one-third of the annulus fibrosus. Therefore, in patients with discogenic pain, the dye is often seen to extravasate from the nucleus pulposus to the outer third of the annulus fibrosus.

There are five grades of potential fissuring that may be seen on post-discography injection. Grade 0 is the absence of a fissure. Grade I is a fissure that penetrates to the inner third of the annlus. Grade II penetrates the middle third of the annulus. Grade III penetrates to the outer third of the annulus. Grade IV penetrates circumferentially around the rim of the annulus.

To diagnose sacroiliac joint disease, intra-articular blocks of the joint may be performed under fluoroscopic guidance. By temporarily blocking the nerve fiber transmission of pain from the joint, a patient with sacroiliac joint disease should experience pain relief following an intra-articular block.

Controlled blocks of the Z-joints may be performed for diagnosing Z-joint disease. It is important to perform controlled blocks of the joint(s) because single blocks have a high false-positive rate. Z-joints may be blocked with either an intra-articular injection or by blocking the medial branches of the dorsal rami that innervate the joint(s).

Treatment

Patients with straightforward, acute low back pain may be treated with rest, ice, and NSAIDs. Patients should also be enrolled in a physical therapy program that emphasizes lumbar stabilization and specifically targets tight or weak muscles with stretching and strengthening exercises. Ergonomic training and instructions on good back hygiene, including sleeping supine with a pillow underneath the knees, may be beneficial for patients. Patients with trigger points may gain some relief from a trigger point injection with anesthetic and/or steroid. Many physicians also offer patients epidural steroid injections or intra-articular Z-joint injections depending on the suspected site of pathology.

Patients with low back pain that is found to be discogenic may benefit from many of the aforementioned therapies. In addition, intradiscal electrothermal therapy (IDET) may improve symptoms. IDET is a minimally invasive procedure in which a catheter is introduced into the annulus of the disc under fluoroscopic guidance. The catheter is then heated, dennervating the nerves and denaturing the collagen. The rationale behind IDET is the thermal effect decreasing mechanical and chemical nociceptors and coagulation of intradiscal/posterior annular nociceptive pain fibers. Nucleoplasty (intradiscal decompression) is another minimally invasive percutaneous option to treat discogenic low back pain. For patients who fail to respond to these comprehensive conservative measures, artificial disc replacement or interbody fusion surgery may be necessary, although data regarding the efficacy of artificial disc replacement and fusion surgery remain somewhat controversial.

Patients with low back pain that is found to originate from Z-joint disease may be treated with radiofrequency neurotomy of the involved nerves. This is a percutaneous procedure performed under fluoroscopic guidance that essentially severs the nerves innervating the painful joint with radiofrequency energy. The nerves may regenerate, and the procedure may need to be repeated periodically if pain returns.

Patients with low back pain that is found to originate from the sacroiliac joint are more difficult to treat. Because the nerves supplying the sacroiliac joint are numerous and do not run in a predictable pattern, it is difficult to simply sever them. Intra-articular anesthetic and steroid injections may provide only temporary pain relief.

Lumbosacral Radiculopathy

Background

Lumbosacral radiculopathy is caused by compression or ischemia of a nerve root and results in a condition of loss. As in the cervical spine, because radicular pain often accompanies radiculopathy, the two conditions are described together in this section. The most common cause of lumbosacral radiculopathy is a disc bulge, protrusion, extrusion, or sequestration, accounting for as much as 98% of all cases. Other causes of lumbosacral radiculopathy include osteophytes, Z-joint hypertrophy, cyst, tumor, or other causes of foraminal stenosis.

History

Patients typically complain of numbness, tingling, burning, and/or electric, radiating pain shooting down the thigh and/or leg in a band-like manner. The distribution of symptoms depends on the level of nerve root involvement. In the lumbar spine, it is important to recall that the nerve exits *under* the vertebra of the same number. For example, the L4 nerve root exits between the L4 and L5 vertebrae. *See* Table 2 for a list of nerve root levels with associated sensory, motor, and reflex deficits. Patients with discs causing the symptoms may complain of exacerbation of symptoms with forward flexion (this position increases pressure on the disc). Patients with symptoms from posterior element (e.g., Z-joint) hypertrophy may have worsening symptoms with extension (this position increases pressure on the posterior elements).

Physical Examination

Gait evaluation may reveal a Trendelenberg gait in a patient with a L5 radiculopathy and resulting weakness in the gluteus medius. Sensory, muscle, and reflex testing should be performed and may reveal dysethesia, weakness, and/or diminished reflex in the involved segment(s) (*see* Table 2).

Dural tension signs should be evaluated in a patient with a suspected radiculopathy. These may be performed with the patient in the seated or supine position. In the sitting position, the patient leans forward and tucks the head to the chest as the examiner extends the patient's knee and dorsiflexes the patient's ankle. In the supine position, the examiner flexes the patient's hip with leg extended. In both maneuvers, the dural tension sign is positive if the patient experiences radicular symptoms in response to the maneuver. Tightness or stretching in the back of the thigh does *not* represent a positive sign. In the supine test, at 35 to 70° of hip flexion, the nerves become maximally stretched.

When the femoral nerve is implicated as being potentially involved, the patient may be placed in the prone position and the reverse straight-leg raise performed. In this test, the patient's hip is put into extension with the knee in flexion. If radicular symptoms are reproduced, the test is considered positive.

Imaging and Diagnostic Procedures

Standing AP and lateral X-rays may be obtained. MRI may also be obtained, and is optimal for evaluating the soft tissues that may be involved. It is important to remember that more than one-third of all asymptomatic people will have MRI findings of disc abnormalities. However, when the patient's symptoms, straight-leg raising test, and MRI findings are correlated, the specificity of the diagnosis of radiculopathy caused by the disc is increased dramatically. Therefore, it is important to treat the patient, not the MRI findings.

Table 2
Neurological Evaluation of the Lower Limb

Root	*T12–L3*	*L4*	*L5*	*S1*	*S2, S3, S4*
Function	• Hip flexion (T12–L3) • Hip adduction (L2–L4)	• Knee extension • Dorsiflexion	• Toe extension • Foot inversion • Hip abduction	• Foot eversion/ plantar flexion • Hip extension	• Toe clawing—no testing
Myotome	• Iliopsoas (T12–L3) • Adductor brevis, longus, and magnus (obturator n. L2–L4)	• Tibialis anterior • Quadriceps	• Extensor digitorum longus • Extensor hallucis longus • Gluteus medius	• Peroneus longus and brevis • Gastroc-soleus • Gluteus maximus • Posterior tibialis	• Intrinsic foot muscle—no testing
Dermatome	• L1-inguinal ligament • L2-Mid-thigh • L3-Medial side of knee	• Medial leg and medial site of foot (Saphenous n. and superficial peroneal n.)	• Lateral leg and dorsum of foot (lateral sural cutaneous n. and superficial peroneal n.)	• Lateral side of foot (Sural n.)	• S2—posterior thigh • S3, S4—anal area
Reflex	• None	• Patellar	• Tibialis posterior	• Achilles	• Superficial anal reflex

Treatment

Conservative treatment is often successful and includes rest, NSAIDs, heat, and physical therapy that targets the involved muscles and emphasizes stretching and strengthening. Ergonomic training is also helpful. In addition, fluoroscopically guided epidural steroid and anesthetic injections are a very effective, adjunctive, minimally invasive treatment. The injectate may be delivered via either a caudal, interlaminar, or transforaminal approach. Failure to use fluoroscopic guidance may result in a relatively high rate of needle misplacement. Percutaneous nucleoplasty using fluoroscopic guidance is another minimally invasive option for patients with radicular symptoms.

When patients fail to respond to aggressive nonoperative treatment and there is a surgically definable lesion, surgery should be considered. Progressive neurological symptoms are another indication for surgery.

Hip OA

Background

OA is the most common form of joint disease. It is a primarily degenerative disorder that probably has an inflammatory component. Changing biomechanical forces, preexisting congenital, and/or developmental hip disease play an important role in its pathogenesis. The result of OA is the breakdown of synovium, articular cartilage, and subchondral bone of joints.

History

Patients are typically older and present with pain localized to the groin and anterior or lateral thigh. The pain may or may not refer to other areas, such as the low back or knee. Patients typically report that the pain is worse after prolonged activity. Pain may also be worse when the patient goes to lie down at night. As the disease process progresses, patients note increasing pain and stiffness. Patients may also complain of a limp resulting from pain. Uncomfortable prolonged sitting, having additional pain when patients rise from a seated position, and difficulty walking on inclines are some of the characteristic features of hip joint pathology. It is important to exclude the other periarticular disorders, such as trochanteric bursitis, piriformis syndrome, and even low back pain, before attributing the pain to hip OA. The American College of Rheumatology classification criteria for the hip OA is hip pain and at least two of the following three items:

1. Erythrocyte sedimentation rate (ESR) less than 20 mm per hour.
2. Radiographic femoral or acetabular osteophytes.
3. Radiographic joint-space narrowing.

Physical Examination

Evaluation of the patient's gait may reveal an antalgic gait. ROM, particularly flexion and internal rotation, may be limited by pain. Often, the patient may keep the affected leg in external rotation and adduction. The Fabere or Patrick's test (described in the Section entitled, "Axial Low Back Pain") may be positive.

Imaging and Diagnostic Procedures

AP and lateral views of the pelvis are typically obtained. Typical findings of OA on radiographs include decreased joint space, subarticular sclerosis, cyst formation, and ostophytes. However, the severity of symptoms *does not* necessarily correlate with radiological findings. Patients should be treated according to symptoms and not radiographic findings of degeneration.

Treatment

Most patients are treated initially with conservative care. The cornerstone of the conservative treatment is controlling pain and educating patients. Conservative management of OA includes patient education and weight loss (if overweight), activity modification with joint protection and energy conservation, rest, gait aides (e.g., cane in the hand contralateral to the affected hip), heat (especially useful just before exercise), nonimpact exercises (e.g., swimming), and ROM and strengthening exercises. Daily oral glucosamine sulfate and chondroitin sulfate has also been found to decrease symptoms and may slow the progression of OA. An intra-articular injection of anesthetic and steroid may also be helpful. Intra-articular injection(s) of hyaluronic acid may be beneficial to temporarily relieve symptoms. Patients may need assistive devices, such as dressing sticks, raised toilet seats, and bathtub wall bars.

When conservative care is insufficient to control symptoms, surgery may be considered. The decision to treat a patient surgically with a total hip replacement is made on a patient-by-patient basis, and must include consideration of the patient's symptoms, ability to function on daily basis, expectations, and comorbidities. In general, total hip replacement is a very successful procedure in the right patient population, and can considerably improve a patient's quality of life when more conservative measures have failed.

Hamstring Strains

Background

The hamstring muscles are double-joint muscles that extend the hip and knee and are formed by the biceps femoris, semimembranosus, and semitendinosus muscles. These muscles share the same origin at the ischial tuberosity. Injury to the hamstrings occurs when one of these muscles is maximally stretched during an active contraction, especially fast acceleration/deceleration activity related to sports, such as running, water skiing, soccer, football, or sprinting. A strain or tear of the muscle usually occurs during early stance or the last half of the swing phase of the gait.

History

Patients typically report a sudden posterior thigh pain or tightness during muscle loading. Patients may report that they "felt a pull" or "heard a pop" followed by immediate pain and loss of function. Pain may increase with straight-leg raising. Hearing an audible "pop" is associated with a higher-grade injury. Associated risk factors include preexisting poor flexibility, insufficient warm-up, quadricep/hamstring strength imbalance, and, most importantly, previous hamstring injury.

Physical Examination

Patients may have edema and ecchymosis. The hamstring muscles should be palpated from their shared origin at the ischial tuberosity inferiorly to the maximal tender area. Localized ischial tuberosity tenderness is significant for a potential avulsion fracture. Patients with significant swelling, ecchymosis, and knee flexion weakness may show complete rupture at the hamstring origin. Assessing bilateral ROM and strength will provide the examiner information regarding flexibility deficit and severity of injury. Neurovascular testing of the limb is important to rule out acute posterior thigh compartment syndrome.

Imaging and Diagnostic Procedures

This is usually a clinical diagnosis. Plain pelvis radiograph confirms the diagnosis of avulsion fracture when there is a suspicion. In recalcitrant cases and/or for prognostication, MRI or CT may be utilized.

Treatment

Because of the recurrence and career-ending possibility for an elite athlete, recognition, prevention, and treatment of this injury is essential. Most hamstring tears may be treated conservatively. Initially, rest, ice, compression wraps, and elevation help prevent further edema and hemorrhage. Pain control is also important. Usually, after the first 3 to 7 days, rehabilitation should focus on gentle stretching and progressive strengthening exercises with adjunctive aquatic therapy and exercise on the stationary bike. The duration of rehabilitation depends on the patient's previous activity level and degree of injury. Elite athletes usually require a more aggressive rehabilitation program. Surgery may be attempted in cases of complete hamstring rupture or bony avulsion with a 2-cm displacement. Patients can return to their previous level of activities when they regain their normal flexibility, endurance, and coordination.

Osgood-Schlatter Disease

Background

This disorder is usually seen in preadolescent athletes who participate in activities such as jumping or running. The disorder is a result of recurring microtrauma from the quadriceps contracting and, via the patellar tendon, repetitively pulling on the skeletally immature cartilage of the tibial tubercle. Because of the secondary muscular tightness, fast growth may worsen the symptoms. Other potential injuries to consider in the differential diagnosis include pes anserinus bursitis, patellar tendonitis, quadriceps tendon avulsion, patellafemoral disorder, and tibial plateau fracture.

History

Patients typically complain of pain and sometimes swelling over the tibial tubercle. The patients typically report worsening of symptoms during participation in sports. Pain may be unilateral or bilateral

Physical Examination

There may be tenderness and/or swelling over the tibial tubercle. Resisted knee extension may result in pain.

Imaging and Diagnostic Procedures

AP, lateral, and sunrise X-rays may be obtained to rule out a more serious underlying pathology. However, the diagnosis is generally based on clinical findings.

Treatment

Treatment is conservative and includes ice, rest, and infrapatellar strap during exacerbating activities, and physical therapy that emphasizes stretching and strengthening the quadriceps and hamstring muscles.

Knee Ligament and Meniscus Injury

Background

The knee joint is supported by its surrounding capsule, ligaments, and menisci. The menisci serve as a shock absorber for the knee, redistributing the weight of the body. The constant twisting, cutting, turning, and colliding make the knee a common source of injury in athletes.

History

Patients with a ligament injury will typically report a deceleration injury that led to immediate pain and swelling. Up to half of all patients with a ligament injury will recall having heard or felt a "pop" at the time of injury.

Patients with a meniscus injury will usually recall a history of trauma, but symptoms will not begin until minutes to hours after the injury. Older patients with a meniscus injury may report a more gradual onset of symptoms.

The precise mechanism of injury will offer further information about the probable injury. For example, a patient who was tackled from the side and suffered a valgus stress is likely to have a medial collateral ligament injury.

Patients with meniscus or ligament injuries may report "giving way" of the knee. Patients with meniscus injury may report catching or locking of the knee. Because the medial meniscus is responsible for approximately 90% of the load-bearing of the knee, and because it is attached to the joint capsule (making it less mobile), the medial meniscus is injured more often than the lateral meniscus.

Physical Examination

Inspection of the knee may reveal an effusion. The joint line will be tender over the portion of the knee that is injured. In a meniscus injury, knee flexion and extension may result in a palpable or audible clicking. In anterior cruciate ligament (ACL) injury, the patient will likely have a negative pivot shift, positive anterior drawer sign, and Lachman's test. Lachman's test is the most sensitive test for an ACL tear. To perform this test, the examiner flexes the patient's knee to 30° and evaluates the AP glide of the tibia. A loose end point suggests an ACL tear. To perform the anterior drawer test, the examiner flexes the patient's knee to 90° and stabilizes the patient's lower extremity by sitting on the patient's foot. The AP glide is then evaluated and compared with the opposite side. The other ligaments—the medial collateral ligament (MCL), lateral collateral ligament, and posterior cruciate ligament—are all evaluated in a similar way: assessing for a loose end point when the ligament is stressed. For example, to evaluate for a MCL tear, the examiner applies a valgus stress on the knee while palpating the medial joint line. Excessive gapping suggests an MCL injury.

The Apley compression and distraction test is a good additional examination tool to evaluate for meniscus and ligamentous injury. In this test, the

patient lies in the prone position and the examiner flexes the patient's knee to 90°. The examiner then compresses the patient's leg while simultaneously turning it into external and internal rotation. Pain produced on the medial side may be a medial meniscus injury, MCL injury, or both. Likewise, pain at the lateral side may be a lateral meniscus injury, lateral collateral ligament injury, or both. The examiner then applies traction to the leg while simultaneously putting the leg into internal and external rotation. By putting the leg into traction, pressure is taken *off* the menisci. If pain disappears in traction, the pain generator is more likely to be coming from the meniscus and not the ligament. However, if pain persists in both compression and distraction, the culprit is more likely the ligament.

Imaging and Diagnostic Procedures

AP, weight-bearing AP, lateral, and tunnel X-rays should be obtained for most cases. MRI should also be obtained, especially in suspected ligamentous or meniscus injuries.

Treatment

An ACL injury is treated with rest, ice, NSAIDs, physical therapy, and bracing. If an associated meniscus or ligament injury is present, surgery may be necessary. Surgical reconstruction may also be necessary for patients who wish to return to competitive sports.

MCL injury is treated with ice, rest, hinged knee brace, and physical therapy.

Small meniscus tears (<10 mm) and partial-thickness tears with no other pathological conditions are treated with ice, rest, NSAIDs, and physical therapy. Larger tears that fail conservative treatment and any acutely locked knee may require surgery. In addition, tears in the avascular portion of the meniscus typically require partial meniscectomy. Arthroscopic meniscus repair may be performed for tears in the vascular portion.

Knee OA

Background

Knee OA increases in prevalence and severity with increasing age. For a further discussion on osteoarthritis, *see* the Background subheading under the Hip OA heading.

History

Patients usually complain of progressive knee pain that is worse after prolonged, weight-bearing activity. As the disease progresses, patients complain of morning stiffness and increasing pain. Nighttime pain may increase, and this is a sign of significant disease progression. Rest typically helps ease symptoms. The American College of Rheumatology criteria for diagnosis of knee OA requires the presence of knee pain *and* osteophytes plus at least one of the following:

1. Age over 50 years.
2. Crepitus.
3. Morning stiffness for less than 30 minutes.

Physical Examination

Patients may have an anatalgic gait. Crepitus is a common but nonspecific finding in the knee.

Imaging and Diagnostic Procedures

AP, lateral, and skyline patella X-rays should be obtained. It is important to remember that osteoarthritic radiographic findings are nonspecific and *do not* necessarily correlate with severity of disease. Therefore, it is important to treat the patient and not the radiograph.

Treatment

Conservative care of knee OA is similar to that of hip OA, and includes activity modification, ambulatory aides (e.g., cane), weight reduction (this is more important than in hip OA in overweight patients), nonimpact exercises, NSAIDs, heat modalities, and rest. Daily glucosamine sulfate and chodrointin sulfate may also be helpful. Intra-articular injections of hyaluronic acid may be used to temporarily improve symptoms. These injections must be repeated periodically (approximately every 6 months). Intra-articular injections of corticosteroid and anesthetic may also be helpful. An unloading brace may be necessary for varus or valgus deformity.

In patients with severe symptoms refractory to further conservative care, surgery should be considered. Total knee replacement may significantly improve patients' quality of life when performed for the right patient population.

Patellofemoral Disorder

Background

Patellofemoral pain may affect as many as one-fourth of all athletes, making it a common source of morbidity. There are many potential causes of patellofemoral disorder. Often, the patella tracks laterally and may be owing to a weak vastus medialis oblique (VMO)

History

Patients typically complain of dull, aching pain in the anterior knee. Patients usually report worsening symptoms with descending stairs and squatting. The movie theater sign is classic for patellofemoral disorder, and occurs when the patient reports needing to extend the leg into the movie aisle because the knee hurts with prolonged sitting with the knee in flexion.

Physical Examination

Patients should be examined in multiple positions, including walking. Observation of the alignment can be checked when the patient is in standing position. VMO evaluation is better when the patient is sitting with the knee bent to 90°. Moving from knee flexion to extension could produce crepitus and the "J shift sign." This sign shows lateral shifting and can be seen in patellar subluxation. Tenderness is often elicited in the patella and retropatellar region. The quadricep angle is often increased. The quadriceps angle is formed by the intersection of a line drawn from the anterior superior iliac spine to the mid-patella, with a line from the tibial tubercle to the mid-patella. Typical angles are up to 14° for males and 17° for females. An increased angle indicates lateral tracking.

Imaging and Diagnostic Procedures

AP, lateral, and sunrise X-rays should be obtained. If the patient is an adolescent, and slipped capital femoral epiphysis or Legg-Calve-Perthes disease needs to be ruled out, X-rays of the hip should also be obtained. CT scan could be a useful tool for femur and tibia rotational misalignment evaluation. MRI may provide additional information on the patellofemoral joint and its surrounding structures.

Treatment

Conservative care is usually successful in treating patellofemoral disorder. Conservative care includes patella bracing, NSAIDs, ice, and physical therapy that emphasizes ROM exercises, proprioceptive exercises, and strengthening (particularly the VMO). Intra-articular injections of corticosteroid and anesthetic may be considered for patients not responding to treatment. Surgery is reserved for patients with an identifiable lesion, such as acute patella dislocation, or occasionally in patients with a chronic patella-tracking disorder that has been resistant to prolonged conservative treatment. In these patients, a tibial tubercle osteotomy may be performed.

Ankle Sprain

Background

Ankle sprains are ubiquitous in sports, and are the most common athletic injury. Ankle sprains almost always occur on the lateral side. The anterior talofibular ligament is the most vulnerable ligament, and is the most commonly injured. The calcaneofibular is the second most commonly sprained. The posterior talofibular ligament is only sprained in severe injuries. The strong medial deltoid ligament is rarely injured. Ankle sprains are categorized as grade I, which is an intact but stretched ligament; grade II, which is a partial ligament tear; or grade III, which is a complete ligament tear.

History

Patients typically report a history of falling over the ankle; for example, stumbling over an already inverted foot. Subsequent to the injury, the patient reports pain and swelling. At the time of injury, patients may hear a "pop." In a grade-I injury, the patient will be able to bear weight with mild pain. In a grade-II injury, the patient will report difficulty with weight-bearing; and in a grade-III injury the patient will be unable to bear weight on the affected side. Previous lateral ankle sprains and natural hypermobility contribute to ankle laxity and are important risk factors for ankle sprain. The most common cause of chronic pain after an ankle sprain is a missed associated injury.

Physical Examination

Tenderness and swelling over the involved ligament(s) should be noted on physical exam. The anterior drawer test should be performed. In this test, with the ankle in 20° of plantarflexion, the examiner stabilizes the ankle and brings the calcaneus anteriorly. Excessive AP glide reveals a positive anterior drawer test, and suggests an ankle sprain. The talar tilt test may also be performed. In this test, the examiner inverts the ankle and compares the laxity with the unaffected ankle. This maneuver tests both the anterior talofibular ligament and calcaneofibular. Bilateral comparison is important.

Bony tenderness should also be assessed. Bony tenderness, particularly of the medial malleolus, is an indicator of a possible underlying fracture and requires further evaluation with radiographs. External rotation stress test should be performed to rule out syndesmosis injury.

Imaging and Diagnostic Procedures

The Ottawa ankle rules were developed as a guide for deciding which patients with a suspected ankle sprain require radiographs and which patients do not. Using these rules as a guide, patients *without* bony tenderness who can also bear weight for four consecutive steps do *not* require radiographs. If the history or physical examination is suspicious for an injury other than a sprain, or if the patient is not responding to proper conservative management, X-rays should be obtained. Because of the variability, stress radiographs are not suggested. MRI is helpful for ruling out other etiologies and for best evaluating subtalar joint ligamentous injury.

Treatment

Ankle sprains are generally managed with rest, ice, compression, and elevation. A protective device, such as an air cast, high-top sneakers, and/or ankle taping, may also be helpful. Physical therapy should emphasize aggressive ROM and proprioceptive exercises (e.g., balance board). A good, simple exercise is to have the patient repetitively spell his or her name with the foot. Standing on the injured foot in the neutral position and using a wall for support is another good proprioceptive exercise. The patient slowly looks away from the foot, gradually closes the eyes, and relies on proprioception for balance. Strengthening exercises should also be performed.

Grade III ankle sprains in competitive athletes, and patients with chronic ankle instability, may require surgery. A general rule of thumb is that patients may return to sport when they can run, jump 10 times on the injured foot, stand on the injured foot for 1 minute with eyes closed, and pivot on the injured foot without significant pain.

Achilles Tendon Injury

Background

The Achilles tendon is the largest and strongest tendon in the body. The tendon may become inflamed, fibrotic, and eventually rupture. Repetitive stress on the tendon from running and jumping, particularly in athletes who suddenly begin to exercise after prolonged periods of inactivity, may lead to Achilles tendonitis. Achilles tendon rupture may also result from a sudden stress on the Achilles.

History

Patients typically report gradually increasing pain in the Achilles tendon that is brought on by activities such as running. The pain may be described as having a burning quality. If a patient complains of a sudden audible "popping" in the Achilles followed by pain and plantarflexion weakness, the patient may have a ruptured Achilles tendon.

Physical Examination

The Achilles tendon is typically tender. Plantarflexion and dorsiflexion may be painful. Calcaneal tenderness and, classically 2 to 6 cm from the tendon insertion site, palpable tender defect ("Hatchet strike" defect) may also be present. If a rupture is suspected, the Thompson test is performed. In this test, the patient lies in the prone position and the examiner squeezes the patient's Achilles tendon. Failure of the ankle to plantarflex is a positive Thompson's test and a diagnosis of Achilles tendon rupture.

Imaging and Diagnostic Procedures

Not generally necessary in uncomplicated tendonitis. If surgery is being contemplated, MRI should be obtained. In patients with a suspected Achilles rupture, lateral radiographs should be obtained to rule out a calcaneal avulsion fracture. Although ultrasound is valuable for identifying soft-tissue inflammation, tendinosis, or rupture, MRI is the best diagnostic test in chronic degenerative changes and incomplete tendon tear.

Treatment

Patients with Achilles tendonitis may be treated with rest, ice, compression, and elevation. Physical therapy should focus on stretching and strengthening exercises. Orthotics should be used, including heel cups and/or arch supports. NSAIDs are helpful in reducing inflammation. Patients who do not respond to conservative care may require debridement of the tendon. Patients with Achilles tendinosis are generally not treated with surgery.

Patients with Achilles tendon rupture may be treated with surgery or bracing. Surgical results tend to be better when an open procedure is used.

Plantar Fasciitis

Background

The plantar fascia is a band of fibrous tissue on the plantar surface of the foot. This fascia may become inflamed from repetitive trauma (such as from walking on a hard surface) or increased load-bearing (e.g., during pregnancy).

History

Patients typically complain of insidious medial plantar heel pain that is worst when taking the first step of the day in the morning. The pain may improve during the course of the day, but then worsen toward the evening.

Physical Examination

Passive dorsiflexion will provoke pain. Location of tenderness provides valuable information on the differentials. Tenderness will usually be present over the medial part of the heel, at the insertion of the fascia, and along the course of the fascia. However, lateral heel tenderness can be seen in a calcaneal stress fracture. When tenderness is present in the midportion of the abductor hallucis, then medial plantar nerve compression (Jogger's foot) should be suspected.

Imaging and Diagnostic Procedures

None necessary. This is a clinical diagnosis. However, if there is a clinical suspicion of calcaneal stress fracture, then a lateral weight-bearing X-ray is indicated.

Treatment

Activity modification, stretching the fascia, orthotics, and NSAIDs are the cornerstones of therapy. If these measures fail to alleviate the symptoms, a corticosteroid and anesthetic injection may be performed. However, care must be taken when injecting corticosteroids into this region because plantar fat pad atrophy and plantar fascia rupture have been reported. Rarely, cast immobilization or surgical intervention may be necessary.

Interdigital Neuroma (Morton Neuroma)

Background

Shoes with narrow toe boxes have the potential for causing multiple foot problems. One of these potential problems is an interdigital neuroma in which the interdigital nerve is compressed beneath the intermetatarsal ligament.

History

Patients typically complain of burning pain, numbness, and/or tingling between in their second or third web spaces.

Physical Examination

Tenderness is found in the involved web space.

Imaging and Diagnostic Procedures

Imaging is not generally necessary. X-rays may be used to rule out a stress fracture. An anesthetic injection aids in the diagnosis.

Treatment

Changing shoes to a wider toe box if the patient has a narrow toe box, using a metatarsal pad, and rest are common conservative treatments. An interdigital corticosteroid and anesthetic injection is often useful. Patients with symptoms that do not respond to these conservative measures may require surgical excision of the neuroma. However, as many as 20% of neuromas may recur after excision.

Key References and Suggested Additional Reading

Bogduk N. Clinical Anatomy of the Lumbar Spine and Sacrum, 4th ed. New York: Churchill Livingstone, 2005.

Braddom RL. Physical Medine and Rehabilitation, 2nd ed. Philadelphia: Saunders, 2000.

Fardon DF, Gaffin SR. Orthopedic Knowledge Update Spine, 2nd ed. American Academy of Orthopedic Surgeons. Illinois. 2002.

Greene WB. Essentials of Musculoskeletal Care, 2nd ed. Rosemont, IL: American Academy of Orthopedic Surgeons, 2001.

Lillegard WA, Butcher JD, Rucker KS. Handbook of Sports Medicine: A Symptom-Oriented Approach, 2nd ed. Boston: Butterworth-Heinemann, 1999.

Mellion MB, Putukian M, Madden CC. Sport Medicine Secrets, 3rd ed. Philadelphia: Hanley & Belfus, 2003.

12 Electrodiagnostic Medicine

Joseph Feinberg, Jennifer Solomon,
Christian M. Custodio, and Michael D. Stubblefield

Introduction

Electrodiagnostic medicine is an extension of the patient history and physical examination. Electrodiagnostic studies (EDX) consist of two entities: (1) nerve conduction studies (NCS) and (2) needle electromyography (EMG). These studies measure the electrical properties of neuromuscular function and can be helpful in (1) confirming a suspected diagnosis, (2) excluding other possible diagnoses, (3) identifying subclinical disease processes, (4) localizing abnormalities, (5) defining disease severity, (6) defining pathophysiology, and (7) defining disease evolution and guiding prognosis and treatment options. Whereas imaging studies define *anatomy*, NCS and EMG define the *physiology* and *function* of the peripheral nervous system (PNS). This chapter is intended to provide a basic overview of electrodiagnosis, including a review of the PNS anatomy and physiology, an analysis of different wave form parameters, and a discussion of the common pathologies referred for EDX.

Basic Neuroanatomy/Neurophysiology

There are two main types of neurons: unipolar and multipolar. In the human nervous system, sensory nerves consist of unipolar neurons arising from a dorsal root ganglion (DRG) that forms the sensory spinal nerves. The motor nerves are comprised of multipolar neurons that travel through the anterior horn.

From: *Essential Physical Medicine and Rehabilitation*
Edited by: G. Cooper © Humana Press Inc., Totowa, NJ

There are several different types of nerve fibers based on size and function (*see* Table 1). Electrodiagnostics only evaluate Ia fibers. The motor unit is the basic functional element of the neuromuscular system. Each motor unit has several components. The α motor neuron, a Ia fiber, is located in the anterior horn region of the spinal cord, and supervises the output of the entire motor unit. The cell body or soma is the metabolic center of the α motor neuron. The axon (spinal nerve) is the neural branch of the cell body. The cytoskeleton resides in the axon and consists of microtubules, neurofilaments, and microfilaments. Its function is twofold: to propagate current flow and axonal transport of metabolic material (glycoproteins, neurotransmitters, toxins, viruses) to and from the cell body to the nerve terminals. The speed of conduction is dependent on the diameter of the axon and degree of myelination. The larger the diameter, the lower the internal resistance of the axon; the less the internal resistance, the more rapidly current spreads down the axon, and the more quickly the membrane potential at a distant site is brought to threshold. The transport system consists of slow anterograde (1–3 mm/day) cytoskeletal elements along microtubules and faster retrograde (150–200 mm/day) large vesicles derived from endocytosis at nerve terminals.

Axons can be unmyelinated or myelinated. Myelin is formed by a Schwann cell in the PNS. Glial cells are in the central nervous system (CNS). Myelin functions as an axon insulator, which reduces membrane resistance and capacitance, allowing for faster conduction of action potential. Nodes of Ranvier are located every 1 to 2 mm along the axon and house an increased concentration of voltage gated sodium channels. At each node, the action potential is capable of regenerating via depolarization, and conduction occurs in a saltatory fashion. In unmyelinated nerves, the conduction velocity (CV) varies in proportion to the square root of the fiber diameter. Therefore, large-diameter myelinated fibers are capable of faster conduction compared with unmyelinated fibers. When nerve conduction velocities are performed, they are assessing primarily the function of large-diameter myelinated fibers.

Living cells have a transmembrane potential across their cell membranes. Resting membrane potential is the difference in electrical potential between the inside and outside of the cell, resulting from the balance between intracellular anions and extracellular cations. In nerve and muscle, the resting membrane potential is usually around –70 mV. Na^+–K^+ ATP-dependent pumps assist in maintaining a negative potential inside the cell by actively exporting three ions of Na^+ and importing two ions of K^+ through a semipermeable membrane. If these sodium channels were not

Table 1
Neuron Anatomy/Fiber Classification

Lyod and Hunt (sensory)	*Erlanger and Gasser (sensory and motor)*	*Diameter (mm)*	*Velocity (m/s)*	*Function*
Ia fibers	A-α fibers	10–20	50–120	Motor: α motor neurons largest, fastest; sensory: muscle spindle
Ib fibers	A-α fibers	10–20	50–120	Sensory: golgi-tendon organ, touch, pressure
2 fibers	A-β fibers	4–12	25–70	Motor: intrafusal and extrafusal muscle fibers; Sensory: muscle spindle, touch, pressure
3 fibers	A-γ fibers	2–8	10–50	Motor: γ motor neurons, muscle spindle
	A-δ fibers	1–5	3–30	Sensory: touch, pain, temperature
4 fibers	B-fibers	1–3	3–15	Motor: preganglionic autonomic fibers
	C-fibers	<1	<2	Motor: postganglionic autonomic fibers; Sensory: pain, temperature

present, a negative resting potential could not be maintained. This system keeps each ion against a concentration gradient with a deficit of positive ions inside the cell.

Axon depolarization can be artificially generated when an outside current is applied to a nerve by a stimulator consisting of a negative pole (cathode) and a positive pole (anode). The membrane potential is then lowered owing to the attraction of the positive charges on the axon to the negative charges of the cathode. The membrane becomes increasingly permeable to Na^+, which rushes into the cell through the opened voltage-gated channels toward an equilibrium. This process of sodium conductance is the most important initiating event in generating an action potential, which is one of the primary functions of neurons. The task of the neuron is to transmit signals over long distances rapidly and with preservation of the characteristics of the signal. The threshold is the membrane potential at which the all-or-none action potential is generated. Once this occurs, the electric impulse propagates along an axon or muscle membrane. The all-or-none response travels in both directions along the axon. Once reached, the action potential generated remains at a constant size and configuration. If it is below this threshold, no potential will occur. A stimulus intensity that is greater than the threshold will not generate a larger potential.

After the action potential is generated, there is a period in which an action potential cannot be formed, no matter how strong the stimulus. This period is called the absolute refractory period, and pertains to the time of inactivation of the ion channels. Shortly thereafter, there is a period that requires a more intense stimulus to produce an action potential, referred to as the relative refractory period.

A number of physiological factors—temperature, sex, age, height, and circulation—have direct effects on action potential propagation. Only temperature can be modified. As temperature of the nerve is lowered, the amount of current required to generate an action potential increases. A decrease in temperature affects the protein components and causes a delay in opening and closing of the gates. In turn, this leads to an increase in the action potential's amplitude, latency, and CV. The surface temperature of the arm or leg can be recorded using a surface temperature-recording electrode. In general, surface temperature in the arms should be more than 32°C and more than 30°C in the legs. If the limbs are too cold, they should be warmed using a heating lamp or hot compress.

The neuromuscular junction (NMJ) is the location where a "synapse" occurs. This is the site at which the neuron transmits information or exerts influence on the activity of another cell (muscle). The cell sending the information is presynaptic, and the cell receiving the information is postsynaptic. The distal portion of the motor axon (presynaptic) has small projections that innervate individual muscle fibers (postsynaptic). The axon terminal contains various neural structures, including mitochondria and synaptic vesicles with acetylcholine (ACh). This portion of the nerve and single muscle fiber forms the motor endplate. They are separated by a synaptic cleft. If the communication is between a motor neuron and a muscle cell, the cleft is called the NMJ. In response to an action potential, chemical neurotransmitters are released from the presynaptic cell, diffuse across the synaptic cleft, and bind to receptors on the postsynaptic cell.

A "motor unit" begins as an anterior horn cell in the spinal cord and exists as a continuum through the nerve root, to the plexus, then peripheral nerve, and then the NMJ and individual muscles fibers the nerve terminals innervate. The muscle fibers of one motor unit fire in near synchrony in response to the CNS activation of the anterior horn cell. The action potential is propagated through the axon and its nerve terminals to the muscle fibers. When the fibers fire synchronously, the resulting motor unit action potential (MUAP) will be a large, triphasic action potential.

Equipment

Electrodes are used to stimulate nerves and record from the skin, directly over the nerve, or from the muscle. The two sites from which the electrode is used to record are the active and reference sites. The active site used when performing motor nerve studies is over the region called the *motor point*. This roughly corresponds to the motor endplate region of the muscle. The reference site is usually over an electrically inactive location, such as a tendon, or can be several centimeters distal to the recording electrode over the muscle itself. The recorded response from the muscle is called the compound muscle action potential (CMAP). When sensory nerves are studied, the active electrode is placed directly over a sensory nerve or over the skin surface it supplies. The reference is 3.5- to 4-cm distal along the course of the nerve. This recorded response is called a sensory nerve action potential (SNAP). Mixed nerve studies include both motor and sensory nerves. They are also recorded directly over a nerve and are called mixed nerve action potentials. A third electrode, the ground electrode, is usually placed between the stimulus and recording electrodes, and drains off electric noise (artifact) from the recording electrodes. To obtain a proper reading, the impedance (resistance) between electrode and skin must be kept low by removing skin lotions, oils, gels, etc.

Electrical stimulation of the nerve provides a clearly defined, reproducible response for NCSs. A potential is generated by a superficial cutaneous stimulation, but this can also be performed subcutaneously when indicated. A stimulator is used to excite the axons and consists of a cathode that is negatively charged and an anode that is positively charged. Stimulation depolarizes the nerve under the cathode and hyperpolarizes it under the anode. Larger myelinated axons are more easily stimulated than smaller unmyelinated axons. As the intensity of stimulation increases, more axons are stimulated until a point where all of the motor or sensory axons being studied are excited. A stronger stimulus will not increase the recorded response, and the stimulus is termed supramaximal. This is an electrical stimulus at 20% above the maximal stimulus and is typically used for NCSs. Threshold stimulus is an electrical stimulus occurring at an intensity level just sufficient enough to produce a detectable evoked potential from the nerve. An electrical stimulus at an intensity below the maximal level but above the threshold level is labeled as a submaximal stimulus. This can lead to a falsely lower recorded amplitude and prolonged latency reading because all the axons of the nerve are not being discharged. The duration of the stimulus should be 0.1 to 0.3 ms. If it is higher, it can falsely prolong the distal latency. When performing sensory nerve studies, averaging is often used.

This process extracts the desired neurophysiological signal from larger noise and interference signals. These unwanted signals can occur from biological or environmental sources, such as EMG audio feedback, needle artifact, 60-Hz cycles, preamplifier proximity to the machine, fluorescent lights, or the patient. Averaging improves the signal-to-noise ratio by a factor that is the square root of the number of averages performed. The number of averages must be increased by a factor of four to double the signal-to-noise ratio.

A differential amplifier is a device that responds to alternating currents of electricity. It cancels waveforms recorded at both the active and reference pick-ups and amplifies the remaining potentials. Filters help to remove electrical noise from the environment with as little effect on the electrophysiological signals as possible. Filters are designed to reduce the frequencies above (high-frequency or low-pass filters) and below (low-frequency or high-pass) the frequency of the electrophysiological signals we wish to record. Elevation of the low-frequency filter typically decreases peak latency and amplitude of SNAPs and CMAPs. Reduction of the high-frequency filter increases onset and peak latency and slightly decreases the amplitudes of SNAPs. However, reduction of the high-frequency filter may not affect the amplitude of CMAPs. Typical settings are as follows: sensory NCS, 20 Hz to 2 kHz; motor NCS, 2 Hz to 10 kHz; and EMG, 20 Hz to 10 kHz.

Once a signal has been recorded, amplified, and filtered it is digitally converted and displayed on a cathode ray tube. A grid is projected on the monitor with divisions consisting of a horizontal axis (*x*-axis), allocated as sweep speed, and a vertical axis (*y*-axis), allocated as sensitivity. Both of these parameters can be adjusted to manipulate the recorded waveform for an accurate measurement. The sweep speed pertains to the time allocated for each *x*-axis division, and is measured in milliseconds. Sensitivity pertains to the height allocated for each *y*-axis division, and is measured in millivolts or microvolts. The term *gain* is sometimes used interchangeably with sensitivity. The gain is actually a ratio measurement of output to input and does not have a unit value, such as millivolts or microvolts.

Nerve Conduction Studies

NCSs are used to determine the speed with which the nerve conducts and the number of axons that are functioning. This will be an introduction to basic techniques. Motor conduction studies consist of stimulating the nerve at two or more points along its course, and recording muscle action potentials with the active and reference surface electrodes: an active lead (G1) placed on the belly of the muscle and an indifferent lead (G2) placed on the tendon. Depolarization of the cathode results in the generation of a CMAP. The action potential gives rise to a simple, biphasic waveform with the initial negative deflection. A small, negative potential may precede the negative peak with inappropriate positioning of the recording electrode. If G1 is not placed over the motor point, it records multiple motor points that may alter the onset of the action potential. A stimulation (shock) artifact becomes problematic if it is larger than the response or overloads the amplifier.

Sensory studies consist of stimulating a nerve and the signal propagating to the active electrode (G1) and the reference electrode (G2) at a remote site. An initially positive triphasic waveform characterizes the orthodromic potential with G1 on the nerve and G2 at a remote site. In conduction studies, there are two directions in which an action potential can travel: orthodromic and antidromic. An orthodromic stimulus is one in which the action potential monitored is traveling in the direction of its typical physiological conduction. The normal physiological conduction of sensory fibers is toward the spinal cord, whereas motor fibers conduct from the spinal cord distally. In antidromic studies, the action potential is monitored in the opposite direction from the physiological nerve conduction. Most motor nerve studies are performed orthodromically, whereas sensory studies are more commonly performed both antidromically and orthodromically. Mixed nerve studies by definition must be both orthodromic and antidromic.

Waveforms of CMAPs are generally configured as biphasic or triphasic, depending on the location of the motor point and the recording site. The onset latency is defined as the interval between the onset of a stimulus and the onset of a response. This measures the fastest conducting fibers. On the other hand, the peak latency is the interval between the onset of a stimulus and a specified peak of the evoked potential, which measures the onset of slower conducting fibers. The distal latency is typically determined using a fixed distance. Onset latencies are more commonly used both in motor and sensory studies. Similarly, a proximal latency can be obtained with stimulation of the nerve more proximally. Latency is expressed in milliseconds and reflects nerve conduction speed. Amplitude is the maximum voltage difference between two points. It reflects the number of axons functioning. It can be measured from base to negative peak in biphasic waveforms, or positive peak to negative peak in triphasic waveforms.

The amplitude is proportional to the number and size of the fibers under the recording electrode, and is dependent on the distance between the active tissue and the recording electrode. The amplitude provides an estimate of the amount of functioning, active tissue. The units of amplitude are millivolts for CMAPs and microvolts for SNAPs. The "area" is defined as the area under the waveform, and is a function of amplitude and duration. Although amplitudes of motor and sensory responses are typically what are reported, the more accurate measurement of the number of axons measured is the absolute area-under-the-curve of the waveform. Termination is the time it takes for the wave to finally return to baseline. The duration is the time from onset to termination. The total duration measures the dispersion of all components and, thereby, differences in the time-of-onset and CV of the components. Analysis of the shape and duration of a waveform can provide an estimate of the distribution of CVs of the fibers contributing to the potential.

CV is the speed an impulse travels along a nerve, and is primarily dependent on the integrity of the myelin sheath. It is calculated by dividing the change in distance (proximal stimulation site in mm – distal stimulation site in mm) by the change in time (proximal latency in ms – distal latency in ms). Normal values are 50 m per second in the upper limbs and 40 m per second in the lower limbs. Nerve compression and demyelinating neuropathies lead to conduction slowing. When this affects a nerve in a heterogenous manner, as is the case in most compressive and systemic demyelinating neuropathies, there is widening of the waveform. This is otherwise known as temporal dispersion. CV can be affected by age and temperature. CV is 50% of an adult for newborns, 80% of an adult by 1 year, and equal to an adult by 3 to 5 years. Temperature measurements are important to ensure that proper CV is accurately calculated so that a demyelinating process is not under- or overdiagnosed. The normal is approximately 32°C for the upper limbs and 30°C for the lower limbs. CV decreases 2.4 m per second per 1°C dropped.

Motor Studies

A CMAP is the action potential recorded from muscle when stimulation anywhere along the motor pathway is sufficient to activate some or all of the muscle fibers in that muscle. It is the summated response of the activity of all the muscle fibers innervated by the axons and motor units represented in that muscle. A CMAP provides assessment of the descending motor axons in the pathway below the level of stimulation, the NMJ, and the muscle fibers activated by the stimulus. The CMAP amplitude is a reflection of the number of functioning muscle fibers. The CMAP amplitude is reduced in neural disease if there is a loss of motor units or anterior horn cells, or if the rate of denervation of muscle fibers exceeds the rate of reinnervation. It is also reduced in muscle disease if muscle fiber loss exceeds repair. As previously mentioned, the CMAP is measured in millivolts.

Late responses are recordable potentials that can occur after a CMAP is generated. They can provide information about proximal nerve segments in the evaluation of neurological diseases. Late responses, such as F-waves, A-waves, and H-reflexes, assess the function of the peripheral nerve and the spinal cord. F-waves are CMAPs that are activated antidromically by action potentials that travel, initially, proximally from axons to the anterior horn cells, causing activation of a small variable percentage of anterior horn cells. This results in an orthodromic volley, which is recorded by the recording electrodes distally. The F-wave latency, therefore, includes the time required for the action potential to travel from the site of stimulation antidromically to the spinal cord, plus the time to travel orthodromically back to the muscle. Because the percentage of anterior horn cells that are stimulated is variable, the F-wave amplitude and latency is also variable.

A-wave latencies, if present, generally lie between that of the CMAP and F-wave. They also result from an antidromic action potential, but differ from F-waves in that they are mediated by a peripheral collateral branch from the primary axon, causing propagation of an orthodromic action potential in an adjacent axon. A-waves are thus evidence of branched motor axons, commonly seen in peripheral nerve disorders. They are more constant than F-waves in occurrence and appearance.

The H-reflex is a monosynaptic reflex response elicited by submaximal stimulation of Ia muscle spindle afferents that directly activate anterior horn cells. It is similar to a tendon reflex, except that it bypasses the muscle spindle. It is usually easily recorded from the soleus or flexor carpi radialis muscles, and its major application is in identifying a delayed or reduced response in patients who may have an S1 or C7 radiculopathy.

Repetitive stimulation allows the electromyographer to generate multiple stimulations in rapid succession to the same site. This allows analysis of the resulting CMAP potentials for consistency of amplitude, area, and duration.

Repetitive stimulation is an advanced technique used in assessing the function of the neuromuscular junction in the evaluation of associated disorders, such as myasthenia gravis or the Lambert-Eaton myasthenic syndrome. A discussion on the anatomy and physiology of the NMJ and how it applies to repetitive stimulation studies will not be briefly reviewed. The NMJ consists of the distal portion of a motor axon, which has small projections that innervate individual muscle fibers. The motor endplate is formed from the distal portion of the nerve and a single muscle fiber. The axon terminal contains various neural structures, including mitochondria and synaptic vesicles with ACh. The terminal itself does not contact its muscle fiber, but rather, it remains separate from it by primary and secondary synaptic clefts. The terminal endings of the axon consist of presynaptic bulbs, which encompass three storage compartments containing ACh. They are contained in packets called *quanta* consisting of approximately 5000 to 10,000 molecules. The ACh migrates from the main and mobilization storage compartments to replenish the immediate storage compartment, which is depleted in the process of generating each action potential. This migration of ACh takes approximately 4 seconds. The zone between the axon and the muscle fiber is called the *synaptic cleft*. This is a gap where ACh crosses from the presynaptic region toward receptors on the postsynaptic region. It contains an enzyme, ACh esterase, which degrades ACh into acetate and choline as it crosses the cleft. The postsynaptic region is a membrane lined with ACh receptors. It has convolutions to increase its surface area by approximately 10 times the surface of the presynaptic membrane. At the apex of each fold, receptors are located across from the presynaptic active zones, which are the sites of ACh release. Each postsynaptic ACh receptor requires two molecules of ACh to become activated.

ACh is continuously released, even in the so called "resting state." During periods of inactivation, a quantum (5000–10,000 molecules) is released approximately every 5 seconds, which is defined as a miniature endplate potential (MEPP). During the periods of activation, a nerve depolarization opens voltage-gated calcium (Ca^{2+}) channels. Ca^{2+} floods the nerve terminals and remains there for approximately 200 ms. This leads to the release of multiple quanta into the synaptic cleft, which increases the amount of MEPPs. These MEPPs summate and form an endplate potential (EPP), which generates a MUAP. Normally, the EPP's amplitude is four times the amount needed to initiate an action potential. However, the EPP's amplitude drops each time the EPP is produced owing to a drop in immediately available ACh. This initial excess amplitude of the EPP is called the safety factor, and allows time for ACh to move from the main and mobilizing storage compartments to replenish the immediate storage compartment. This avoids a drop of the EPP's amplitude below the threshold needed to cause an action potential. The safety factor depends on two parameters: the amount of ACh quanta released with each depolarization and the ability of the ACh receptors to respond to the ACh molecules.

Neuromuscular disorders hinder the production, release, or uptake of ACh. A low safety factor leads to reduction of the amplitude of the EPPs to fall below the threshold needed to generate a muscle fiber action potential. This occurs as a result of an alteration of the amount of quanta released or the amount of ACh in each quanta. Myasthenia gravis is a disorder of the postsynaptic membrane in which there is a lack of response owing to loss of ACh receptors. This leads to reduced MEPP amplitudes, but their frequency remains normal. Eaton-Lambert syndrome (myasthenic syndrome) is a disorder resulting in decreased quanta content leaving normal MEPP amplitudes, but with decreased frequency. Repetitive stimulation is thus utilized to aid in the diagnosis of neuromuscular disorders.

Sensory Studies

A SNAP is recorded from a sensory nerve or mixed nerve when stimulation is sufficient to generate a propagated action potential along the course of the nerve, and is measured in microvolts. It is useful in determining whether a lesion is present proximal or distal to the DRG. The DRG is the cell body of the sensory nerve. From the DRG, two axons arise; one travels distally and one travels centrally. If a patient complains of sensory loss and the SNAP is reduced or absent, that would imply a postganglionic lesion. If the SNAP is normal, this would indicate a lesion proximal to the DRG. SNAPs are also helpful in brachial plexus and peripheral injury localization.

Electromyography

Needle EMG is used to identify and characterize disorders of the motor unit, including pathology involving the anterior horn cell, peripheral nerves, NMJs, and muscles. Performing EMG requires learning specialized skills, including auditory pattern recognition and semiquantization. The needle exam should only be performed by a physician.

Equipment

Needle electrodes are inserted directly into muscle and record electrical activity. Standard concentric needles and monopolar needles are most commonly used for diagnostic EMG. The needle electrode is attached via a cable to the preamplifier. Concentric needles are composed of a bare needle shaft, which acts as a reference electrode; and a central fine wire insulated from the shaft, which acts as the active electrode. Monopolar needles are Teflon®-coated, and a separate surface electrode is needed for a reference electrode. The recording surface is usually larger than that of a concentric needle, which results in different characteristics of the recorded potentials. Monopolar needles are more commonly utilized by some electromyographers because they are less expensive and possibly less uncomfortable for patients. A ground electrode is utilized to eliminate ambient electrical noise.

EMG Waveforms

Insertional activity is provoked by movement of the needle electrode through muscle tissue and can be described as normal, increased, or decreased. Normal insertional activity is a single burst lasting less than 300 ms after cessation of needle movement. Activity that continues for more than 300 ms after cessation of needle movement is defined as increased activity. Decreased activity is few, if any, electrical potentials detected following needle movement. Spontaneous activity is electrical activity recorded with the muscle at rest, not related to needle movement. Normal resting activity should be electrically silent after a needle is inserted into normal muscle. However, if a needle is placed into the NMJ, two waveforms can occur: MEPPs and EPPs. Needle placement in this area is painful. End plate spikes are characterized by moderate amplitude, short duration, and an irregularly firing biphasic waveform with an initially negative deflection that sounds like frying bacon. End plate noise arises from MEPPs and is characterized by small amplitude, short duration, and continuous noise, sounding similar to seashell noise.

Abnormal activity is defined as electrical activity at rest and is pathological. This activity can be generated from a muscle or neural source. Fibrillation potentials are spontaneously firing action potentials originating from denervated muscle fibers secondary to uncontrolled ACh release. Its hallmark sign is its regularity of firing. They sound like raindrops falling on a rooftop. Positive sharp waves are spontaneous firing action potentials stimulated by needle movement of an injured muscle fiber that is also denervated. *See* Table 2 for grading classification.

Fasciculations represent irregular nonvolitional firing of a motor unit, which is variable in duration and amplitude, and results in intermittent muscle fiber contraction. Fasciculations sound like popcorn popping. If associated with fibrillation potentials or positive sharp waves (PSWs) they are considered pathological. Its hallmark sign is a slowed, irregular-firing

Table 2
Grading Classifications

Grade	*Characteristic*
0	None
1+	Persistent single runs <1 second in two areas
2+	Moderate runs <1 second in three or more areas
3+	Many discharges in most muscle regions
4+	Continuous discharges in all muscles areas

motor unit. Normal voluntary motor unit firing does not occur at the slow rates seen with pathological fasciculations.

Complex repetitive discharges (CRDs) are a bizarre, spontaneously firing group of action potentials that start and stop abruptly, with continuous runs of waveform patterns that repeat regularly at 10 to 100 Hz. CRDs are initiated from muscle fibers in which there is a principal pacemaker orchestrating muscle fibers to fire in near synchrony. The current spreads to the other muscle fibers by ephaptic transmission. CRDs result from denervated muscle fibers that are reinnervated by collateral sprouting. CRDs sound like a motor boat.

Myotonic activity resembles continuous PSWs waxing and waning in frequency and amplitude. They are single muscle fiber action potentials triggered by needle movement, percussion, or voluntary contraction. They are caused by an alteration of the ion channels in the muscle membrane, and can be seen with or without clinical myotonia. Its hallmark sign is the smooth change in rate and amplitude. This abnormal activity sounds like a dive bomber.

Myokymic activity is regularly firing bursts of motor unit potentials (MUPs), with regularly occurring silent periods between bursts. This sounds like marching soldiers. They can be associated with a clinical myokymia, which presents as slow, continuous muscle fiber contractions. This gives a rippling appearance to the overlying skin.

Neurotonic activities are high-frequency (100–300 Hz) discharges originating from motor axons, and are associated with continuous muscle fiber activity. They may be continuous for long intervals or recur in bursts. They are classically seen in neuromyotonia (Isaac's syndrome). This is a disorder associated with continuous muscle fiber activity, resulting in the appearance of muscle rippling and stiffness secondary to irritable nerves. The progressive decrement of its waveform is the result of single muscle fiber fatigue and drop off.

Cramps are sustained, often painful, muscle contractions of multiple motor units lasting seconds to minutes. They are usually abrupt-onset and -cessation, and typically, increasing numbers of potentials are recruited as the cramps develop, and then drop out as the cramp subsides.

Motor Unit Morphology

The MUAP is the recorded, summated electrical depolarization of the muscle fibers innervated by a single motor neuron. Rise time is the time from the initial positive peak to the initial negative peak. It is the fastest component of the MUAP. It is a function of the distance of the recording electrode from the fibers of the motor unit. A short (<0.5 ms) rise time indicates that the needle electrode is in the immediate vicinity of the motor unit, and accurate assessment of the motor unit is possible. The duration of a MUAP is the time from the initial shift of the MUAP from the baseline until its final return to the baseline. It is proportional to the number of muscle fibers in the range of the recording electrode. The durations of MUAPs in a given muscle have a normal distribution that can be described by a mean and standard deviation. Normative data have been established for individual muscles.

The amplitude is measured from the maximum negative peak to the maximum positive peak (peak to peak). Because the MUAP amplitude is a function of needle electrode proximity, as well as the motor unit itself, it is more variable for any single motor unit than the duration. Therefore, normal values for amplitude are not available. The number of phases of a MUAP is determined by adding 1 to the number of times the potential crosses the baseline. MUAPs are typically triphasic; they may be complex, and if the number of phases exceeds four, then they are referred to as "polyphasic." The number of phases is proportional to the synchrony of muscle fibers and the total number of fibers comprising the MUAP. Normal muscles will demonstrate a small (5–15%) proportion of polyphasic potentials. Turns are potential reversals in slope that, unlike phases, do not cross the baseline. Electrophysiologically, they mean the same thing as phases and contribute to the complexity of the MUAP.

Pathophysiology

Peripheral Nerve Injuries

Peripheral nerve injuries may cause an extensive amount of disability. To determine the appropriate diagnosis, localization, severity, prognosis, and treatment of peripheral nerve injury, it is essential to understand the classification, mechanism of the injury, and the implications of the electrodiagnostic test.

The two most commonly used classifications for nerve injuries are the Seddon and Sunderland classifications. Seddon's classification is characterized by neuropraxia, axonotemesis, and neurotmesis.

Neurapraxia (first-degree Sunderland, first-degree Seddon) is the mildest injury that affects only myelin without Wallerian degeneration or axonal cell death. Compression injury and/or ischemia are the main etiologies that cause motor and sensory loss without Wallerian degeneration (dying back phenomenon). In a pure neurapraxic lesion, the CMAP will show change immediately after the lesion. When recording from the distal muscle and stimulating distal to the lesion, the CMAP will be normal. However, when stimulating proximal to the lesion, a conduction block secondary to demyelination will cause a decreased or temporally dispersed waveform. This proximal amplitude drop should be more than 20% of the distal amplitude to consider conduction block.

Focal nerve conduction slowing can also occur from a conduction block. This is commonly seen with ulnar neuropathies at the elbow. Similar changes in the SNAP can also be seen after focal nerve injury. Because there is no axonal injury in neurapraxia, EMG will be normal, although decreased recruitment may be seen with conduction block. Neurapraxia has a good prognosis, taking several weeks to three or more months post-injury for recovery.

Axonotmesis (Sunderland's and Seddon's second degree) is usually seen in traction (i.e., falls and motor vehicle accidents), crush, or percussion injuries (i.e., gunshot wounds). Wallerian degeneration occurs distal to the lesion. Both axons and myelin are injured; however, the endoneurium, perineurium, and epineurium are preserved. Wallerian degeneration is a length-dependent process that starts at approximately the third day and is completed by about day 9 post-injury.

NCSs may reveal results similar to a severe neuropraxia when stimulating distal to the injury. EMG testing may reveal similar findings in severe neuropraxia and axonotmesis. It may be difficult to differentiate neurapraxia from axonotmesis or initially complete neurotmesis even as late as 6 months. Typically, complete axonotmesis will show no response proximal and distal to the site of injury in CMAP 9 days and SNAP 11 days post-injury. Partial axonal loss will lead to a drop in amplitude. Side-to-side SNAP comparisons are useful if the other limb is not injured. Comparison is significant when a 50% or greater difference in amplitude is noted.

EMG will show PSWs and fibrillation potentials in 10 to 30 days, depending on the distal nerve stump length. The shorter the stump is, the faster the appearance of fibrillation potentials. Therefore, timing of the injury is important for the electromyographer to make the correct estimation of severity and prognosis.

The presence of abundant fibrillations and absent MUAPs should not be prematurely concluded as complete denervation. In this case, a partially preserved CMAP would suggest there is a partial neuropraxic component. A complete axonotmesis injury will yield no CMAP response once Wallerian degeneration has taken place; however, both neuropraxias and axonotmesis may lead to detectable decreases in motor unit recruitment and an increase in single motor unit firing rate (>15 cycles per second). Motor unit configuration changes (high amplitude, long duration, and/or polyphasia) may also be seen in chronic injuries.

Recovery in axonotmesis depends on axonal regeneration and terminal collateral axonal sprouting. The amplitude of the CMAP helps to estimate the prognosis. Patients usually have initially fast recovery followed by a slow additional recovery. Sensory healing takes more time to recover compared with motor healing. A complete lesion has the worst prognosis. The length of the axonal loss is also important to determine the recovery period; axonal re-growth is generally 2 to 3 mm per day.

Recovery from axonal injury occurs via two mechanisms: (a) collateral sprouting and (b) axonal re-growth. Collateral sprouting is the process by which an intact axon from an intact motor unit innervates a denervated muscle fiber of an injured motor unit. The connecting "sprout" contains smaller terminal branches, thinner myelin, and weaker neuromuscular junctions. As a result of collateral sprouting, the muscle fibers become a part of the new motor unit and take on its characteristics, increasing the size of the fiber type's territory. Remodeling results in motor units with poor firing synchronicity secondary to the immature terminal sprouts. This process results in polyphasic waveforms with increased amplitudes.

The second mechanism of repair occurs from axonal re-growth. Axons will regrow down their original pathway toward their muscle fibers. This development occurs 2 to 3 mm per day or 1 in. per month, if the supporting connective tissue remains intact. These axons will have a decreased diameter, thinner myelin, and shorter internodal distance. As a result of reinnervation, low amplitude, long duration, and polyphasic potentials known as nascent potentials are formed. If the connective tissue is not intact to guide proper nerve re-growth, a neuroma can form with failure to reach the final end organ. If both axonal regeneration and collateral sprouting occur, the strongest neuromuscular junction will triumph.

Neurotmesis (Seddon's third degree, and third through fifth degrees of Sunderland) is a complete severance of the nerve trunk involving the endoneurium, perineurium, and epineurium. Sharp injury, severe traction injury, percussion injuries, and even noxious drug injections may cause neurotmesis. Electrodiagnostic findings are the same as complete axonotmesis. There is a complete loss of motor and sensory functions. There is no recovery unless surgical repair is undertaken.

Sunderland's classification is divided into the following five categories:

1. Type 1: Focal conduction block resulting from local myelin injury with axonal continuity (neuropraxia).
2. Type 2: Loss of nerve conduction at the injury site and distally from axonal degeneration with Wallerian degeneration. Endoneurium, perineurium, and epineurium are intact. Axonal regeneration is required for recovery. Prognosis is good.
3. Type 3: Loss of nerve conduction at the injury site and distally from disruption of axonal continuity and endoneurial tubes. Perineurium and epineurium are intact. Poor prognosis because the disruption of endoneurial tubes leads to axonal misdirection with re-growth.
4. Type 4: Loss of nerve conduction at the injury site and distally from disruption of axonal continuity endoneurial tubes and perineurim. Epineurium is intact. Poor prognosis with disorganization, intraneural scarring, and axonal misdirection.
5. Type 5 (neurotmesis): Severance of the entire nerve. Treatment requires surgical modification and prognosis is guarded.

Optimal Electrodiagnostic Timing

To obtain optimal information, it is important to perform the electrodiagnostic studies at the appropriate time. Electrodiagnostic testing may localize and differentiate conduction block from axonotmesis as early as 7 to 10 days from the time of injury. This is especially true of distal nerve injuries, where precise anatomic localization can be done even right after injury. However, because of the delay in the appearance of fibrillation potentials and PSWs, EDX evaluation after 3 to 4 weeks post-injury will give a better indication of the degree of axonal injury. For follow-up on recovery, testing can be done a few months post-injury, and then repeated every few months when axonal regeneration is being monitored.

Median Mononeuropathy

Background

The median nerve is the most commonly compressed nerve in humans. The most common injury site is at the carpal tunnel. The anterior interosseous nerve (AIN), the median nerve passing between the heads of pronator teres (PT) muscle, and the median nerve passing under the ligament of Struther's, are all uncommon but reported sites of entrapment. There are also reports of iatrogenic injuries to the brachial plexus during the injection of local anesthesia that involve the fascicles of only the median nerve. In these cases, denervation patterns suggest a more distal median nerve injury; however, distal NCSs reveal no focal signs of slowing or conduction block.

Anatomy

C5, C6, C7, C8, and T1 roots make the median nerve's origin; medial and lateral cords of brachial plexus form the median nerve. The nerve does not innervate any muscle in the arm. It passes through the ligament of Struther's at the medial epicondyle of elbow, then between the two heads of the PT muscle to arrive at the forearm. It innervates the PT, flexor carpi radialis (FCR), palmaris longus, and flexor digitorum superficialis (FDS); the nerve continues with a pure motor division AIN that innervates flexor digitorum profundus (FDP; second and third fingers), flexor pollicis longus (FPL), and pronator quadratus. At the wrist, it goes through the carpal tunnel and innervates the "LOAF" muscles (Lumbricals [first and second], Opponens pollicis, Abductor pollicis brevis, and Flexor pollicis brevis [superficial]). The palmar cutaneous branch of the median nerve is the last branch given off by the main trunk in the forearm, and it provides cutaneous sensation to the bases of the thenar eminences. It does not pass through the carpal tunnel. The main trunk passes through the carpal tunnel and divides into the first common palmar digital nerve and then divides into the proper digital nerves. These branches have variable extensions to the first, second, and third digits. Median nerve sensory fibers originate from the C6 and C7 nerve roots.

Ligament of Struther's Syndrome

Background

Ligament of Struther's is a fibrous band between the supracondylar process (bony spur) and medial epicondyle of humerus; it is present in 1% of the population.

Clinical Findings

Patients may present with paresthesia along the median sensory distribution in the hand including the thenar eminence. In advanced cases, weakness in wrist flexion (FCR weakness) and grip strength (FDP and FDS weakness) occur. Because of FDP weakness, patients may show difficulty in bending the second and third fingers (Benediction sign). Involvement of all median innervated muscles is not uncommon. Weakness of pronation helps to differentiate between ligament of Struther's and pronator syndrome. When the brachial artery runs with the median nerve under the ligament, then the brachial pulse will be decreased.

Electrodiagnostic Findings

Reduced CV or conduction block in the upper arm to the elbow is found in median NCSs. EMG shows neurogenic changes (spontaneous activity, abnormal MUPs, and abnormal recruitment) in median innervated muscles.

PT Syndrome

Background

The median nerve is compressed between the heads of the PT or by a tight band of the FDS muscle. Because of the innervation pattern, the PT muscle whose branch comes off proximally is typically spared.

Clinical Findings

Patients should have pain over the PT muscle, especially exacerbated by pronation (PT) or making a fist (FDS). They may present with paresthesia in a median sensory location, including the palm and thenar eminence, which clinically separates this syndrome from carpal tunnel syndrome (CTS) (the palmar cutaneous branch is spared in CTS). Weakness and atrophy can be observed in median innervated muscles distal to the PT muscle.

Electrodiagnostic Findings

These include reduced CV or conduction block in the elbow-to-wrist section of the median nerve with an abnormal activity in median innervated muscles distal to PT muscle.

AIN Syndrome

Background

The anterior interosseous nerve is the largest and is a "pure" motor branch of the median nerve. However, it does contain some sensory fibers to wrist and hand joints. The AIN innervates the FPL, pronator quadratus, and FDP (second and third fingers). A mnemonic is "four P muscles." AIN syndrome could be a manifestation of idiopathic brachial plexus (Parsonage Turner syndrome). Trauma or compression may also cause AIN syndrome.

Clinical Findings

Acute onset of first- and second-digit weakness without any sensory deficit is a characteristic presentation. Because of FPL and FDP weakness, patients may exhibit a positive "OK sign" (inability to make an "O" with the thumb and index digits) or inability to make a fist. When there is a superimposed Martin-Gruber anastomosis, ulnar nerve fibers travel with the AIN; patients also may have intrinsic hand muscle atrophy.

Electrodiagnostic Findings and Approach

Routine nerve conduction studies are usually normal. Extensive arm and shoulder muscle testing is very important to rule out idiopathic brachial plexopathy. All SNAPs in the affected limb are normal. EMG finding is neurogenic pattern in "four P muscles," unless there is a superimposed Martin-Gruber anastomosis.

Carpal Tunnel Syndrome

Background

This is the most common entrapment neuropathy. CTS is often bilateral and usually affects the dominant hand more severely. Women are more prone to this disorder. Enlarged canal volume (pregnancy, thyroid disease, congestive heart failure, mass), diminished canal volume (rheumatoid arthritis, amyloidosis, fractures), idiopathic process, or double crush syndrome (diabetes, cervical radiculopathy, and "true" thoracic outlet syndrome) may cause the nerve injury.

Clinical Findings

Patients complain of numbness, parasthesias, and pain in the median nerve distribution. These symptoms are typically intermittent early on in the process and are worse at night. Symptoms are typically relieved with shaking of the hand or the "flick" sign. Individuals may complain of difficulty buttoning their clothes. Patients may have difficulty localizing the sensory abnormalities to the median nerve distribution. Common physical examination testing includes Phalen's test and Tinel's sign, which are abnormal in approximately 60% of patients with CTS.

The LOAF muscles can be affected. Two-point discrimination may be damaged before pain and temperature sensation. C6 or C7 cervical radiculopathy may occur because of the numbness and/or pain of first, second, or third digits; "true" thoracic outlet syndrome owing to thenar atrophy; peripheral polyneuropathy; proximal median neuropathies, which are usually present with FPL, arm pronation weakness should be considered as differentials. Sensory loss or paresthesia over the thenar eminence, in addition to the usual distribution of sensory changes in fingers, is also suggestive of a more proximal median nerve involvement. For more information, *see* Chapter 11

Table 3
Electrodiagnostic Classification of Carpal Tunnel Syndrome

Severity	*Mild*	*Moderate*	*Severe*
Sensory NCS	• Slowed conduction velocity • Normal amplitude	• Slowed conduction velocity • Decreased amplitude	• Absent
Motor NCS	• Normal • Normal amplitude	• Prolonged latency • Decreased amplitude	• Prolonged latency
EMG	• No abnormal activity	• No abnormal activity	• Abnormal activity

Electrodiagnostic Findings and Approaches

In order to make a CTS diagnosis, one should demonstrate abnormal EDX findings in the wrist segment of the median nerve. Focal slowing of median sensory nerve CV at the wrist, prolonged distal latency of the median motor nerve, median sensory and/or motor nerve action potentials with low amplitude(s), and abnormal spontaneous activity in abductor pollicis brevis (APB) muscle are some of the distinctive EDX findings. Although each lab has its own standard values, CV less than 50 m per second across the tunnel is usually pathological slowing.

SNAPs are affected first and are abnormal more often than motor studies. Median sensory and motor distal latencies are the most commonly used measuring techniques in the diagnosis. However, because of less sensitivity and specificity of these studies on mild and early cases, a number of other techniques have been advocated and widely used, such as median–ulnar sensory latency difference between the wrist and ring finger, median–radial sensory latency difference between the wrist and digit, palmar mixed nerve studies, and median nerve inching techniques.

In severe CTS, absent median-digit sensory and median–APB motor responses may cause difficulty in diagnosing CTS, and in these cases, one must rely primarily on the needle exam. Then, median NCSs should include the comparison to same-side ulnar nerve. The median–ulnar second lumbrical interosseous test may also be useful. A decreased sensory amplitude on the affected side could indicate either an axonal lesion of the median nerve or a conduction block across the carpal tunnel (if proximal amplitude is <50% of distal mid-palm amplitude). More than 50% amplitude difference (as compared with median sensory amplitude on the unaffected side) is felt to be a significant difference.

Late responses (F-wave and H-waves) are not useful in CTS.

Electromyographic testing is important to demonstrate if there is any axonal loss from active (increased spontaneous activity and fibrillation potentials/PSWs) denervation or decreased recruitment. When there is chronic axonal loss, giant MUPs may be present.

Muscle testing requires not only APB, but also more proximal median-innervated muscles to exclude a more proximal median neuropathy. It is also important to consider a non-median-innervated C8 muscle testing to help rule out "true" thoracic outlet syndrome, a brachial plexopathy or radiculopathy. This should include testing of the paraspinal muscles.

CTS can be described as mild, moderate, and severe. *See* Table 3.

Ulnar Neuropathy

Background

Ulnar neuropathy is the second most common compressed neuropathy. Even though the nerve can be injured at any level, injury at the elbow is by far the most common entrapment site. Pathology at the wrist is the second most common site.

Three ulnar compressive syndromes at the elbow are relatively common:

1. Cubital tunnel syndrome.
2. Ulnar nerve subluxation from condylar groove (retrocondylar groove).
3. Tardy ulnar palsy.

When the compression happens at or beneath the proximal edge of the flexor carpi ulnaris (FCU) aponeurosis or arcuate ligament, it is called cubital tunnel syndrome. The most accepted etiopathological explanation of this syndrome is that during elbow flexion, the distance between the olecranon and medial epicondyle increases and tightens the FCU aponeurosis over the nerve. In the retrocondylar groove, the nerve is located between bone and skin and is subject to chronic compression. The nerve can be rolled over the medial epicondyle. This is seen in approximately 16% of the population. Tardy ulnar palsy may occur years after a distal humerus fracture owing to bone overgrowth or scar formation, and is associated with valgus deformity at elbow.

The ulnar nerve can be damaged at Guyon's canal; however, it is not common. There are three types of lesions based on physical examination, signs, and symptoms. Type I occurs proximal to or within the canal, and affects the superficial and deep branches with a combined sensory and motor loss. Patients complain of diminished sensation on the volar aspect of the fifth and fourth digits, as well as the medial palmar surface. The dorsal ulnar cutaneous nerve is spared. Type II affects the deep branch only with preserved sensation. Type III affects only the superficial sensory branch and patients complain of diminished sensation in the volar aspect of the hypothenar eminence and the fourth and fifth digits. These can be seen in cyclists as a result of resting on the handlebars (cycler's palsy).

Anatomy

The ulnar nerve is derived from the roots of C8 and T1. The fibers pass through lower trunk and medial cord and then form the ulnar nerve. The ulnar nerve innervates the following: the adductor pollicis, one-half of the flexor pollicis brevis (FPB; deep head), FCU, one-half of the FDP (fourth and fifth digits), the fifth digit and half of the fourth digit sensation. There are no branches in the arm and there is no sensory innervation above the wrist. In the arm, the nerve is located in a groove with the medial triceps and is covered by a fascial plane referred to as the arcade of Struthers. At this point, the nerve is tightly bound to the medial head of the triceps muscle and by the arcade of Struthers. At the elbow, the ulnar nerve presents posterior and superficially. Consequently, the ulnar nerve is vulnerable to injury at this level. After passing dorsally to the medial epicondyle, it enters the cubital tunnel. In the forearm, the nerve gives off the first motor branch to the FCU followed by the FDP and two cutaneous sensory branches, the palmar and dorsal ulnar cutaneous. The palmar branch innervates the proximal medial part of the palm, whereas the dorsal branch innervates the dorsal surface of the fifth and ulnar side of the fourth digit, as well as the ulnar side of the dorsal surface of the hand. At the wrist, the ulnar nerve passes through Guyon's canal (created by the hook of the hamate and pisiform) and it breaks up into the superficial (primarily sensory), deep palmar, and hypothenar branches. The deep palmar branch has pure motor fibers and nerves to the palmaris brevis, four Dorsal interossei ("DAB" for abduction), three Palmar interossei ("PAD" for adduction), two lumbricals (medial), one adductor pollicis, and one-half of the FPB (deep head). The hypothenar branch is mainly motor fibers, which innervate the opponens, abductor, and flexor digiti minimi muscles.

Clinical Findings

Patients usually present with numbness and tingling of the fifth digit. Hand weakness may also be present, but pain is not common. Inspection may reveal ulnar clawing. Ulnar claw hand occurs because of an unopposed pull of extensor digitorum communis that creates an extension of the metacarpophalangeal, which results from fourth and fifth finger partial proximal interphalangeal and distal interphalangeal joint flexion. A lesion at the elbow may cause ulnar-innervated muscle atrophy at the hand, which is most apparent in the interossei, especially the first dorsal interosseous muscle. A positive Froment's sign indicates adductor pollicis (ulnar-innervated) weakness and substituted normal FPL (median-innervated). In these cases, the patient is unable to hold a piece of paper between the thumb and index finger with pure thumb adduction. Patients compensate by utilizing the FPL muscle causing thumb interphalangeal joint flexion. Patients may also demonstrate the inability to adduct the fifth digit secondary to interosseous weakness, and therefore their fifth digit is in an abducted position. (Wartenberg's sign is abduction of fourth and fifth digits). Tinel's sign, produced by percussion of the nerve at the elbow, is often positive; however, it is not specific.

The sensory exam may be normal even with sensory symptoms. However, there may be a sensory loss in the fifth and medial part of the fourth digits (it is characteristic of an ulnar nerve lesion). It is important to remember that the dorsal ulnar cutaneous branch contains sensory fibers to the dorsum of medial aspect of the hand. This nerve does not pass through Guyon's canal. Consequently, a lesion at or distal to Guyon's canal will spare the dorsal ulnar cutaneous branch and, therefore, spare sensory innervation to the dorsum of the medial aspect the hand. Presence of sensory loss of more than 2 to 3 cm above the wrist suggests that the etiology is not isolated to the ulnar nerve. Abnormalities in this territory suggest a lower plexus, C8 or T1, or medial cutaneous nerve of forearm lesion.

Electrodiagnostic Findings and Approaches

Electrodiagnostic studies can assist in confirming the diagnosis, localizing the lesion for some surgical cases, excluding other conditions (e.g., C8 radiculopathy), and even providing prognostic data. Because surgical treatments of cubital tunnel syndrome and tardy ulnar palsy may be different, localization and diagnosis of these conditions are vital. However, EDX studies do not always offer gratifying lesion localization at the elbow, even with short-segment incremental studies. In these cases, one may need to rely on other clinical information, such as magnetic resonance imaging or physical exam findings.

Sensory NCSs should include ulnar SNAP at the fifth finger and dorsal ulnar cutaneous nerve. Because the dorsal ulnar cutaneous nerve branches off at mid-forearm, ulnar neuropathy at the elbow would influence ulnar sensory response at the fifth digit and dorsal ulnar cutaneous SNAP; however, lesion at the wrist level or after the dorsal ulnar cutaneous nerve (e.g., Guyon's canal) will show normal dorsal ulnar cutaneous SNAP with decreased or absent ulnar sensory response at the fifth digit. Keep in mind that dorsal ulnar cutaneous SNAP amplitudes are asymmetric in one-fifth of normal individuals. Side-to-side SNAP amplitude difference of more than 50% indicates considerable axonal loss.

Motor NCSs are mostly recorded at the abductor digiti minimi. When there is a strong suspicion of ulnar nerve injury and standard studies are inconclusive, then the American Association of Neuromuscular and Electrodiagnostic Medicine Quality Assurance Committee recommends recording from the first dorsal interosseus (FDI), which may show the pathology. Delayed latency and/or decreased CV can signify a demyelinating process. Low CMAP amplitude is indicative of axonal loss. However, if there is more than a 20 to 30% decrease in amplitude distally (wrist) compared with the amplitude proximally (elbow), it should raise the consideration of Martin-Gruber anastomosis versus conduction block. (Martin-Gruber anastomosis is an anomalous connection between the ulnar and median nerves and is sometimes bilateral. It is present in 20% of the population.) When conduction block is present, it is important to define the exact location of the lesion. Therefore, short segmental studies ("inching") are necessary. When short segmental studies are abnormal, they can exhibit focal slowing, conduction block, or both. Most authors believe that elbow should be flexed when performing ulnar NCSs, but there is no consensus on optimal degree of flexion.

Late responses (F-wave and H-wave) are not specific, but comparison of the median and ulnar F-waves may support other EDX findings.

Because of limited muscle innervation at the arm (and their localization), EMG studies can be difficult to evaluate. Abductor digiti minimi and FDI are the most commonly tested ulnar-innervated muscles. FCU is commonly spared with lesions around the elbow, and FDP (fourth and fifth digits) are typically affected. Therefore, normal FCU EMG results cannot exclude proximal ulnar nerve pathology. In this case, NCS is more valuable than EMG study.

Treatment of ulnar neuropathy at the elbow/wrist may be conservative or surgical. Early recognition of ulnar neuropathy and correcting predisposing factors while avoiding repetitive compression are very important and can prevent more axonal damage. Activity-specific or night splinting may be helpful.

Radial Mononeuropathy

Background

The radial nerve is the largest nerve in the upper extremity. The nerve can be injured at any level; however, certain sites are more commonly injured.

The most common site is at the spiral groove (Saturday night palsy or honeymooner's palsy). The accepted common mechanism for the nerve injury is having placed and compressed the arm against the humerus on a solid surface for a long time. Other sites include the axilla (improper crutch use), arcade of Frohse (posterior interosseous nerve [PIN] syndrome or supinator syndrome), and at the wrist (tight watchband or hand-cuffs). Nerve compression at the arcade of Frohse or compression at the radial head secondary to dislocation in a Monteggie fracture can lead to PIN syndrome.

Anatomy

The radial nerve originates from the C5, C6, C7, C8, and T1 roots. The fibers pass through the upper, middle, and lower trunks and posterior cord to form the radial nerve. From the axilla to the spiral groove, the nerve is located posteriorly and sends branches to the triceps and ancenous muscles, as well as sensory branches, such as the posterior cutaneous and lower lateral cutaneous nerves of arm. At the spiral groove, the nerve lies directly on the humerus. The nerve then travels to the anterior compartment and supplies the brachioradialis, extensor carpi radialis longs, and extensor carpi radialis brevis. Near the formation of the brachialis muscle's tendon, the radial nerve transverses the elbow joint and divides into the PIN and superficial radial nerves just before the supinator muscle. PIN, a motor nerve, first innervates the supinator muscle and then travels through the arcade of Frohse and supplies the extensor digitorum communis, extensor digiti minimi, extensor carpi ulnaris, abductor pollicis longus, extensor pollicis longus, extensor pollicis brevis, and extensor indicis. The superficial radial sensory branch supplies the dorsolateral surface of the hand.

Clinical Findings

Radial nerve lesions usually appear with acute onset. Patients' clinic presentations depend exclusively on the location of the lesions. Patients with lesions at the spiral groove present with elbow flexion, supination, and wrist and finger extension weakness. Innervation of the anconeus and most of the triceps muscles is intact, and therefore, elbow extension is present. Sensory deficit can occur on the dorsal surface of the hand and the posterior aspect of the arm.

In the majority of patients with PIN syndrome, the nerve is affected after the ECL, and usually the extensor carpi radialis brevis is innervated and the superficial radial nerve has branched off. The patient may present with wrist and finger drop, but typically presents with a dull or sharp pain in the deep extensor mass distal to the radial head. On physical examination, sensation is preserved. Similar presentation can take place in posterior cord lesions and severe cervical radiculopathies (C7 and C8 radiculopathies). Patients with PIN syndrome display radial deviation with wrist extension. In complete neural loss, finger extensors are absent, and partial paralysis of the nerve leads to pseudo-claw hand deformity.

In superficial radial neuropathy, or cheiralgia paraesthetica, wristwatch syndrome, or handcuff palsy, the only complaint is sensory deficit in the hand surface without weakness.

Electrodiagnostic Findings and Approaches

A superficial radial nerve with a demyelinating lesion will show delayed distal latency when the lesion is distal to the stimulation site. In axonal injuries, after 4 to 7 days, the SNAP amplitude may be decreased. In superficial radial nerve injury, radial CMAP should be normal.

Motor Nerve Conduction Studies

If PIN is affected, radial CMAP may be abnormal, but radial SNAP should be normal (PIN syndrome).

The extensor indicis is the most distal radial-innervated muscle and, therefore, is commonly the first muscle tested. The deltoid muscle evaluation is important in differentiating radial neuropathy from posterior cord lesions.

When compressing the radial nerve, the supinator is spared because its branch comes off the radial nerve proximally and before the nerve has been passed under the supinator. For exclusion of a C7 radiculopathy and a brachial plexopathy, other nonradial nerve-innervated C7-innervated muscle (e.g., PT or FCR) testing is recommended, including the cervical paraspinals. These muscles should be normal in radial nerve lesions. In a spiral groove lesion, typical EMG findings are brachioradialis and/or ECR denervation (spontaneous activity, decreased recruitment, and large MUAPs) with sparing of the deltoid. There may be some involvement of the distal triceps (medial or lateral heads).

Peroneal Neuropathy

Background

Peroneal nerve injuries are the most frequent peripheral nerve injuries in the lower limbs. The majority of peroneal nerve injuries occur at the fibular head region. The etiologies are usually compression, traction, laceration, or metabolic. There are also common predisposing factors in compressive peroneal nerve injuries at fibular head, such as habitual leg-crossing (associated with weight loss), recent surgery, anesthesia, and prolonged hospitalization, maladaptive braces, extended repetitive squatting occupations, mass, diabetes, and peripheral polyneuropathy.

Anatomy

The peroneal nerve originates from the roots of L4, L5, S1, and S2. They travel through the lumbosacral plexus and sciatic nerve. The sciatic nerve divides into the tibial nerve and common peroneal nerve at approximately the middle to distal one-third of the thigh region (although the separation starts about mid-thigh, they continue in a sheath until the popliteal fossa). The common peroneal nerve innervates the short head of the biceps femoris muscle. Proximal to the fibular head, the common peroneal nerve gives off two branches: the sural communicating branch and the lateral cutaneous nerve of the calf. The common peroneal nerve then courses around the fibular head and passes through an opening in the superficial head of the peroneus longus and brevis muscle. Distal to this fibular tunnel, it divides into the deep and superficial peroneal nerves. The superficial peroneal nerve innervates the peroneaus longus and brevis and then becomes the superficial sensory peroneal nerve to innervate the lateral lower two-thirds of the leg and the dorsum of the foot. The deep peroneal nerve innervates the tibialis anterior (TA), extensor hallucis longus, extensor digitorum longus, peroneus tertius, and extensor digitorum brevis (EDB) muscles, and a sensory branch to the web space between the first and second digits.

Clinical Findings

The majority of patients with peroneal nerve injury presents with acute foot drop. Foot drop can also be caused by upper motor neuron lesions, spinal cord injury, radiculopathy (commonly L5, rarely L4), plexopathy, mononeuropathy (sciatic or peroneal neuropathies), or muscle disorders. Therefore, a detailed history and physical examination is essential to make an accurate diagnosis for optimal treatment. Symptoms and findings usually depend on the location of the nerve injury. A steppage gait or foot slap may be seen with ambulation. Weakness occurs in the ankle dorsiflexors, toe extensors (TA, extensor hallucis longus, and extensor digitorum longus), and ankle everters (peroneus longus and brevis). L5 radiculopathy would also produce ankle invertor weakness, as well as proximal weakness in L5 innervated muscles. Tinel's sign may be positive at the fibular head or shaft. Sensory loss may be found over first web space (deep peroneal) and/or lower lateral leg and dorsal foot area (superficial peroneal). Pain is not a common symptom.

Electrodiagnostic Findings and Approaches

Like other mononeuropathies, EDXs aid in identifying the location of the lesion, the severity, the type (axonal, demyelinating, or mixed), and the prognosis. Bilateral studies are essential.

The superficial peroneal SNAP is helpful in determining if the superificial peroneal nerve is involved or spared. A loss in amplitude implies that there has been some axonal loss affecting its superficial division.

When peroneal injuries are present, it is essential to perform conduction studies in the leg, as well as across the fibular head. Motor NCSs, which exhibit "pure" conduction block (>20–50% decrease in amplitude and/or area) across fibular heads, are classically demyelinating lesions. Prognosis is much better with pure conduction blocks compared with axonal loss. When axonal injury is present, then CMAP amplitudes would be decreased or absent, representing pathology involving the deep peroneal motor component. EDB is generally used as the recording site for motor peroneal studies. However, EDB can often be atrophied (tight shoes) so the TA is also recommended as another recording site.

Late responses are nonspecific; however, the F-wave could be absent or prolonged on the affected side. H-reflexes are checked to rule out other pathologies and should be normal in peroneal neuropathy.

Needle EMG may show decreased MUAP recruitment with normal morphology in demyelinating lesions. However, spontaneous activity, PSWs, fibrillation potentials, and MUAP-decreased recruitment are seen in axonal injuries in peroneal neuropathies. In chronic axonal loss, MUAP morphology changes (increased amplitude, long duration, and polyphasia) may be demonstrated.

EMG plays a crucial role in differentials of other neuropathies, radiculopathies, or plexopathies. Sampling other L5 innervated muscles (i.e., gluteus medius, FDL, tibialis posterioror) with paraspinals is important to rule out L5 radiculopathy. These muscles are normal in peroneal neuropathy. The short head of the biceps femoris (the most proximally peroneal innervated muscle) is another key muscle (innervated by sciatic nerve peroneal division) in deciding if the lesion is proximal (i.e., foot drop post-hip surgery). Abnormal EMG findings in this muscle are supportive of sciatic neuropathy.

Cervical and Lumbar Radiculopathies

Background

A radiculopathy is defined as an axonal and/or demyelinating disorder affecting the nerve fibers of one spinal nerve root. The typical cause in young adults (<40 years of age) is a herniated disk, whereas a combination of foraminal narrowing and arthritic changes are common in older patients. Although root compression is a common cause, a noncompressive etiology can occur. In order to diagnose and confirm radiculopathy or exclude neurological weakness and other causes for a patient's complaints, electrodiagnostic testing is useful as an extension of the physical examination. However, not all patients with radiculopathy require elctrodiagnostic testing. Radiculopathy is the second most common reason for referral for electrodiagnostic evaluation (CTS being the first). The most common radiculopathies seen in an electrodiagnostic lab are L5 at lumbar and C7 at cervical levels.

Anatomy

There are 31 spinal nerves that are derived from the merger of the ventral and dorsal rootlets within the spinal cord. After the foramina, spinal nerves are separated to dorsal (posterior) and ventral (anterior) rami. The posterior ramus innervates the paravertebral skin and paraspinal muscles, whereas the ventral ramus innervates the anterolateral aspect of the trunk and limb muscles. The dorsal root axons are originated from DRG sensory neurons within intervertebral foramen, before the merger of the dorsal and ventral roots. The cell bodies of the ventral roots are located within the anterior horn cells (motor fibers) within the spinal cord, as opposed to dorsal roots, which have cell bodies outside of the spinal cord in DRG (sensory fibers).

Dorsal (sensory) root compression usually appears in the spinal canal proximal to DRG and causes preganglionic injury, but spares postganglionic sensory fibers. Therefore, SNAPs are usually normal in radiculopathy.

Except for C8, cervical roots exit over matching vertebrae, whereas thoracic, lumbar, and sacral roots leave the spinal canal caudal to their matching vertebra. For example, although a C6–C7 foraminal disc herniation would result in a C7 radiculopathy, an L5–S1 foraminal disc herniation would cause an L5 radiculopathy. It is also important to keep in mind that one disc level pathology may compromise more than one root (i.e., L4–L5 disc level pathology may cause L4, L5, and less commonly, S1 radiculopathies).

A ventral root-innervated muscle is known as a myotome. The majority of muscles are innervated by more than one myotome. The rhomboid is innervated only by the C5 nerve root, and is the exception to the rule. A dermatome is defined as a single nerve root sensory distribution.

Clinical Findings

Patients usually present with neck or back pain in a dermatomal distribution. The onset may be acute, subacute, or chronic with or without sensory symptoms. Patients may complain of paresthesia in a corresponding dermatome, but negative sensory examination findings are not uncommon. Patients may also have weakness in corresponding myotomes and decreased or absent deep tendon reflexes. Even though there are multiple different presentations, paresthesia and weakness are suggestive of a radiculopathy. Certain symptoms and signs aid the exact location of pathology. For example, a

C7 radiculopathy may present with triceps weakness, C5 radiculopathy with supra and infraspinatus weakness, and C8 radiculopathy with weakness of hand intrinsics. Please refer to Table 4 for detailed information.

Electrodiagnostic Findings and Approaches

EDXs are particularly important to observe root compression findings, rule out any other pathological causes, and determine if the root lesion is at one or multiple levels. For example, spondylotic changes may cause compression of more than one root.

Sensory NCSs are usually normal in radiculopathies, except when there is a co-existing pathology or other etiology, such as a brachial plexopathy and/or peripheral neuropathy. Foraminal compression of the DRG can lead to a drop in sensory amplitude in certain cervical or lumbar radiculopathies.

Commonly tested lower extremity SNAPs, when evaluating for a possible radiculopathy, are the sural for S1 and the superficial peroneal for L5.

Motor nerve conduction studies typically have normal CMAP amplitudes in mild-to-moderate radiculopathies. However, in severe axonal lesions, decreased CMAP amplitude should be expected.

Generally, both sensory and motor NCSs should be normal.

Late Responses

The H-reflex can be helpful in differentiating L5 from S1 radiculopathies. The H-reflex assesses afferent and efferent S1 fibers. Clinically, L5 and S1 radiculopathies may appear similar on EMG owing to overlapping myotomes. The H-reflex latency side-to-side difference that is more than 1.5 ms with an amplitude difference of 60% or more indicates pathology in the S1 root. However, normal H-reflex does not exclude S1 radiculopathy. Also, keep in mind that an absent H-reflex is not uncommon in polyneuropathies and the elderly.

F-waves are usually not very helpful to diagnose radiculopathies.

The most specific and reliable part of the EDX to identify a radiculopathy is the presence of normal SNAPs and denervation in two muscles from different peripheral nerves innervated by the same root with paraspinal muscle denervation. Common EMG findings in radiculopathies are spontaneous activity, decreased recruitment (neurogenic MUP firing pattern), and large/polyphasic MUPs with sprouting and reinnervation. Spontaneous activity (fibrillation potentials, PSWs, fasciculations) is the main finding for an acute denervation. They appear after motor axonal loss in proximal paraspinal muscles in 5–7 days and then in the limb muscles (in 3 weeks). They resolve after nerve reinnervation or fiber fatty degeneration. Dener-

Table 4
Clinical and Electrodiagnostic Correlation of the Radiculopathies

Root level	*Clinical findings*	*Myotome(s) involved (nerve)*	*Common resemblances and some important points*	*Common NCS/EMG findings*
C5	• Shoulder abduction weakness • Lateral arm parasthesia • Hypo- or areflexic biceps	• Rhomboid (dorsal scapular) • Spinati (suprascapular) • Deltoid (axillary) • Teres minor (axillary) • Biceps brachii (musculocutaneous) • Brachialis (musculocutaneous)	• Upper trunk lesion • C6 radiculopathy • Neurological amyotrophy • Owing to limited innervated muscles and SNAP, it is difficult to make a definitive diagnosis	• Paraspinal muscle fibs/PSWs • Rhomboid and other muscle fibs/PSWs; decreased recruitment; large/polyphasic MUPs
C6	• Wrist extension, elbow flexion weakness • Lateral forearm and thumb/index fingers parasthesia • Hypo- or areflexic brachioradialis	• Pronator teres (median) • FCR (median) • ECR longus and brevis (radial) • Deltoid (axillary) • Teres minor (axillary)	• Upper trunk lesion • CTS paraspinal fibs/PSWs	• Normal median (thumb/index recorded) and lateral cutaneous of forearm SNAP • At least two innervated muscles from same root with fibs/PSWs; decreased recruitment; large/polyphasic MUPs
C7	• Arm extension, wrist flexion, and/or finger extension weakness • Middle finger parasthesia • Hypo- or areflexic triceps	• Triceps (radial) • Pronator teres (median) • Anconeus (radial) • EDC (radial) • EIP (radial) • FCR (median) • FCU (ulnar)	• CTS (common) • Middle trunk brachial plexopathy (rare) • The most common cervical radiculopathies	• Normal index and middle finger recorded median SNAP • Paraspinal fibs/PSWs • At least two innervated muscles from same root with fibs/PSWs; decreased recruitment; large/polyphasic MUPs

Continued

Table 4 *(Continued)*
Clinical and Electrodiagnostic Correlation of the Radiculopathies

Root level	*Clinical findings*	*Myotome(s) involved (nerve)*	*Common resemblances and some important points*	*Common NCS/EMG findings*
C8	• Finger flexion weakness • Medial forearm and/or little finger parasthesia	• FCU (ulnar) • FPL (median) • FDS (median) • FDP (median/ulnar) • EIP (radial) • EPB (radial) • FDI (ulnar)	• Lower trunk lesion • Ulnar neuropathy • Owing to overlapping myotomes, differentiating C8 from T1 is difficult • When there is triceps innervation, consider C8 radiculopathy, rather than T1	• Normal fifth finger recorded ulnar and medial antebrachial SNAP • Paraspinal fibs/PSWs • At least two innervated muscles from same root with fibs/PSWs; decreased recruitment; large/polyphasic MUPs
L2/L3	• Hip flexion and abduction weakness • Mid-thigh and knee medial site parasthesia	• Iliacus (femoral) • Vastus medialis (femoral) • Adductor longus (obturator) • Gracilis (obturator)	• Lumbar plexopathy • Less common (because of their short courses) • Owing to limited muscle innervation, its diagnosis is very difficult	• Paraspinal fibs/PSWs • At least two innervated muscles from same root with fibs/PSWs; decreased recruitment; large/polyphasic MUPs
L4	• Foot inversion and dorsiflexion weakness • Medial leg and foot parasthesia • Hypo- or areflexic patella	• Tibialis anterior (deep peroneal) • Vasuts medialis (femoral) • Rectus femoris (femoral)	• Lumbar plexopathy • Diabetic proximal neuropathy • Difficulty in SNAP evaluation (especially in obtaining saphenous SNAP in elderly)	• Paraspinal fibs/PSWs • At least two innervated muscles from same root with fibs/PSWs; decreased recruitment; large/polyphasic MUPs

Continued

Table 4 ***(Continued)***
Clinical and Electrodiagnostic Correlation of the Radiculopathies

Root level	*Clinical findings*	*Myotome(s) involved (nerve)*	*Common resemblances and some important points*	*Common NCS/EMG findings*
L5	• Toe extension and hip abduction weakness • Lateral leg and/or dorsum of foot parasthesia • Hypo- or areflexic tibialis posterior	• EDL (deep peroneal) • EHL (deep peroneal) • Gluteus medius (superior gluteal)	• S1 radiculopathy	• Both normal superficial peroneal SNAP • Paraspinal muscle fib/PSWs • At least two innervated muscles from same root with fibs/PSWs; decreased recruitment; large/polyphasic MUPs
S1	• Foot eversion and plantar flexion weakness • Foot lateral parasthesia • Hypo- or areflexic Achilles	• Peroneus longus and brevis (superficial peroneal) • Gluteus maximus (inferior gluteal) • Gastrocnemius/soleus/ FHB (tibial)	• L5 radiculopathy • S2 radiculopathy (because of their overlapping myotomes, they are difficult to separate) • Peripheral polyneuropathy (common; especially bilateral S1 and S2 radiculopathies)	• Normal sural SNAP • Common absence or asymmetrically abnormal H-reflex • Paracervical fibs/PSWs • At least two innervated muscles with same root fibs/PSWs; decreased recruitment large/polyphasic MUPs

CTS, carpal tunnel syndrome; ECR, extensor carpi radialis; EDC, extensor digitorum communis; EDL, extensor digitorum longus; EHL, extensor hallucis longus; EIP, extensor indicis; EPB, extensor pollicis brevis; FCR, flexor carpi radialis; FCU, flexor carpi ulnaris; FDI, first dorsal interosseus; FDP, flexor digitorum profundus; FDS, flexor digitorum superficialis; fibs, fibrillation potentials; FPL, flexor pollicis longus; MUPs, motor unit potentials; PSWs, positive sharp waves; SNAP, sensory nerve action potential.

vated muscle fiber reinnervations follow the same model (proximally 2–5 months, distally 3–7 months after lesion).

In general, muscle sample groups for radiculopathy evaluation should cover two muscles for each root and major nerve. Table 5 shows the group of muscles for EMG evaluation for cervical radiculopathy and Table 6 for lumbosacral radiculopathy.

Normal EMG studies do not rule out a radiculopathy, especially in acute radiculopathies. Neuropraxic root lesions present with both normal NCS and EMG findings and, therefore, are difficult to identify. There is also the problem of the 3- to 4-week time delay before PSWs and fibrillation potentials can be identified. For this reason, EDX can never completely rule out a radiculopathy.

EMG studies 3 to 4 weeks after injury can provide useful prognostication. For example, no abnormal spontaneous activity with decreased recruitment suggests a moderate-to-severe neurapraxia, whereas abnormal spontaneous activity with normal recruitment is the evidence of mild neurapraxia and mild-to-moderate axonal injury.

Brachial Plexopathies

Background

The diagnosis of a plexopathy can be difficult secondary to the anatomic complexity, relative anatomic inaccessibility, and numerous etiologies. However, EDXs can provide an appropriate anatomic diagnosis, localization, and severity. This can aid in prognostication, rehabilitation, and surgical planning. The most common etiologies are trauma, which includes traction, stretch, obstetrical injuries, transection, compression, and hemorrhage, idiopathic (neuralgic amyotrophy), tumor, and radiation therapy.

Among all plexopathies, brachial plexus disorders are most commonly seen. Because of its clinical relevance for incidence, severity, and prognosis, brachial plexus lesions are classified as supra and infraclavicular. Supraclavicular plexus lesions are more common and have more severe lesions with worse prognosis. Etiologies include closed-traction injuries (motor vehicle accident, obstetric, and Stinger syndrome), cancer, true neurogenic thoracic outlet syndrome, median sternotomy, malpositioning on the operating table, and backpack palsy. Common etiologies of the infraclavicular plexopathies are trauma (e.g., radiation, gunshot and stab wounds, humeral head fractures, clavicular fractures, and shoulder dislocations), iatrogenic causes (shoulder operations, arthroscopies, and regional anesthetic blocks), and inappropriate crutch use.

Table 5
Recommended Muscles in EMG Screening for Cervical Radiculopathy

Muscle	*Root*	*Nerve*
Midcervical paraspinals	C5–C6	Posterior rami
Low cervical paraspinals	C7–C8	Posterior rami
Deltoid	C5–C6	Axillary
Biceps	C5–C6	Musculocutaneous
Pronator teres	C6–C7	Median
EDC	C7–C8	Radial
FDI	C8–T1	Ulnar

EDC, extensor digitorum communis; EMG, electromyography; FDI, first dorsal interosseus.

Table 6
Recommended Muscles in EMG Screening for Lumbosacral Radiculopathy

Muscle	*Root*	*Nerve*
Midlumbar paraspinals	L4–L5	Posterior rami
Low lumbar paraspinals	L5–S1	Posterior rami
Vastus lateralis	L3–L4	Femoral
Tibialis anterior	L4–L5	Deep peroneal
EDB	L5–S1	Deep peroneal
Gluteus medius	L5–S1	Superior gluteal
Medial gastrocnemius	S1–S2	Tibial
FDL or Tibialis posterior	L5–S1	Tibial

EDB, extensor digitorum brevis; EMG, electromyography; FDL, flexor digitorum longus.

Anatomy

The brachial plexus is formed from the combination of the fifth, sixth, seventh, and eigth cervical anterior rami and the first thoracic anterior ramus. Contribution from C4 and T2 differs in each individual. In the posterior triangle of the neck, trunks are named for their relationship to each other: upper, middle, and lower. The upper trunk is formed by blending of the C5 and C6 anterior rami; the middle trunk is a continuation of the C7 anterior ramus; and the lower trunk results from the union of the C8 and T1 anterior rami. The upper trunk proximally gives off two motor branches: the suprascapular nerve and the nerve to subclavius muscle. After passing the clavicle, the trunks form anterior and posterior divisions to become cords. While the anterior divisions of the upper and middle trunk form the lateral cord, the medial cord is made by the lower trunk anterior division. Three posterior divisions of the upper, middle, and lower trunks create the posterior cord.

The lateral pectoral nerve is a branch of the lateral cord. The median nerve is formed from the combination of a branch from the lateral cord and the medial cord. The musculocutaneous nerve is also a branch from the lateral cord. The posterior cord branches to form the radial and axillary nerves. The medial cord gives off the following branches: the medial pectoral nerve, the medial brachial cutaneous nerve, the medial antebrachial cutaneous nerve, the ulnar nerve, and a branch to the median nerve.

A common rule to remember: median sensory fibers bypass the lower plexus; median motor fibers to thenar muscles generally skip the upper plexus. However, ulnar sensory and motor fibers run together while traversing the plexus.

Clinical Findings

The presentation varies depending on the pathology and injury-involved site of the plexus. Brachial plexus injury can result in motor, sensory, and sympathetic disturbances. Impairments can be temporary, such as burner injuries in football players, or they may be intractable. A patient with an upper trunk lesion usually complains of numbness over the lateral aspects of the arm, forearm, and hand. He or she may also present with weakness similar to Erb's palsy—shoulder and upper arm weakness with no hand involvement. A reduced or absent biceps reflex can be found. Middle trunk lesions appear with decreased sensation or numbness in the middle or, sometimes, index finger, and weakness in generally radial nerve-innervated muscles. Triceps reflex may be reduced. Lower trunk-injured patients present with loss of sensation in the medial part of the arm, forearm, and hand in the fourth and fifth digits and weakness similar to Klumpke's palsy—intrinsic hand and finger flexor muscles with no upper arm and shoulder involvement.

In brachial neuritis (Parsonage Turner syndrome), patients typically present with sudden onset of severe pain followed by proximal shoulder weakness. Electrodiagnostic findings may include involvement of the suprascapular nerve, long thoracic nerve, axillary nerve, AIN, spinal acessory nerve, or a diffuse plexus injury.

A brachial plexopathy caused by a carcinomatous lesion generally presents with pain plus lower trunk symptoms. However, radiation-induced plexopathies usually do not present with pain, but with parasthesia that progresses slowly, and involve the upper trunk.

On physical examination, look for asymmetry, atrophy, skin changes, and fasciculations. Proximal weakness generally affects activities of daily living, including feeding, grooming, and dressing.

Electrodiagnostic Findings and Approaches

Sensory NCS provides more information in brachial plexopathy than motor NCS. SNAPs can be useful to differentiate a presynaptic lesion from a postsynaptic lesion and to help determine the severity of a plexus lesion. SNAPs are absent in postsynaptic lesions, although they are present with presynaptic ganglionic lesions, such as radiculopathies and root avulsions. Although pre- and postganglionic lesions may present with sensory loss, because of no spontaneous regeneration and limited surgical options, root avulsion (presynaptic) generally has a poor prognosis. SNAPs are also extremely sensitive to axonal loss with their decreased amplitude, but no change in distal latency and CV.

CMAPs are affected if there is a severe brachial plexus lesion. CMAPs are better indicators for axonal loss extension than SNAPs, when they are affected. Contralateral side comparison is also important when you find decreased amplitude. Although motor latencies and distal CVs are not changed in brachial plexopathies, when there is a demyelinating pathology in brachial plexus, Erb's point stimulation may show slowing.

Late responses are nonspecific.

Electromyography

When performing the needle portion of the exam, it is important to screen each root level, and at each root level, different peripheral nerves should be tested. Cervical paraspinal muscle testing should be normal because paraspinal muscles are innervated by posterior rami, whereas the plexus is innervated by anterior rami.

Please refer to Table 7 for the recommended motor NCS, sensory NCS, and muscle groups to make the appropriate diagnosis.

Generalized Peripheral Neuropathies

Background

Peripheral neuropathy is a common manifestation of various systemic diseases. In developed countries, diabetes, alcohol abuse, and their associated nutritional factors are the most common etiologies, whereas leprosy is the most common treatable neuropathy in the world.

Table 7
Recommended Motor, Sensory, and Needle EMG Muscle Groups With Their Lesion Sites

Site of lesion	*Sensory NCS*	*Motor NCS*	*EMG*	*Root*
Upper trunk	• Lateral cutaneous of forearm	• Axillary (recording deltoid)	• Supraspinatus	C5, C6
	• Median (recording thumb)	• Musculocutaneous (recording biceps)	• Infraspinatus	C5, C6
	• Radial (recording base of thumb)		• Pectoralis major	C5, C6, C7
			• Pronator teres	C6, C7
			• Brachioradialis	C5, C6
			• Biceps	C5, C6
			• Triceps	C7, C8
			• Deltoid	C5, C6
Middle trunk	• Median (recording third and fourth digits)	• Radial (recording EDC)	• Latissimus dorsi	C6, C7, C8
			• Teres major	C5, C6, C7
			• Triceps	C7, C8
			• Anconeus	C7, C8
			• Pronator teres	C6, C7
			• EDC	C7, C8
			• FCR	C6, C7
Lower trunk	• Medial cutaneous of forearm	• Ulnar (recording hypothenar and FDI)	• EDC	C7, C8
	• Dorsal ulnar cutaneous	• Median (recording thenar)	• EPB	C8, T1
	• Ulnar (recording fifth digit)	• Radial (recording EDC)	• FCU	C7, C8, T1
			• FDP (3rd and 4th digits)	C7, C8, T1
			• APB	C8, T1
			• ADM	C8, T1
			• FDI	C8, T1

Continued

Table 7 *(Continued)*

Recommended Motor, Sensory, and Needle EMG Muscle Groups With Their Lesion Sites

Site of lesion	*Sensory NCS*	*Motor NCS*	*EMG*	*Root*
Lateral cord	• Lateral antebrachial	• Musculocutaneous (recording biceps)	• Biceps	C5,C6
	• Median (recording thumb)		• Brachialis	C5, C6
			• Pronator teres	C6, C7
			• FCR	C6, C7
Posterior cord	• Radial	• Axillary (recording deltoid)	• Latissimus dorsi	C6, C7, C8
		• Radial (recording ECU)	• Teres major	C5, C6, C7
			• Deltoid	C5, C6
			• Triceps	C7, C8
			• Brachioradialis	C5, C6
			• ECR	C6, C7
			• EDC	C7, C8
			• ECU	C7, C8
			• EPB	C8, T1
			• EIP	C7, C8
Medial cord	• Medial antebrachial	• Ulnar (recording ADM)	• FCU	C7, C8, T1
	• Ulnar (recording fifth digit)	• Median (recording APB)	• FDP (3rd and 4th digits)	C7, C8, T1
			• FPL	C8, T1
			• ADM	C8, T1
			• FDI	C8, T1
			• APB	C8, T1

ADM, abductor digiti minimi; APB, abductor pollicis brevis; ECU, extensor carpi ulnaris; EIP, extensor indicis; EDC, extensor digitorum communis; EMG, electromyography; EPB, extensor digitorum brevis; FCR, flexor carpi radialis; FCU, flexor carpi ulnaris; FDI, first dorsal interosseus; FDP, flexor digitorum profundus; FPL, flexor pollicis longus; NCS, nerve conduction study

Anatomy

There are many different classifications of peripheral neuropathies. Typically, neuropathies are described based on the pathology that is caused, axonal versus dymelinating. Another classification utilizes the duration of symptoms, such as acute (<3 months), subacute (3–6 months), or chronic (>6 months). Peripheral neuropathies may also be described by using anatomic localization, such as symmetric, asymmetric, distal, proximal to distal, and diffuse (both proximal and distal). Physiological associations are also utilized, such as sensory, sensory to motor, motor to sensory, motor, and autonomic. However, using the combination of anatomical location and physiological association can contract the likely causes (Table 8). Determining a primary and predominating process is helpful in understanding the course of the disorder.

Clinical Findings

A thorough history and physical examination can aid in the differential diagnosis. Classically distal segments are predominantly affected compared with proximal segments, and are a length-dependent process. The duration of symptoms is very important for differential diagnosis. For example; a subacute onset could be suggestive of acute inflammatory demyelinating polyneuropathy, Lyme's disease, or acute arsenic intoxication, whereas an insidious onset of a chronic neuropathy may raise a red flag for hereditary neuropathies. Frequently, patients with peripheral neuropathies initially have distal sensory changes and may develop weakness. Patients may also have an associated hypo- or areflexia. Patients presenting with symptoms and signs of autonomic dysfunction are not uncommon. The physical examination should also include careful evaluation for autonomic dysfunction, facial nerve involvement, and neurocutaneous manifestations.

Electrodiagnostic Findings and Approaches

Electrodiagnostic testing aids in the differential diagnosis. An appropriate peripheral neuropathy evaluation requires at least two limb sensory and motor nerves with F-wave testing, as well as an array of muscles tested on the needle examination.

SNAP amplitudes are typically decreased or unobtainable when there is sensory axonal neuropathy. In demyelinating type sensory neuropathy, SNAPs will show slow CVs.

CMAP amplitudes may be decreased or unobtainable in motor axonal neuropathy. If the motor neuropathy is of demyelinating character, then CMAP response may reveal a delayed latency and/or slowed CV (usually

Table 8
Generalized Peripheral Neuropathies (PNs) With Their Electrodiagnostic Findings

EDx Findings	*Axon loss motor> sensory PN*	*Axon loss sensory PN*	*Axon loss sensory motor PN*	*Diffuse demyelinating sensory motor PN*[a]	*Multifocal demyelinating motor to sensory PN*[b]	*Mixed (axonal and demyelinating) sensory motor PN*
Common disorders	• Lead PN • HMSN-II • Dapson PN • Porphyria • AIDP • Paraneoplastic motor neuropathy	• Paraneoplastic syndrome • HSN • Cisplatinum toxicity • Friedreich's ataxia • Spinocerebellar degeneration • Primary biliary cirrhosis • Paraproteinemias • Amyloidosis	• Alcoholic PN[c] • B12/folate deficiency[c] • Vincristine-induced • Metal (gold, thallium, mercury) intoxication • RA/SLE/sarcoidosis • Gout neuropathy • Hypothyroidism • HIV/AIDS-induced • Lyme's disease	• HMSN I/III/IV • Metachromatic leukodystrophies • Tangier disease	• AIDP • CIDP • Leprosy • Amiodarone toxicity • Arsenic intoxication • HNPP	• Diabetic PN[c] • Uremia[c]
Distal latency	• Normal	• Normal	• Normal	• Increased	• Increased	• Increased
CMAP amplitude	• Decreased	• Normal	• Decreased	• Normal	• Decreased as a result of dispersion or conduction block	• Decreased

Continued)

Table 8 ***(Continued)***
Generalized Peripheral Neuropathies (PNs) With Their Electrodiagnostic Findings

EDX Findings	*Axon loss motor > sensory PN*	*Axon loss sensory PN*	*Axon loss sensory motor PN*	*Diffuse demyelinating sensory motor PN*[a]	*Multifocal demyelinating motor to sensory PN*[c]	*Mixed (axonal and demyelinating) sensory motor PN*
SNAP amplitude	• Decreased	• Decreased	• Decreased	• Normal	• Normal or decreased	• Decreased
Nerve CV	• Normal	• Normal	• Normal	• Decreased	• Decreased	• Decreased
Abnormal spontaneous activity	• Present	• Normal	• Present	• Normal	• Normal	• Present
Recruitment	• Decreased	• Decreased	• Decreased	• Normal or decreased	• Decreased	• Decreased

[a]Usually genetic disorders.

[b]Usually acquired disorders.

[c]Distal symmetric weakness.

AIDP, acute inflammatory demyelinating polyneuropathy; CIDP, chronic inflammatory demyelinating polyneuropathy; CMAP, compound muscle action potential; CV, conduction velocity; HMSN, hereditary motor sensory neuropathy, HNPP, hereditary neuropathy with liability to pressure palsies; HSN, hereditary sensory neuropathy; RA, rheumatoid arthritis; SLE, systemic lupus erythematosus; SNAP, sensory nerve action potential.

Table 9
Some Important Myopathic Disorders With Their Classifications

Toxic myopathies	*Steroid-, AZT (azidothymidine)-, alcohol-, vincristine-, colchicine-, chloroquine-induced myopathies*
Endocrine myopathies	Thyroid, parathyroid, adrenal, and pituitary myopathies, including critical illness myopathy
Inflammatory myopathies	HIV-associated myopathy, inclusion body myositis, infectious, dermatomyositis, polymyositis
Muscular dystrophies	Duchenne, Steinert's (myotonic), Becker, Emery-Dreifuss, ocular pharyngeal, facioscapulohumeral, limb girdle muscular dystrophies
Congenital myopathies	Centronuclear myopathy, central core disease, nemaline rod myopathy
Metabolic myopathies	Pompe's disease, McArdle's disease, debrancher deficiency myopathy.

<40 m/second in the lower limbs and <45 m/second in the upper limbs). Significant slowing (<80% than normal of the lower limb) usually suggests a demyelinating neuropathy.

Late Responses

F-wave studies are essential when acute demyelinating neuropathies are considered (usually >125% of upper limit of normal).

Needle EMG studies are helpful for the decision on chronicity by evaluating MUAP (increased duration, large amplitudes, and polyphasic), diffuse or multifocality, or symmetricity.

Myopathy

Background

Myopathies have a broad range of causes. The list of the common myopathic disorders is shown in Table 9. Diagnosis or confirmation of the myopathies usually requires high serum creatine kinase, EMG, and muscle biopsy. It is important to keep in mind that EMG primarily evaluates Type I fibers.

Clinical Findings

Most patients present with proximal muscle weakness and commonly complain of trouble rising from a chair. In hereditary distal myopathies, patients may complain of hand weakness and instability in the ankles and tripping or falling owing to distal muscle weakness. Myopathy weakness is usually symmetric and painless without sensory symptoms. If patients complain of pain, it is typically secondary to cramping and is not well localized. Inspection for muscle atrophy, hypertrophy, body posture, and contracture and evaluation of muscle strength is very important in the physical exam. Some muscular dystrophy patients may present with calf hypertrophy. For more information, please refer to Chapter 8.

Facioscapulohumeral dystrophy is one of the most common types of muscular dystrophy. The usual presentation is between the first and third decades. Ninety-five percent of patients show clinical features before age 20 years. Initial weakness is seen in facial muscles, starting in the orbicularis oculi, orbicularis oris, and zygomaticus. Patients may have difficulty with labial sounds, whistling, or drinking through a straw. Weakness may be asymmetric and, typically, extraocular and pharyngeal muscles are spared. Shoulder weakness is the presenting symptom in more than 82% of patients with symptoms, and scapular fixation is weak from the onset. Winging of the scapula is the most characteristic sign. TA muscle weakness is highly characteristic, whereas posterior muscles of the leg are spared. In a few patients, a foot-drop gait is the presenting complaint. In more than 50% of patients, the pelvic girdle muscles are never involved. Life expectancy is normal in most patients.

Electrodiagnostic Findings and Approaches

Sensory NCSs are normal in myopathies. Motor NCSs are generally normal in myopathies, unless there is severe muscle atrophy or myopathies with hand and foot involvement because routine CMAPs are recorded from distal muscles. These conditions show only reduced CMAP amplitudes. Late responses are not specific.

Needle EMG aids in diagnosing a number of abnormalities and the severity of the disease process. It also may aid in determining the location of the muscle biopsy. Often, the needle examination is restricted to one arm and leg, with both proximal and distal muscles tested. The biceps and vastus lateralis muscles are commonly biopsied. When the needle EMG shows pathology on one side, then the equivalent muscle on the other side can be recommended for biopsy.

PSWs and fibrillation potentials may be found in myopathies, especially in inflammatory myopathies. However, the electrodiagnostic hallmarks are short-duration, small-amplitude polyphasic MUAPs with early recruitment. Unlike the pattern seen in neuropathic disorders, early recruitment is a large number of small motor units firing for a weak contraction. Unlike most myopathies, myotonic muscular dystrophy has distal muscle involvement, and myopathic motor units are seen distally and proximally on needle

EMG. Myotonic discharges, which are waxing and waning character, are prominent in myotonic muscular dystrophy but can also be seen in other conditions, such as hyperchloremic periodic paralysis, acid maltase deficiency, hyperthyroidism.

The most common myopathy in the elderly is inclusion body myositis. Typically, the needle examination demonstrates occasional fibrillation potentials and CRDs. Like myotonic dystrophy, it generates significant distal muscle damage, and the distal muscles demonstrate usual myopathic units.

Clinical Pearls

Critical illness myopathy may show some fibrillation potentials and normal to mildly myopathic units. Because steroid myopathy affects Type II fibers significantly, EMG is generally normal in steroid myopathy. McArdle's disease develops characteristically muscle contractures, which are silent on needle studies. Polymyositis and dermatomyositis show prominent, complex repetitive discharges, especially in the paraspinal muscles.

Motor Neuron Diseases

Background

Motor neuron diseases affect mainly the anterior horn cells with motor axonal distal degeneration, and typically spare bowel/bladder and extraocular muscle functions. In general, there are no major sensory and cognitive changes. The majority of the motor neuron diseases are amyotrophic lateral sclerosis (ALS), progressive lateral sclerosis, poliomyelitis, and spinal muscular atrophies (SMAs). Motor neuron disease diagnosis requires detailed history/physical exam with electrodiagnostic testing, neuroimaging, and laboratory testing.

Anatomy

The motor cortex, corticospinal (motor) tracts, and the anterior horn cells are usually affected sites.

Clinical Findings

Patients with motor neuron disease may present with upper and lower motor neuron findings. Patients may have muscular weakness and atrophy with varying corticospinal tract signs. Generally, SMA and poliomyelitis present with lower motor neuron signs (atrophy, flaccidity, hyporeflexia, and fasciculations—uncommon in SMA). Patients with progressive lateral sclerosis and ALS have upper motor neuron signs (weakness, spasticity, hyperreflexia, and up-going plantar response).

Electrodiagnostic Findings and Approaches

Because there is no DRG damage, sensory NCSs should be classically normal.

Motor NCSs show generally normal CMAP latency, amplitude, and CV. If there is significant muscle weakness and atrophy, CMAP amplitude will be decreased or absent. Also, in severe axonal loss, motor CVs may show decreased CV, but this slowing should not be more than 20% of normal.

Late responses may be useful for excluding other pathologies.

To make the diagnosis of motor neuron disease, abnormal findings in at least two different nerve distributions (peripheral nerve, plexus, or root) in each of three limbs or two limbs and bulbar muscles is required. For ALS diagnosis, The El Escorial criteria (needle abnormalities in two of four regions: bulbar, cervical, thoracic, and lumbar). Two abnormal muscles innervated by different roots and peripheral nerves are required for cervical and lumbosacral regions. The thoracic and bulbar regions need only one abnormal muscle and can be utilized as well. Paraspinal muscle testing would help for excluding radiculopathies. Because thoracic radiculopathies are rare, when thoracic paraspinal muscles show abnormal findings, they can be more suggestive of motor neuron disease; however, abnormal findings may also be present in patients with diabetes mellitus.

Needle EMG will show PSWs and fibrillation potentials in affected muscles. Fasciculations are commonly observed and are a hallmark feature of motor neuron disease. MUAPs typically have a neuropathic (polyphasic with increased complexity when there is reinnervation or decreased recruitment; sometimes, there may be giant motor units) pattern.

Key References and Suggested Additional Reading

Campbell WW. AAEM Quality Assurance Committee. Literature review of the usefulness of nerve conduction studies and electromyography in the evaluation of patients with ulnar neuropathy at the elbow. Muscle Nerve, 1999: 22(Suppl 8): S175–S205.

Daube JR. Clinical Neurophysiology, 2nd ed. New York: Oxford University Press, 2002.

Dumitru D. Electrodiagnostic Medicine, 2nd ed. Philadelphia, PA: Hanley & Belfus, 2002.

Ferrante MA. Electrodiagnostic approach to the patient with suspected brachial plexopathy. Neurol Clin North Am, 2002; 20:423–450.

Frontera WR. Essentials of Physical Medicine and Rehabilitation, 1st ed. Philadelphia, PA: Hanley & Belfus, 2002.

Greenberg SA, Amato AA. EMG Pearls, 1st ed. Philadelphia, PA: Hanley & Belfus, 2004.

Katirji B. Electromyography in Clinical Practice, 1st ed. St. Louis, MO: Mosby, 1998.

Wilbourn AJ. AAEM minimonograph #32: electrodiagnostic examination in patients with radiculopathies. Muscle Nerve 1998; 21:1612–1631.

Index

D

L

M

P

R

S